Laboratory Tests for Clinical Nursing

Jane Onstad Lamb, RN, BA, PNP

ROBERT J. BRADY CO.
BOWIE, MARYLAND 20715
A Prentice-Hall Publishing and Communications Company

Executive Editor: Richard A. Weimer
Production Editor: Karen A. Zack
Art Director: Don Sellers, AMI
Assistant Art Director: Bernard Vervin
Typesetting by: Harper Graphics, Inc., Waldorf, MD
Typefaces: Palatino (text) and Century Schoolbook (display)
Printed by: R. R. Donnelley & Sons Co., Harrisonburg, VA

Laboratory Tests for Clinical Nursing

Library of Congress Cataloging in Publication Data

Lamb, Jane Onstad.
    Laboratory tests for clinical nursing.

    Bibliography: p.
    Includes index.
    1. Diagnosis, Laboratory.   2. Nursing. I. Title.
[DNLM: 1. Diagnosis, Laboratory—Nursing texts.
2. Diagnostic tests, Routine—Nursing texts.
QY 4 L1237]
RB37.L285   1983   616.07'56   83-12237
ISBN 0-89303-265-4 {PBK.}

ISBN 0-89303-616-1

Prentice-Hall International, London
Prentice-Hall Canada, Inc., Scarborough, Ontario
Prentice-Hall of Australia, Pty., Ltd., Sydney
Prentice-Hall of India Private Limited, New Delhi
Prentice-Hall of Japan, Inc., Tokyo
Prentice-Hall of Southeast Asia Pte. Ltd., Singapore
Whitehall Books, Limited, Petone, New Zealand
Editora Prentice-Hall Do Brasil LTDA., Rio de Janeiro

Printed in the United States of America

83 84 85 86 87 88 89 90 91 92 93 10 9 8 7 6 5 4 3 2 1

For Tina M. Wallis
    and for Mom and Dad
Those who have taught me about humor
    and courage and dignity.

CONTRIBUTING AUTHORS:

Suzanne Weyland Canale, RN, BSN, MSN
Instructor of Nursing
Lane Community College
Eugene, Oregon

Glenna Sandgathe Clemens, RN, BSN, MN
Instructor of Nursing
Lane Community College
Eugene, Oregon

David George Everett, BS, MT, (ASCP), CLS
Director
Everett Medical Laboratory
Ashland, Oregon

Janice Brown Kinman, RN, BSN
Instructor of Nursing
Lane Community College
Eugene, Oregon

Susan Ulrich, RN, BSN, MSN
Instructor of Nursing
Lane Community College
Eugene, Oregon

Anne Kieran Westerman, RN, BS
President, Western Institute of
Continuing Education
Ashland, Oregon

Contents

L

M

O

P

R

S

Preface

Laboratory Tests for Clinical Nursing is a quick, easy-to-use reference guide for the most frequently ordered laboratory tests. The nursing process format is used to define the nurse's role and responsibility to the patient before and after testing. Nurses must have some knowledge of laboratory tests, of the various influences that may alter test values, and of the specific role the nurse plays in providing an environment that promotes accurate test results. Nurses should have a basic understanding of what the nurse can do to improve abnormal test values.

Laboratory Tests for Clinical Nursing lists tests alphabetically by name and lists most common medical abbreviations. The tests are cross-referenced in the index by name, abbreviation, and most common medical grouping—electrolytes, isoenzymes, chemistry screen, etc. A short glossary, preceding the index, defines unfamiliar laboratory terminology.

The structure of each page is designed to give information easily. The format is simple and direct. Syntax is purposely concise. Each test discussion includes the most popular national value range and type of specimen used. The procedure of collection is outlined. Laboratory methodology is not discussed, as method varies from laboratory to laboratory. A brief description follows that includes source, function, excretion, and purpose of the substance measured.

The scientific rationale underlying the conditions related to increases and decreases in laboratory results is given. Drugs and the effects that may influence laboratory test results are listed. The drugs are listed generically with examples of trade names in parentheses. Pertinent related laboratory tests are mentioned just before the nursing care section.

Nursing care is divided into pretest and posttest sections. The pretest section is concerned with factors related to the test. The pretest nursing goal is to achieve a therapeutic environment to promote accurate test results. The nursing process format is used to guide planning of nursing care connected with preparation for the test. The posttest section deals with factors related to the results of the test. The posttest nursing goal is to promote a homeostatic environment. Nurses have a responsibility to the patient beyond recognizing abnormal test results because specific nursing action can correct or begin to correct some abnormal test values. Considerations for specific nursing care that will have a direct influence on abnormal test results are discussed. Considerations for nursing care are specific only to the influence it may have on the test result. Repetition within the nursing care sections is necessary because it reduces the number of places the nurse must look for information. Each test is complete. Only specific information regarding related tests requires the nurse to refer to another part of the book.

This is not a physiology text or a general nursing care book. The aim of this book is to present information about laboratory tests and the way nursing care directly influences laboratory results. The nursing care sections are specific to nursing procedure that relates to nursing influence on tests. Because of this approach, this book should become a necessary companion in the practice of nursing.

Acknowledgment

To Jerry and Kate for support and love during the best and worst of times.

To Laura Dysart Marcy, Executive Editor, Robert J. Brady Company, for her remarkable patience and keen eye.

To Charles Corrigan Brown, MD, for his wit, wisdom, and encouragement.

To Sacred Heart Hospital Medical Library staff, Eugene, Oregon, for their help and goodwill.

To David and Sally Everett for books, for information, and for caring.

To Lane Community College Department of Nursing Education, Eugene, Oregon, for helpful suggestions, books, and faculty time.

Thank you to a special support system of Lana McGraw Boldt, Margaret Ruth Evans, Martha Weigel Moehl, and numerous readers. Thank you, too, to Karen Moran, my cheerful, all-hours typist.

Jane Onstad Lamb
Ashland, Oregon

Introduction

Nursing is an eclectic profession. As such, it requires the nurse to have a working knowledge of all other health professions. Laboratory technology is just one of the areas the nurse must understand. In the following test-by-test discussions, the nurse will become familiar with the role laboratory testing has in the planning of patient care.

The Laboratory

The clinical laboratory is a carefully controlled microcosm. This control is necessary because a number of variables—altitude, humidity, surges in line voltages, temperature changes—may influence the laboratory environment. Because of laboratory environmental variables and the choice of specific test procedures, each laboratory determines its particular set of reference norms. It is of utmost importance that nursing personnel follow local laboratory directives in ordering the test, preparing the patient, and collecting the specimen. Reference values given in this book are given simply as reference guides. General preparation of the patient is presented with each test and is also intended for use as a guide. Check local clinical laboratory guidelines for specific preparation.

The Laboratory Test

A laboratory test is a tool. By itself, the laboratory test is almost useless, but in conjunction with a pertinent history and physical, it may confirm a diagnosis or provide valuable information about a patient's status and response to therapy.

Just as a laboratory environment is carefully monitored and controlled, the substance to be tested needs to be as free of interfering variables as possible. The nurse working with the patient will minimize these influencing factors. Usually, *it is the nurse who is the pivotal person in laboratory testing*.

Interferences to accurate laboratory testing may begin with the lab slip. The most common errors in filling out lab slips include incompletely filled out lab slip, illegible information, wrong abbreviations, misspelled words, and incorrect patient's name and/or room number.

Or the interference may be due to incorrect specimen collection and handling: wrong preservative or lack of a necessary preservative, slow delivery of a collected specimen to the lab, aging specimens that contain destroyed cells and may increase or decrease test results, incorrect patient preparation, hemolysis of blood samples, incomplete collection, especially timed urine collections, or incorrect labeling of specimen.

There are also patient factors that influence test results that may or may not be controlled. These factors may include diet preparation, current drug history, preexisting conditions such as illness, plasma volume, position, exercise, postprandial status, time of day, pregnancy, age, and lack of patient knowledge.

Knowledge and communication are the keys to prevention of error in laboratory testing. The nurse should be sure of the test ordered and have a basic understanding of that test. Patients and their families (as appropriate) should be knowledgeable about tests to be performed and preparation necessary for correct test results. Any dietary restrictions or collection of multiple or timed specimens should be communicated to patients and staff.

Knowledge of the correct collection and handling of specimens is essential. Blood is collected for analysis on plasma, serum, or whole blood. Blood may be collected in capillary tubes, vacuum tubes, or in a syringe and transferred to a tube containing the correct additive. Blood vacuum collecting tubes come in a variety of sizes: 2 ml, 5 ml, 7 ml, 9.5 ml. Vacuum collecting tubes should be filled completely. The amount of blood needed for different tests varies with the laboratory. Be sure of the amount needed before drawing blood. The amount stated in the Procedure section of each test discussed is a reference amount only and for purposes of patient education.

Vacuum collecting tubes come in a variety of colors. Each color designates a purpose for that tube.

Tube Top color	Tube Interior	Purpose
Blue	Sodium citrate	Prevents clotting; used for coagulation studies
Brown	Minimal lead content	Lead levels
Gray	Glycolytic inhibitor	Used most often for glucose determinations
Green	Sodium heparin	Used for tests on plasma samples (ammonia, cortisol, ACTH, etc.)
Lavender	EDTA	An anticoagulant; used when the need to preserve cells is essential (hematology)
Red	No additive	For serum samples; most chemistries, serology, blood bank studies
Red and black	No additive but contains silicone gel	Silicone gel separates the cells from serum, so serum can be poured off easily. Gel coats cells so this tube is not used for blood bank studies
Yellow	Sterile	Blood culturing

After collection of blood in a vacuum tube that contains an additive, it is important to rotate the tube gently for complete mixing of the additive into the specimen.

Hemolysis of a blood sample is a problem that is preventable. Specific precautions can decrease the chance of a hemolyzed specimen. Leaving a tourniquet on too long, skin wet with antiseptic, and probing about the venipuncture site can cause hemolysis. Forceful withdrawing of blood, withdrawing the blood too slowly, or shaking or roughly agitating the specimen also cause destruction of red blood cells. In the very old or very young these precautions are particularly important as blood vessels in the extremes of age are small or fragile.

The most concentrated urine specimen is generally the first morning specimen. As a rule this is the best specimen for analysis. There are, of course, exceptions to this rule and these exceptions are noted in the discussion of a particular urine test. Clean-catch urine specimens are a good idea routinely, though the patient or nurse must be careful to rinse the soap used in cleaning free of the genitalia or the soap may contaminate the specimen. Collected urine specimens that will have a wait before being sent to the lab should be refrigerated.

Timed urine specimens are often collected with great difficulty. It is essential to collect *all* urine within a collection period. If one or part of one specimen is discarded, the collection must be restarted. As a general rule, urine collected during a timed collection period should be refrigerated during the entire collection time. Before collection begins, the correct collection container must be obtained, as some collections require a preservative in the collection container.

Certain blood and urine tests are performed at the nursing unit by nursing personnel. It is essential that the correct directions are used with the testing method being performed. Color charts are not interchangeable. If testing kits are kept dry, in air-tight containers, and directions are followed precisely, testing values become far more reliable.

The Nurse's Responsibility

Nurses collect data and formulate nursing diagnoses in order to prepare and carry out individualized patient care. The nursing process is the methodical and dynamic method that helps the nurse focus on the patient. Each patient has a unique history, physical exam, and list of needs. In this book the discussion of implications and considerations for nursing care includes a possible nursing diagnosis. The nursing responsibilities in the Pretest phase of laboratory testing include:

1. Ordering tests correctly
2. Coordinating patient activities and testing
3. Recognizing and correcting or minimizing interfering factors
4. Preparing the patient properly
5. Educating patient and family about the test(s)

These actions help to achieve a therapeutic environment for accurate laboratory testing.

The nursing responsibilities in the Posttest phase of patient laboratory testing include:

1. Recognizing abnormal test results and possible effects on the patient
2. Defining nursing actions and instituting appropriate intervention around the needs of the patient in conjunction with findings of the nursing assessment, as well as laboratory test results
3. Determining if nursing actions can have a positive influence on abnormal results

These actions promote a homeostatic environment.

Presenting the implications and considerations for nursing care in a nursing care plan format is done to show how laboratory testing should be a natural part of patient care planning.

The Format

The book format is designed to provide information easily. If a section is not applicable to the test, it is omitted. This is the only variance to the format. The format is organized as follows:

Name of test
Abbreviation

Reference Values
Specimen
Description
Procedure
*Conditions Related to Increases
*Conditions Related to Decreases
Drug Influences
Related Lab Studies
Pretest Implications
Posttest Considerations

---

*Conditions are not necessarily listed according to frequency of occurrence.

Test:	Acid Phosphatase
Abbreviation:	ACP
Reference Values:	*Adults* (11)

0.13–0.63 U/L
0.0–0.8 IU/L

Children (23)
Newborn—2 weeks   10.4–16.4 King-Armstrong (KA) U/ml
2 weeks–13 years   0.5–11.0 KA U/ml

Specimen: Serum

Description: Acid phosphatases (ACP) are a group of related enzymes that are active in an acid environment. These enzymes are found in many tissues, including bone, liver, spleen, kidney, erythrocytes, and the prostate gland. The prostate gland contains a high concentration of the enzyme. The prostatic ACP isoenzyme can now be measured. Mode of excretion is unknown. ACP is measured to detect metastatic prostatic cancer and to follow the response to treatment. Because of the high acid phosphatase concentrations in seminal fluid, a vaginal aspirate for ACP becomes a significant part of an investigation of alleged rape.

Procedure: (red top tube)   2–5 ml venous blood is drawn from the patient.

Conditions Related to Increases

1. Metastatic carcinoma of the prostate

2. Vigorous prostatic massage

3. Gaucher's disease

4. Hyperparathyroidism
   Paget's disease
   Multiple myeloma
5. Sickle-cell crises
   Thrombocythemia
   Thrombocytosis
   Thrombophlebitis

Rationale

1. The prostate begins to release ACP as soon as there is metastasis beyond the gland. In nonmetastatic prostatic carcinoma or benign prostatic hypertrophy, there is little or no rise in serum ACP. ACP levels drop within 3–4 days after surgery if the tumor is successfully removed. Levels drop 3–4 weeks after estrogen therapy. ACP usually increases with the onset of relapse.

2. The release is from release of ACP from prostatic manipulation.

3. Caused by spillage into bloodstream from tissue accumulation, especially from the spleen.

4. The bone marrow cells show varying degrees of ACP activity that is reflected in increased values.

5. From release of erythrocytic ACP into serum.

Arterial embolism
Pulmonary embolism
Hemolysis of specimen
6. Acute myelogenous leukemia

7. Impaired kidney function
   Renal insufficiency
8. Liver damage

6. Auer bodies, found in this disease, are strongly ACP-positive.
7. Release of ACP from renal tissue into serum.
8. Release of ACP from liver tissue into serum.

Conditions Related to Decreases

1. Environmental conditions; high temperature

Rationale

1. High temperatures increase pH and inactivate the enzyme.

Drug Influences: The following drugs may influence test results. The drugs are listed alphabetically by generic name and divided into columns according to the effect of the drug. Examples of trade names are in parentheses.

The following drugs may cause an increase in test results:

Androgenic effect (in female)
   danazol (Cyclomen)
   ethylestrenol (Maxibolin)
   fluoxymeterone (Android-F)
   methandrostenolone (Dianabol)
   methyltestosterone (Android-5)
   nandrolone deconoate (Anabolin)
   oxandrolone (Anavar)
   oxymetholone (Adroyd)
   stanozolol (Winstrol)
   testosterone (Android-T)
   testosterone cypionate (Andro-Cyp)
   testosterone enanthate (Testostroval-PA)
   testosterone propionate (Androlin)

Miscellaneous
   clofibrate (Atromid-S)

The following drug may cause a decrease in test results:

In Vivo inhibition
   fluorides (sodium fluoride)

Related Lab Studies: Monitor response to treatment or progress of disease and adjust nursing care accordingly. See individual tests for information.

Metastatic Prostatic Carcinoma
   acid phosphatase (for assessing status of therapy)
   alkaline phosphatase (↑ , indicating bone involvement)
   *bone scan (to determine extent of metastasis)

---

*Not discussed in this book.

IMPLICATIONS FOR NURSING CARE
PRETEST: Factors related to the test
Nursing Diagnosis: Potential for injury related to changes in biochemical balance

Guide to assessment	Guide to planning and intervention	Guide to evaluation
1. Drug history of receiving clofibrate (Atromid-S) (See Drug Influences) 2. Preexisting conditions (See Increases/Decreases)	1. Indicate on lab slip if patient has received clofibrate within last 24 hours. 2. Record preexisting conditions on lab slip.	1. The patient's history of receiving clofibrate is indicated on lab slip. 2. The patient's preexisting conditions pertinent to test are noted on lab slip.
3. Lack of patient knowledge	3. Explain test to patient: a. Define ACP (See Description). b. Explain procedure (See Procedure).	3. The patient demonstrates knowledge of test by defining test and explaining procedure.

Patient Preparation Checklist

1. √ Drug history (See Drug Influences).
2. √ Preexisting conditions and note on lab slip (See Increases/Decreases).
3. √ Patient knowledge; explain test to patient (See Description/Procedure).

CONSIDERATIONS FOR NURSING CARE RELATED TO ABNORMAL TEST RESULTS
POSTTEST: Factors related to the results of the test
Nursing Diagnosis: Potential for injury related to changes in biochemical balance

Guide to assessment	Guide to planning and intervention	Guide to evaluation
Prostatic massage	1. Do not perform vigorous prostatic massage during physical exam immediately prior to ACP being drawn. 2. Note on lab slip if this occurs within 24 hours prior to test.	1. The patient is protected against an increase in ACP levels due to vigorous prostatic massage.

Test: Alanine Aminotransferase
Serum Glutamic Pyruvic Transaminase

Abbreviation: ALT, SGPT

Reference Values: Infant   below 54 U/L
Children   1–30 U/L
Adults   0–48 U/L

Specimen: Serum

Description: Alanine aminotransferase (ALT), also known as glutamic pyruvic transaminase (GPT), is a necessary enzyme in the Kreb's cycle. It is essential for tissue energy production. ALT is present in highest amounts in the liver, with smaller amounts in the kidneys, heart, and skeletal muscle. When damage to these tissues occurs by toxins, infections, or hypoxia, enzyme activity increases. Measurement of ALT is a rather specific indicator of hepatocellular damage. It is also used in conjunction with AST (SGOT) measurements to help distinguish between cardiac and hepatic damage. With cardiac damage, the AST (SGOT) levels are very high, with only mildly elevated ALT levels. ALT can be used to differentiate between hemolytic jaundice (in which case there would be no rise in ALT) and jaundice due to liver disease (ALT levels would be high). ALT levels are now being used to monitor treatment of hepatitis, cirrhosis, Reye's syndrome, and treatment with drugs known to be toxic to the liver.

Procedure: (red top tube)
1. The patient should abstain from alcohol for 24 hours prior to the test; otherwise, no food or fluid restrictions.
2. 0.5–3 ml of venous blood is drawn from the patient.
3. Observe the puncture site for bleeding or evidence of hematoma.

Conditions Related to Increases

Rationale

1. Liver disease
   Hepatitis
   Cirrhosis
   Liver tumor

1. Damaged liver cells release increased amounts of ALT (SGPT).

2. Reye's syndrome

2. In this disease, ALT (SGPT) is increased to 500–800 U/L. This increase is due to dramatic cellular changes in the liver. Inflammation and necrosis of the liver are not part of this disease. The cellular liver changes are usually reversible.

3. Diseases that often involve the liver
   Amebiasis
   Disseminated tuberculosis
   Brucellosis
   Septicemia
   Psittacosis
   Infectious mononucleosis
   Actinomycosis
   Histoplasmosis
   Schistosomias
   Regional enteritis
   Sarcoidosis

3. These conditions often have associated liver involvement. Damaged liver cells release increased amounts of ALT (SGPT).

4. Biliary tract obstruction
   Cholecystitis
   Pancreatitis
   Cholelithiasis
   Dubin-Johnson syndrome

4. Obstruction causes backup of bile into the liver and hepatic congestion that leads to increased release of hepatic enzymes.

5. Myocardial infarction
   Congestive heart failure

5. Both of these conditions may decrease the normal blood flow to the liver, causing liver congestion and damage. Also, small amounts of ALT (SGPT) are present in the myocardial tissue and released during damage.

6. Leukocytic disorders
   Reticulum cell carcinoma
   Lymphosarcoma
   Hodgkin's disease
   Leukemia
   Gaucher's disease
   Nieman-Pick disease

6. Elevated enzyme levels in these conditions are a sign of systemic cellular damage or indicate liver involvement common to these disorders.

7. Alcoholism or drug dependence

7. Often there is some hepatocellular damage after long-term use.

8. Some musculoskeletal diseases
   Progressive spinal muscular atrophy
   Progressive muscular dystrophy
   Myotonia atrophica
   Dermatomyositis
   Polymyositis

8. ALT (SGPT) is present in skeletal muscle and released in increased amounts when there is damage to muscles.

9. Renal disorders
   Chronic renal failure
   Renal infarction

9. Small amounts of ALT (SGPT) are found in kidneys.

10. Systemic lupus erythematosus

10. SLE often affects major organs such as the liver and kidneys.

11. Conditions causing trauma or hypoxia
    Crushing injury
    Hypothermia
    Shock
    Burns
    Delerium tremens
    IM injections
    Radiation damage
    Heat stroke

11. Trauma or hypoxia causes increased release of ALT (SGPT) from muscles and major organs.

12. Preeclampsia and eclampsia

12. The hypertension involved can cause tissue hypoxia. If convulsions occur, acidosis often follows, and the toxicity of acidosis can cause increased release of tissue enzymes. One theorist also states that toxemia may be caused by malnutrition and that concurrent liver damage may be occurring with the malnutrition (53).

13. Hemolysis

13. Since RBCs contain higher concentrations of ALT than plasma, hemolysis will cause falsely elevated results (13).

Conditions Related to Decreases

1. None

Rationale

1. None

Drug Influences: Many drugs affect ALT (SGPT) values. Listed below are some of the drugs that influence test results. The drugs are listed alphabetically by generic name and divided into columns according to the effect of the drug. Examples of trade names are in parentheses.

The following drugs may increase test results:

Hepatic necrosis
   acetaminophen

Hepatotoxicity
   allopurinol (Zyloprim)
   antifungal agents (Fungizone, Mysteclin-F)
   asparaginase (Elspar)
   aspirin
   azathioprine (Imuran)
   carbenicillin (Geocillin)
   clofibrate (Atromid-S)
   colchicine
   cycloserine (Seromycin)
   erythromycin
   flurazepam (Dalmane)
   gentamicin (Garamycin)
   kanamycin (Kantrex)

  lincomycin
  oral contraceptives
  procainamide (Pronestyl)
  pyrazinamide (Tebrazid)
  rifampin (Rimactane)
  tetracycline, especially pregnant women
  thiothixene (Navane)

Intrahepatic cholestasis
  acetohexamide (Dymelor)
  anabolic steroids (Anavar, Testryl, Drolban)
  desipramine (Norpramin, Pertofrane)
  indomethacin (Indocin)
  isoniazid (INH)
  methyldopa (Aldoclor, Aldomet)
  nalidixic acid (NegGram)
  phenothiazines (Thorazine, Compazine, Prolixin)
  phenytoin (Dilantin)

Miscellaneous
  aminosalicylic acid
  barbiturates
  clindamycin
  codeine
  ethionamide (Trecator-SC)
  guanethidine (Ismelin)
  meperidine (Demerol, Meperagan)
  mithramycin (Mithracin)
  morphine
  mushroom poisoning
  spectinomycin (Trobicin)

Related Lab Studies: Monitor response to treatment or progression of disease and adjust nursing care accordingly. See individual tests for information.

In Liver Disease:
  ↑ serum ammonia
  ↑ serum bilirubin
  ↑ urine bilirubin
  ↓ albumin
  ↓ total protein
  ↑ prothrombin time
  ↑ or ↓ Cholesterol
  ↑ AST (SGOT)
  ↑ GGTP
  ↑ LDH
  ↑ alkaline phosphatase
 * ↓ BSP excretion
 *bile acids radioimmunoassay
_____

  *Not discussed in this book

IMPLICATIONS FOR NURSING CARE
PRETEST: Factors related to the test
Nursing Diagnosis: Potential for injury related to changes in biochemical balance

Guide to assessment	Guide to planning and intervention	Guide to evaluation
Assess patient factors that may influence test results:		
1. Comprehensive drug history	1. Report drugs the patient is receiving that may influence lab results to the patient's physician and to the lab:	1. Drugs and/or alchohol patient is currently receiving that may influence test results are identified and the proper people are notified.
a. See Drug Influences	a. Withhold hepatotoxic or cholestatic drugs prior to the test if possible (narcotics, salicylates, chlorpromazine, methotrexate).	
b. Alcohol ingestion	b. Instruct patient to abstain from alcohol for 24 hours prior to the test.	
c. Multiple IM injections	c. Note on lab slip if patient is receiving IM injections.	
2. Preexisting conditions	2. Record preexisting conditions on lab slip.	2. Patient's preexisting conditions are noted on lab slip.
3. Knowledge deficit	3. Explain test to patient: a. Define ALT (SGPT) (See Description). b. Explain procedure (See Procedure).	3. Patient demonstrates knowledge of test by defining test and stating procedure.

Patient Preparation Checklist

1. √ Influencing drugs and/or alcohol ingestion noted and reported (See Drug Influences).
2. √ Preexisting conditions noted on lab slip (See Increases/Decreases).
3. √ Patient knowledge; explain test and procedure (See Description and Procedure).

CONSIDERATIONS FOR NURSING CARE RELATED TO ABNORMAL TEST RESULTS
POSTTEST: Factors related to the results of the test
Nursing Diagnosis: Alterations in biochemical balance

Guide to assessment	Guide to planning and intervention	Guide to evaluation
Assess patient factors that may be influencing tests results. Nursing history and/or physical exam indicative of:		
1. Liver dysfunction Liver enlargement Jaundice Clay-colored stool Dark urine Water retention/ascites Level of consciousness Irritability Seizure activity Bleeding tendencies	1. Prevent further liver damage by: a. Protecting patient from excessive liver palpation by students and staff. b. Measuring and adjusting nutritional intake according to water retention and ascites. c. Increasing protein and carbohydrate intake if status allows.	1. The patient is protected against further liver damage: a. Liver palpation is minimized. b,c. Water retention and ascites are controlled by the measurement and adjustment of patient intake; intake and output are balanced; abdominal girth is decreased or stable.
d. Alcoholism/drug dependence	d. Teaching patient importance of abstinence from alcohol; encouraging participation in an alcohol rehabilitation program as appropriate.	d. Patient states understanding of importance of abstaining from alcohol.
e. Infectious diseases involving liver	e. Administering antiinfective agents as ordered.	e. Patient receives medications.
f. Systemic lupus erythematosus	f. Administering adrenocorticosteroids or immunosuppressive drugs as ordered.	f. As above.
g. Pancreatitis	g. Giving prescribed anticholinergic drugs and maintaining NPO, gastric suction, fluid intake, and treatment plan.	g. Patient demonstrates decreased pancreatic stimulation by reduced abdominal distention:
(1) Pancreatic pain that is boring, bandlike, and constant in nature in abdomen and back.	(1) Giving pain medications as needed (not morphine or its derivatives); help patient assume position of comfort.	(1) Statements of diminished pain after pain medication given and position of comfort achieved.
	(2) Administering nitroglycerine, papaverine, or other smooth muscle relaxants as ordered.	(2) Statements of less frequent episodes of pain.

Guide to assessment	Guide to planning and intervention	Guide to evaluation
2. Congestive heart failure Dyspnea Orthopnea Weight gain Edema Distended neck veins Enlarged tender liver Basilar rales	2. Prevent congestion of portal system with subsequent liver damage by: a. Administering diuretics and cardiotonics as ordered. b. Providing and monitoring diet restricted in sodium as ordered. c. Teaching patient the importance of restricting sodium intake, as well as teaching about foods, medicines, and other substances high in sodium that must be avoided.	2. The patient demonstrates positive response to therapy. a. Edema and ascites will be reduced by maintaining decreased sodium and fluid intake. b. As above. c. Patient will verbalize understanding of, and willingness to comply with, dietary restrictions.
3. Myocardial infarction	3. Initiate nursing measures to prevent further myocardial damage from decreased oxygen, decreased coronary blood flow, or secondary thromboemboli.	3. The patient remains adequately oxygenated; does not complain of chest pain or shortness of breath, and demonstrates a negative Homan's sign with no evidence of inflammation in legs.
4. Musculoskeletal diseases Dermatomyositis Polymyositis Trauma Delerium tremens Multiple IM injections	4. Promote decrease in musculoskeletal disease process by: a. Administering prednisone or immunosuppressive drugs as ordered. b. Encouraging patient to rest as much as possible, limiting muscle activity. c. Decreasing the number of IM injections the patient receives.	4. The patient will demonstrate decreased signs and symptoms of the musculoskeletal disease. b. The patient's ALT (SGPT) levels are not increased by unnecessary muscle activity.
5. Renal disorders Chronic renal failure Renal thrombosis	5. Prevent further kidney damage by: a. Administering steroids, chlorambucil, cyclophosphamide, or indomethacin as ordered. b. Assisting with renal dialysis as ordered. c. Administering anticoagulants as ordered.	5. The patient's waste products are adequately removed from the blood and further renal damage does not occur. c. The patient does not experience further renal thrombosis.

Test: Albumin

Abbreviation: None

Reference Values: Premature   2.5–4.5 g/dl
                      Full-term newborn   2.5–5.0 g/dl
                      1–3 months   3.0–4.2 g/dl
                      3–12 months   2.7–5.0 g/dl
                      1–15 years   6.5–8.6 g/dl (46) dye binding
                      Adult   3.8–5.0 g/dl (11) dye binding

Specimen: Serum

Description: Albumin is the smallest protein molecule and makes up the largest portion of total serum protein. It is synthesized almost totally in the liver. The protein is catabolized and excreted as an end product of protein metabolism. Because of its high molecular weight, albumin plays an important role in total water distribution (colloidal osmotic pressure) in the body. Albumin transports and stores many different low molecular weight substances, such as metal ions, fatty acids, steroids, hormones, and drugs (17). In the newborn, albumin has the important functions of binding and detoxification. Because most diseases cause protein breakdown, the serum albumin level is rarely elevated.

Procedure: (red top tube)
                      1. Collection should be prior to high-fat meal.
                      2. 0.5–2 ml of blood is drawn from the patient.
                      3. Observe for bleeding at venipuncture site or appearance of hematoma.

Conditions Related to Increases

1. Dehydration
   Exercise
2. Anxiety and depression

3. BSP dye

4. Hemolysis

Rationale

1. The increase is due to hemoconcentration from loss of body water.
2. The magnitude of the increase and the etiology was not stated (21).
3. The serum specimen for albumin should not be collected until 48 hours after a BSP dye test, as the serum specimen will show a falsely elevated level (5). This is not an influence if immunochemical methods of determining albumin are used (11).
4. Release of hemoglobin due to hemolysis will increase protein values (21).

Conditions Related to Decreases

1. Chronic liver disease, especially cirrhosis

Rationale

1. The decrease is due to deficient synthesis of albumin. The diminished value is not seen in acute liver dis-

ease due to the long half-life of albumin (15–19 days) (11).

2. Ascites
   Cirrhosis
   Right-sided heart failure
   Cancers
   Peritonitis

2. Increased portal pressure forces leakage of plasma proteins into the peritoneal cavity, the diseased liver is unable to synthesize more albumin, and so serum albumin is greatly reduced.

3. Poor nutrition
   Advanced malignancy
   Malabsorption syndromes
   Starvation
   Beriberi
   Alcoholism
   Parasitism

3. Decline in albumin production due to deficient available protein in severe malnutrition. Within 30 minutes of amino acid replacement, albumin levels begin to rise.

4. Toxemia of pregnancy
   Congestive heart failure
   Water intoxication

4. The decrease in serum albumin is from impaired synthesis and dilution from excess body fluid.

5. Kidney disease
   Nephrosis
   Severe nephritis
   Uremia

5. Excessive protein loss through the glomerulus due to increased glomerular permeability.

6. Gastrointestinal tract disease
   Colitis
   Cancer of GI tract
   Sprue
   Celiac disease
   Enteritis
   Allergic gastroenteropathy

6. These are protein-losing enteropathies; serum proteins leak into the intestinal lumen and become lost in the feces (11).

7. Burns
   Exfoliative dermatitis

7. Through loss of protein-rich fluid, there is diminished protein availability.

8. Acute inflammation
   Hodgkin's disease
   Leukemia
   Multiple myeloma

8. The inflammatory process can act to stimulate the synthesis of some proteins. Albumin, a negative acute phase reactant, is sometimes selected by the liver for a decrease in hepatic synthesis. The mechanism of selection is not understood (11).

9. Normal aging

9. Advanced age shows a slight but significant downward trend in serum values due to decreasing synthesis (11).

10. Interfering molecules, especially fats
    Drugs
    Metabolites, especially bilirubin

10. Because of albumin's ability to transport and bind other substances, a falsely low level may result from the already saturated albumin molecule.

This is not an influence in immuno-chemical methods of determination (11).

Drug Influences: The following drugs may influence test results. The drugs are listed alphabetically by generic name and divided into columns according to the effect of the drug. Examples of trade names are in parentheses.

The following drugs may cause an increase in test results:

Drug sensitivity effect
    gallamine (Flaxedil)

The following drugs may cause a decrease in test results:

Hepatotoxic effect
    acetaminophen (Tylenol)
    asparaginase (Elspar)
    azathioprine (Imuran)
    cyclophosphamide (Cytoxan)
    heroin
    niacin (Nicotinex)
    pyrazinamide (Tebrazid)
    thorium dioxide

Hypersensitivity reaction
    nicotinyl alcohol (Roniacol)
    oxyphenisatin

Metabolic effect
    estrogens (Premarin)
    ethinyl estradiol (Estinyl)

Miscellaneous
    dextran (Macrodex); after infusion

Related Lab Studies: Monitor response to treatment and/or progression of disease and adjust nursing care accordingly. See individual tests for information.

    urinalysis
    total protein (protein electrophoresis)
    serum bilirubin
    urine bilirubin
    urobilinogen
    prothrombin time
    cholesterol
    alkaline phosphatase (ALP)
    AST (SGOT)
    ALT (SGPT)
    gamma glutamyl transpeptidase (GGTP)
    electrolytes

IMPLICATIONS FOR NURSING CARE
PRETEST: Factors related to the test
Nursing Diagnosis: Potential for injury related to changes in biochemical balance

Guide to assessment	Guide to planning and intervention	Guide to evaluation
Assess patient factors that may influence test results:		
1. Food and fluids	1. Schedule test prior to high-fat meal.	1. Patient's values are not influenced by diet.
2. Comprehensive drug history (See Drug Influences)	2. Note influencing drugs on lab slip.	2. Patient's drugs that may decrease test values are noted on lab slip.
3. BSP test	3. Schedule test 48 hours after BSP dye test, or note on lab slip.	3. Patient does not have BSP dye test within 48 hours of serum albumin.
4. Jaundice	4. Note on lab slip if patient is jaundiced.	4. Patient's preexisting conditions that may decrease test results are noted on lab slip.
5. Hemolysis	5. Prevent hemolysis by: a. Not saturating skin with antiseptic. b. Not probing venipuncture site or leaving tourniquet on too long. c. Not forcefully withdrawing specimen. d. Not withdrawing specimen too slowly. e. Not agitating or handling specimen roughly.	5. Patient's values are not influenced by staff mismanagement.
6. Knowledge deficit	6. Explain test to patient: a. Define albumin (See Description). b. Explain procedure (See Procedure).	6. Patient demonstrates knowledge by defining test and stating procedure.

Patient Preparation Checklist

1. √ Test scheduled prior to high-fat meal.
2. √ Note cytotoxic drugs on lab slip.
3. √ Test scheduled 48 hours after BSP test, or noted on lab slip.
4. √ Note patient dehydration on lab slip.
5. √ Patient knowledge; explain test to patient (See Description/Procedure).

CONSIDERATIONS FOR NURSING CARE RELATED TO ABNORMAL TEST RESULTS
POSTTEST: Factors related to the results of the test
Nursing Diagnosis: Alterations in biochemical regulatory function

Guide to assessment	Guide to planning and intervention	Guide to evaluation
Assess patient factors that may be influencing test results. Nursing history/physical exam suggestive of:		
1. Dehydration/ overhydration Edema, especially nondependent Ascites Kidney disease Chronic liver disease	1. Demonstrate body water distribution by: a. Keeping ongoing I&O records. b. Taking daily weights. c. Detecting physical signs/ symptoms of fluid imbalance; report and record findings. d. Measuring abdominal girth daily in cirrhotic patient.	1. Patient's colloidal osmotic (oncotic) pressure is measured.
2. Ascites Abdominal girth Protruding umbilicus Dullness and shifting dullness (abdominal waves) on percussion Bulging flanks	2. Control by: a. Detecting early signs of fluid accumulation in peritoneal cavity. b. Initiating nursing measures to encourage fluid and electrolyte balance. c. Implementing medical plan to treat underlying cause of ascites. d. Administering albumin as ordered. e. Assisting with paracentesis or peritoneal-venous shunt. f. Teaching outpatient to monitor weight gain and rapid increase in abdominal girth.	2. Patient demonstrates control of ascites by diminishing signs of ascites and increased urine output.
3. ↓ Serum albumin Ascites/edema Severe malnutrition Burns	3. Replace lost albumin by: a. Providing adequate oral protein as tolerated and as appropriate. b. Providing protein-sparing carbohydrates in diet.	a. The patient receives adequate dietary protein. b. The patient receives adequate carbohydrate calories in diet.

Guide to assessment	Guide to planning and intervention	Guide to evaluation
	c. Providing adequate dietary potassium.	c. The patient receives adequate dietary potassium for protein synthesis.
d. Need for immediate albumin replacement.	d. Administering IV albumin (Albumisol, Albuminar, etc.) slowly as ordered.	d. The patient receives IV albumin, and without complications of circulatory overload.
4. Kidney disease	4. Promote kidney function by: a. Initiating nursing measures to maintain balanced fluid and electrolyte status. b. Administering blood transfusions and IV fluids. c. Encouraging treatment of streptococcal infections. d. Preparing for dialysis as needed.	4. The patient's kidney function is maintained or restored as demonstrated by laboratory tests; excessive loss of albumin is prevented.
5. Cirrhosis	5. Prevent further liver damage by: a. Removing offending agents (alcohol, drugs, toxic chemicals). b. Encouraging well-balanced diet. c. Administering vitamin supplements of thiamine, vitamin C, and folate as ordered.	5. The patient does not experience further liver damage.

Test: Albumin/Globulin Ratio

Abbreviation: A/G Ratio

Reference Values: 1.5:1–2.5:1

Description: This test shows the proportion of albumin to globulin. Though once considered useful, it is now rarely used, as the ratio may be influenced by many diseases.

Related Lab Studies:

albumin
globulin
serum protein electrophoresis

Test: Aldolase

Abbreviation: ALS

Reference Values: Adult   2–8 U/L
Newborn   up to 4 × adult level
Child   up to 2 × adult level (11, 34, 46)

Specimen: Heparinized plasma

Description: Aldolase is a glycolytic enzyme. It is found in nearly all body tissue but most significantly in skeletal, cardiac, kidney, brain, and liver tissue and in erythrocytes and platelets. The greatest activity is in skeletal muscle. Three aldolase isoenzymes have been identified: type A, which is of skeletal and heart muscle origin; type B, which is of liver, kidney, and leukocyte origin; and type C, of brain tissue origin. Aldolase measurement is useful in combination with creatine phosphokinase (CK) in the diagnosis of muscular dystrophy, especially Duchenne's. It is also clinically useful in following some hepatic diseases.

Procedure: (red top tube)
1. No food or fluid restrictions.
2. 2 ml of blood is drawn from the patient.
3. Observe for bleeding at venipuncture site or for evidence of hematoma.

Conditions Related to Increases

Rationale

1. Skeletal muscle disease
   Duchenne's muscular dystrophy
   Polymyositis
   Dermatomyositis
   Myotonic dystrophy
   Trichinosis
   Amyotrophic lateral sclerosis
2. Neoplastic disease
   Carcinomas
   Lymphomas
   Granulocytic leukemia
3. Hepatitis
   Myocardial disease

1. Because of increased cellular permeability, there is diffusion of the enzyme through muscle membrane (48). There is also increased enzyme release from muscle destruction or degeneration.

2. The increase is reflective of an increased tissue source of the enzyme and/or of increased release of the enzyme from the affected tissue.

3. Useful in following the course of disease, plasma aldolase is not usually used as a diagnostic tool. In hepatitis, the enzyme follows the same course as aspartate aminotransferase (AST/SGOT). The increases are reflective of increased enzyme release from necrotic cells.

4. Acute psychoses
   Delirium tremens
   Crush injuries
   Multiple IM injections, same site

4. Aldolase is found in the cytoplasm of cells and enters the plasma through diffusion with relatively slight injury (11).

5. Hemolysis	5. Platelets may release aldolase during the clotting process. Heparinized plasma is the preferred specimen (13).
6. Exercise	6. There is conflicting evidence from various studies, but it is suggested that aldolase levels be collected in a resting state (21).

Conditions Related to Decreases: None.

Drug Influences: The following drugs may influence test results. The drugs are listed alphabetically by generic name and divided into columns according to the effect of the drug. Examples of trade names are in parentheses.

The following drugs may cause an increase in test results:

Hepatotoxic effect
  chlorinated insecticides (Chlordane)
  organophosphorus insecticides (Parathion)
  thorium dioxide

Muscle damage at injection site or muscle origin
  corticotropin (Acthar)
  epinephrine (Adrenalin chloride)
  thiabendazole (Mintezol)

The following drugs may cause a decrease in test results:

Miscellaneous
  phenothiazines (Thorazine)
  probucol (Lorelco)

Related Laboratory Studies: See individual tests for information. The following lab tests may be ordered with plasma aldolase.

Muscular dystrophies:
  ↑ aspartate aminotransferase (AST/SGOT)
  ↑ creatine phosphokinase (CK/CPK)
  ↑ lactic dehydrogenase
  ↓ creatinine clearance
  ↓ serum creatinine
  * muscle biopsy
  * electromyography

---

*Not discussed in this book.

IMPLICATIONS FOR NURSING CARE
PRETEST: Factors related to the test
Nursing Diagnosis: Potential for injury related to changes in biochemical balance

Guide to assessment	Guide to planning and intervention	Guide to evaluation
Assess patient factors that may influence test results:		
1. Recent drug history IM injections	1. Record recent IM injections, especially of steroids or epinephrine.	1. Injections the patient has recently received that may influence test results are recorded on lab slip.
2. Hemolysis	2. Prevent hemolysis of blood specimen by: a. Not saturating skin with antiseptic. b. Not probing venipuncture site or leaving the tourniquet on too long. c. Not forcefully withdrawing specimen. d. Not withdrawing specimen too slowly. e. Not agitating or handling specimen roughly.	2. The patient's lab results are not influenced by staff error.
3. Activity	3. Encourage patient to rest prior to exam, or at least not engage in physical exertion.	3. The patient's physical activity does not influence test results.
4. Knowledge deficit	4. Explain test to patient: a. Define test (See Description). b. Describe procedure (See Procedure).	4. The patient demonstrates knowledge of test by defining test and explaining procedure.

Patient Preparation Checklist

1. √ Recent IM injections (steroids or epinephrine) noted on lab slip.
2. √ Patient knowledge; explain test (See Description/Procedure).

CONSIDERATIONS FOR NURSING CARE RELATED TO ABNORMAL TEST RESULTS
POSTTEST: Factors related to the results of the test
Nursing Diagnosis: Impaired physical mobility

Guide to assessment	Guide to planning and intervention	Guide to evaluation

Assess patient factors that may be influencing test results.
Nursing history and physical exam suggestive of:
1. Skeletal muscular conditions
	1. Encourage independence; conserve muscle strength:
	  a. Help patient learn to organize daily activities.
	  b. Arrange activities with adequate rest times.
	  c. Use aids for ambulation as necessary (wheelchairs, etc.).
	  d. Encourage support of medical-rehabilitative foundations (Muscular Dystrophy Foundation, etc.).
		1. The patient achieves some measure of independence without increasing muscle damage.

Test: Aldosterone

Abbreviation: None

Reference Values: *Plasma* (29)
Sodium intake   10 mEq/day
Fasting, recumbent   12–36 ng/dl
2 hours later, upright   17–137 ng/dl
Sodium intake   100–200 mEq/day
Fasting, recumbent   3–9 ng/dl
2 hours later, upright   4–30 ng/dl

Urine
Sodium intake
10 mEq/day 20–80 mcg/24 hours
100–200 mEq/day 3–19 mcg/24 hours
↑ 200 mEq/day 2–12 mcg/24 hours

Specimen: Plasma, urine

Description: Aldosterone, the principal and most potent mineralocorticoid, is secreted by the zona glomerulosa of the adrenal cortex. It is secreted in response to the renin-angiotensin stimulus. Aldosterone acts on the cells of renal tubules to increase retention of sodium with resultant water retention and excretion of potassium. In this way aldosterone becomes a very important part of the electrolyte fluid balance system. Aldosterone also causes plasma volume expansion by sodium retention. The enzyme circulates loosely bound to albumin (20) and is metabolized in the liver to an inactive compound and excreted by the kidneys. Confirming a diagnosis of primary aldosteronism or renin-secreting hypertension is the usual reason for determining aldosterone levels.

Procedure: (red top tube)

Plasma

1. Diet may be a specified sodium diet or it may be a normal sodium diet for from 2–4 weeks prior to testing. The patient should abstain from licorice ingestion.
2. Medications that influence aldosterone or renin levels are withheld if possible for 2–4 weeks prior to testing (See Drug Influences).
3. While still in bed and before breakfast, 1.0–7 ml of blood is withdrawn from the patient.
4. After 2 hours of standing and moving about, 1.0–7 ml of blood is again withdrawn from the patient.
5. Observe the puncture site for bleeding or evidence of hematoma.

24-Hour Urine Collection

1. Preparation as in 1 and 2 above.
2. Collection bottle must have glacial acetic acid to maintain a pH of 4–4.5. Urine is refrigerated.
3. Collection.
   a. Discard first voided specimen.
   b. Begin timing.
   c. For the next 24 hours, place *all* voidings into specimen container immediately after voiding.
   d. Have patient void just prior to completion of 24 hours and put sample in collection bottle.
4. Record exact start and finish times on lab slip.
5. Send to lab immediately.

Conditions Related to Increases	Rationale
1. Adenoma of adrenal gland	1. There is excessive unregulated secretion of aldosterone from the adenoma, which results in overactivity of zona glomerulosa.
2. Adrenal gland hyperplasia	2. There is excessive unregulated secretion of aldosterone from the hyperplastic adrenal glands. Urine levels are increased on normal salt diet; urine level increase is not consistently detectable. Levels are not reduced by high salt diet or DOCA administration (9).
3. High renin hypertension	3. There is elevated plasma renin due to lesions in the kidney or kidney vascular supply, which leads to an increase in aldosterone production.
4. Low renin hypertension	4. This is characterized either by aldosterone oversecretion from primary (adrenal) or secondary (extraadrenal) origins.
5. Congestive heart failure	5. Possibly due to decreased liver function or to decreased cardiac output, there is a relative decrease in forcible blood volume, which stimulates an increase in aldosterone secretion that produces an increase in total blood volume. Secretion may be 2–3 times normal level in patients with chronic congestive heart failure.
6. Chronic obstructive lung disease	6. Increased plasma potassium concentration, often found in acidotic patients, stimulates the secretion of aldosterone (21).

7. Cirrhosis

7. Aldosterone is metabolized in the liver to an inactive compound. In the cirrhotic liver, aldosterone is inactivated only ⅓ as well as in the normal liver, thereby increasing aldosterone plasma levels (21).

8. Renal disease
   Poststreptococcal glomerulonephritis
   Nephrotic syndrome
   Chronic renal failure

8. Altered renal arterial dynamics stimulates excess renin production. There is a subsequent increase in aldosterone secretion regardless of the actual state of fluid volume within the body (26).

9. Pregnancy
   Preeclampsia
   Eclampsia

9. There may be a threefold increase in aldosterone secretion during pregnancy. This is in response to progesterone competition, increased renin activity, and, possibly, decreased renal clearance of aldosterone (4).

10. Heat stress

10. There is increased sweating (loss of body sodium) to allow for cooling by evaporation. To conserve body sodium replacing that lost through sweat, aldosterone secretion is increased (16).

11. Stress

11. Aldosterone is secreted as part of the adaptation reaction to the initial alarm reaction to stress. It is a response to the general decreased circulating blood volume. Physical or psychological stress, such as burns, trauma, surgery, extreme anxiety, fear or emotional crises, stimulates aldosterone secretion (9).

12. Low sodium diet

12. A low-serum sodium stimulates the secretion of renin, resulting in aldosterone release.

13. Pseudoaldosteronism from licorice

13. Excessive ingestion of licorice (ammonium glycyrrhizate) causes sodium retention, decreased serum potassium, and decreased plasma renin, which present the picture of primary aldosteronism (11, 24).

14. Hemorrhage
    Dehydration
    Upright position with pooling of
       blood in legs

14. There is a decrease in plasma volume blood flow through the kidneys, which stimulates renin-angiotensin secretion, which causes an increase in aldosterone production. Aldosterone stimulates sodium-

water retention that results in resto-
ration of fluid volume.

Conditions Related to Decreases	**Rationale**
1. Diabetes mellitus	1. In patients with long-term diabetes mellitus with neuropathy, catecholamine secretion is reduced, which causes reduction in renin secretion with a decrease in aldosterone secretion (11).
2. High sodium diet	2. Increased concentration of sodium in the diet decreases aldosterone secretion.

Drug Influences: The following drugs may influence test results. The drugs are listed alphabetically by generic name and divided into columns according to the effect of the drug. Examples of trade names are in parentheses.

The following drugs may cause an increase in test results:

Plasma

Post-IV injection response
  angiotensin
  furosemide (Lasix)
  potassium (Invenex)

Miscellaneous
  spironolactone (Aldactone)

Urine

Post-IV, oral, and/or parenteral administration response
  angiotensin
  corticotropin (Acthar)
  lithium (Lithonate-S)
  oral contraceptives

The following drugs may cause a decrease in test results:

Serum

Hormonal effect
  desoxycorticosterone (Percorten)
  glycyrrhiza

Urine

Production inhibition
  aminoglutethimide
  amphenone B
  chorophenothane (DDT)
  glucocorticoids (Celestone)
  propranolol (Inderal)

Miscellaneous
  clonidine (Catapres)
  glycyrrhiza
  heparin (Heprinar)

Related Lab Studies: Monitor response to treatment or progress of disease and adjust nursing care accordingly. See individual tests for information.

Primary Aldosteronism

  plasma electrolytes ($\uparrow$ Na $\downarrow$ K)

  urine sodium and potassium (with low sodium intake, $\downarrow$ Na $\uparrow$ K)

  *EKG for potassium effect ($\downarrow$ K)

  *plasma renin ($\downarrow$ in primary aldosteronism, $\uparrow$ in secondary aldosteronism)

IMPLICATIONS FOR NURSING CARE
PRETEST: Factors related to the test
Nursing Diagnosis: Potential for injury related to changes in biochemical balance

Guide to assessment	Guide to planning and intervention	Guide to evaluation

Patient factors influencing test results:
1. Electrolyte fluid balance
  Sodium/potassium
  Hydration
  Position
  Licorice intake (excessive)
	1. Demonstrate aldosterone secretion by:
	  a. Administering sodium intake as ordered.
	  b. Administering synthetic mineralcorticoid as ordered.
	  c. Positioning patient from upright position to recumbent position 2 hours prior to specimen collection.
	  d. Indicating licorice intake.
		1. Patient's lab tests are within normal limits.

2. Preexisting Conditions (See Increases/Decreases) 3. Comprehensive drug history (See Drug Influences)	2. Record preexisting conditions on lab slip. 3. Consult with physician and inform lab of drugs the patient is receiving that may influence aldosterone level.	2. Patient's preexisting conditions are noted. 3. The patient's pertinent drug history is discussed with physician and lab.

4. Knowledge deficit	4. Explain test to patient:
	  a. Define aldosterone (See Description).
	  b. Explain procedure (See Procedure).
		4. The patient demonstrates knowledge of test by defining test and stating procedure.

*Not discussed in this book.

Patient Preparation Checklist

1. √ Correct test procedure for sodium administration.
2. √ Patient drug history (See Drug Influences).
3. √ Preexisting conditions and note on lab slip (See Increases/Decreases).
4. √ Patient knowledge and explain test to patient (See Description and Procedure).
5. √ Collection procedure (See Procedure).

CONSIDERATIONS FOR NURSING CARE RELATED TO ABNORMAL TEST RESULTS
POSTTEST: Factors related to the results of the test
Nursing Diagnosis: Alterations in biochemical balance

Guide to assessment	Guide to planning and intervention	Guide to evaluation
1. Laboratory measurements Serum sodium above 140 mEq/L Monitor serum potassium Monitor plasma renin	1. Administer aldosterone antagonists such as spironolactone (Aldactone) as ordered.	1. Aldosterone secretion is suppressed as indicated by lab studies.
2. Preoperative for resection of adrenal adenoma	2. Initiate nursing measures to prepare patient for surgery to remove aldosterone-secreting adenoma.	2. Patient is prepared for surgery.
3. Daily weights I&O	3. Provide the physician with accurate account of patient's body water status.	3. Patient's water, sodium intake, and diuretic therapy are adjusted accurately.
4. Psychological stress Fear Anxiety Emotional crises	4. Reduce psychological stresses by: a. Establishing a tranquil environment. b. Showing sensitivity to patient's feelings. c. Maintaining consistent caregivers if possible.	4. The patient's need for adaptation to psychological stress is reduced.
5. Sodium loss Excessive sweating Gains of water in excess of sodium	5. Teach principles of heat stress: a. Explaining sodium loss and aldosterone secretion. b. Replenishing water and salt losses as they occur. c. Discouraging strenuous activity that produces excessive sweating during hot days.	5. The patient is able to give return explanation of sodium/water loss and aldosterone secretion.

Guide to assessment	Guide to planning and intervention	Guide to evaluation
6. Hyper/hypokalemia Observe for symptoms of potassium imbalance Increased B/P associated with hypokalemia Symptoms of alkalosis Symptoms of decreased cardiac output Symptoms of fluid imbalance	6. Be alert to and report aldosterone imbalances promptly.	6. Aldosterone imbalances are corrected promptly.

Test:	Alkaline Phosphatase
Abbreviation:	ALP
Reference Values:	*Adults* (11)
	20–90 IU/L at 30°C
	Children (23)
	Newborn 50–165 U/L
	Child 20–150 U/L
Specimen:	Serum

Description: Alkaline phosphate (ALP) is an enzyme that catalyzes chemical reactions in the body best in an alkaline environment. ALP is found in bone osteoblasts, the liver, intestinal epithelia, kidney tubules, the placenta, and lactating mammary glands (13). Pathway of excretion is unknown (7, 11), but ALP is probably degraded as part of the general protein pool (26). Specific isoenzymes can now be measured. These isoenzymes are of the liver, bone, intestine, kidney, and placenta. Use of this test is beneficial in the differential diagnosis of bone disorders and liver diseases.

Procedure: (red top tube)
1. Restrict food and fluids for 12 hours or as ordered (procedure may vary with institution). The patient may have water.
2. 2–7 ml of venous blood is drawn from the patient.
3. Observe puncture site for bleeding or evidence of hematoma.

Conditions Related to Increases

Bone Origin

Rationale

1. Paget's disease (osteitis deformans)
2. Osteogenic sarcoma
3. Metastatic bone tumors
4. Osteomalacia, rickets
5. Infections involving bone
6. Healing bone fractures
7. Sickle-cell anemia

1. Increase is caused by intense osteoblastic activity in the involved areas.
2. If an osteoblastic sarcoma, elevation is due to extreme increase in osteoblastic activity.
3. May stimulate osteoblastic activity, causing elevation.
4. Parathyroid activity is stimulated by low blood calcium, which induces reabsorption of bone and stimulates increased osteoblastic activity (9).
5. There is increased osteoblastic activity for replacement of damaged bone cells.
6. Slight elevations occur due to osteoblastic activity during bone healing.
7. Increases during crises are due to vaso-occlusive bone injury, as well as liver damage (9).

Liver Origin

8. Metastatic carcinoma of liver
   Intrahepatic biliary atresia

8. Stimulates formation of ALP from hepatic parenchymal cells (11).

9. Gallstones
   Obstructive tumors or space occupying lesions of biliary ducts

9. Stimulates formation of ALP from hepatic ductal cells.

10. Hepatitis
    Infectious mononucleosis

10. Inflammatory changes within the liver stimulate increased enzyme formation.

11. Congestive heart failure

11. Serum levels increase whenever there is obstruction to hepatic blood flow (10). There is an increase in formation of the enzyme by hepatic parenchymal or ductal cells (11).

12. Carcinoma of head of pancreas

12. The tumor compresses and obstructs the common bile duct, which stimulates formation of ALP from ductal cells.

Kidney Origin

13. Proximal renal tubular acidosis
    Acute pyelonephritis
    Nephrotic syndrome
    Chronic renal failure

13. Renal destruction from inflammation results in release of ALP from renal tubular cells into the bloodstream (9).

Miscellaneous

14. Fistula of stomach and duodenum
    Steatorrhea

14. May lead to secondary osteomalacia. See 4 above.

15. Infusion of human albumin

15. If prepared from placental blood because ALP is produced in placenta (27).

16. Meals (most marked in women)

16. It is found that in some subjects food ingestion has increased test results by as much as 25% due to one or a combination of variables. Blood type and type of meal consumed are examples of these variables (10, 11, 21).

17. Infancy and childhood (especially puberty)

17. Osteoblastic activity during periods of bone growth is increased.

18. Pregnancy, third trimester

18. The increase is reflective of placental manufacture of ALP (26).

19. Environmental variable, specimen at room temperature beyond short time interval

19. The activity of ALP may increase at room temperature due to change in pH.

Conditions Related to Decreases	Rationale
1. Childhood hypothyroidism (cretinism)	1. There is reduced osteoblastic activity due to retarded bone growth.
2. Malnutrition, scurvy, celiac disease	2. Impaired hepatic function from protein-calorie malnutrition and nutrient malabsorption causes a decrease in ALP production.
3. Growth retardation	3. Reduced osteoblastic activity reduces ALP secretion.
4. Hypophosphatasia	4. This disease is characterized by a defect in bone formation with diminished osteoblastic activity. This condition is very rare.
5. Meals	5. Significant effect has been observed. Bile acids, some amino acids, and urea act as ALP inhibitors.

Drug Influences (15, 27): The following drugs may cause an increase in alkaline phosphatase. The drugs are listed alphabetically by generic name and divided into columns according to effect of the drug. Examples of trade names are in parentheses.

Hepatotoxic effect
   azathioprine (Imuran)
   colchicine (Colchicine, Novacolchine)
   gentamicin (Garamycin, Cidomycin)
   kanamycin (Kantrex)
   lincomycin (Mithracin)
   nitrogen mustard
   penicillamine
   phenylbutazone (Butazolidin)
   progesterone (Progestin)
   propylthiouracil (PTU)

Cholestatic effect
   amitriptyline (Elavil, Levate)
   carbamazepine (Tegretol)
   imipramine (Antipres, Tofranil)
   indomethacin (Indocin, Indocid)
   isoniazid (INH)
   methyltestosterone (Android, Testred)
   para-aminosalicylic acid (PAS)
   progestin-estrogen combination (Demulen, Enovid, Lo/Ovral, Modicon, Norinyl, Ortho-Novum, Ovulen, Ovral, Zorane)
   sulfadiazine
   sulfamethizole (Thiosulfil)
   sulfamethoxazole (Gantanol)
   tetracycline

Intrahepatic cholestatic effect
  acetohexamide (Dimelor, Dymelor)
  chlorpropamide (Diabinase, Chloronase)
  erythromycin (Ilosone, Erythrocin)
  methyldopa (Aldomet, Dopamet)
  nitrofurantoin (Furadantin, Furatine, Nifuron, Macrodantin)
  novobiocin (Albamycin)
  phenothiazines (Thorazine, Stelazine, Prolixin, Trilafon, Compazine, Mellaril, Sparine)
  tolazamide (Tolinase)
  tolbutamide (Orinase)

Reversible hepatotoxic effect
  allopurinol (Zyloprim, Lopurin)
  papaverine (Pavabid, Pavacin, Sustaverine, Vasocap)
  procainamide (Procan SR, Pronestyl)
  rifampin (Rifadin)
  thiothixene (Navane)

Miscellaneous
  albumin infusion (See 15, Increases)
  fat emulsions; after prolonged infusion
  cephaloridine (Loridine), estrogens (Estrace, Progynon, Gravigen, Foygen, Theelin); mechanism not listed

The following drug may cause a decrease in ALP.

Improves biliary excretion in biliary cirrhosis
  azathioprine (Imuran)

Related Lab Studies: Monitor response to treatment or progress of disease and adjust nursing care accordingly. See individual tests for information.

Liver function studies
  serum bilirubin
  urine bilirubin
  A/G ratio
  albumin
  total protein
  prothrombin time (PT)
  cholesterol
  AST (SGOT)
  ALT (SGPT)
  GTT
  *bile acids radioimmunoassay

Bone studies
  CBC
  hemoglobin electrophoresis
  *bone scan

---

*Not discussed in this book.

IMPLICATIONS FOR NURSING CARE
PRETEST: Factors related to the test
Nursing Diagnosis: Potential for injury related to changes in biochemical balance

Guide to assessment	Guide to planning and intervention	Guide to evaluation
Patient factors influencing test results:		
1. Food and fluids	1. Restrict food and fluids, as ordered, 12 hours prior to collecting specimen (See 16 Increases, 5 Decreases).	1. The patient's diet does not influence test results.
2. Comprehensive drug history a. See Drug Influences b. IV albumin within past 10 days	2. Report drugs the patient is receiving that may influence lab results to the patient's physician and to laboratory.	2. The patient's current medications do not influence test results because they are identified and the proper people are notified.
3. Preexisting conditions (See Increases/Decreases)	3. Record preexisting conditions on lab slip.	3. Patient's preexisting conditions are noted on lab slip.
4. Lack of patient knowledge	4. Explain test to patient: a. Define ALP (See Description). b. Explain procedure (See Procedure).	4. The patient demonstrates knowledge of test by defining test and explaining procedure.

Patient Preparation Checklist

1. √ NPO for 12 hours, or as ordered.
2. √ Patient drug history (See Drug Influences).
3. √ Preexisting conditions and note on lab slip.
4. √ Patient knowledge, explain test to patient (See Description, Procedure).

CONSIDERATIONS FOR NURSING CARE RELATED TO ABNORMAL TEST RESULTS
POSTTEST: Factors related to the results of the test
Nursing Diagnosis: Alterations in biochemical balance

Guide to assessment	Guide to planning and intervention	Guide to evaluation
1. Dietary history, specifically: Calcium intake Vitamin D deficiency Malnutrition	1. Teach principles of balanced essential food intake, specifically protein, calories, calcium, and vitamin D.	1. The patient demonstrates understanding by words and actions that at each meal the diet should include the four basic food groups.

Guide to assessment	Guide to planning and intervention	Guide to evaluation
2. As above	2. Promote balanced essential food intake by: a. Providing attractive, well-balanced meals. b. Providing choice of nutritional foods within limits of prescribed diet.	2. The patient communicates satisfaction by dietary intake.
3. Probable liver origin Nursing history and/or physical exam suggestive of liver dysfunction or bile duct obstruction Enlarged liver Jaundice, urine/stool color Water retention/ascites ↓ Level of consciousness Irritability Seizure activity Bleeding tendencies	3. Protect patient from excessive liver palpation by students and staff. a. Measure and adjust nutritional intake according to water retention and ascites.	3. The patient is protected against liver damage from excessive liver palpation. a. Water retention and ascites are controlled by the measurement and adjustment of patient intake.
4. Probable bone origin Nursing history and physical findings suggestive of bone disease Fever, malaise, past history of bone trauma Sickle-cell disease Bone pain Bone or joint swelling Fracture(s) Bone fragility	4. Facilitate healing by: a. Promoting treatment of bone infection: (1) Administering antibiotics as ordered. (2) Preventing excessive motion of affected part. b. Maintaining adequate hydration. c. Maintaining proper musculoskeletal alignment. d. Maintaining a safe environment to prevent bone trauma or fracture.	a. The patient is free of fever, malaise, and bone pain due to bone infection. b. The agglutination process of sickled cells in the patient with sickle-cell disease is halted or reversed by adequate hydration. c. The patient's correct musculoskeletal alignment and/or bone union is achieved. d. The patient does not experience bone trauma or fracture due to bone fragility.

Test:	Ammonia
Abbreviation:	NH_3
Reference Values:	Values vary widely. Check local laboratory for normal ranges.
Specimen:	Plasma
Description:	Ammonia is produced mainly in the intestines by action of bacteria on proteins, and to some extent from hydrolysis of glutamine in the kidneys. Ammonia is toxic to the body, but it is absorbed into the portal vein where, in the liver, it is converted to urea. Almost no ammonia is left in circulation. After conversion to urea in the liver, it is excreted by the kidneys. Ammonia levels are done to monitor hepatic disease and possible hepatic coma. Serial ammonia levels are more helpful than single levels.
Procedure:	(green top tube)

1. Patient should restrict food and fluids (except water) for 8 hours.
2. The patient should not engage in physical activity prior to blood drawing.
3. If someone other than laboratory personnel draws the blood, inform lab that blood is to be drawn and what time. This must be done prior to blood drawing.
4. Blood may be drawn from skin puncture or venipuncture method. Up to 2 ml of blood is drawn from the patient.
5. Observe puncture site carefully for bleeding or evidence of hematoma.
6. The blood specimen should be iced and sent directly to the laboratory and given to a laboratory technologist.

Conditions Related to Increases

Rationale

Plasma

1. Certain inborn errors of metabolism:
   Familial protein intolerance
   Ornithine transcarbamoylase deficiency

1. The increase in ammonia is due to depressed urea-cycle function. In familial protein intolerance, the diminished urea-cycle function is due to decreased absorption of ornithine and arginine (amino acids). In ornithine transcarbamoylase deficiency, the decreased urea-cycle function is due to the lack of the liver enzyme, ornithine transcarbamoylase (34).

2. Hemolytic disease of the newborn
   Congestive heart failure, severe
   Cor pulmonale

2. Hepatic insufficiency due to hepatic congestion and, possibly, some actual hepatic damage is the cause of increased plasma ammonia.

3. Reye's syndrome

3. Damaged hepatic mitochondria depresses liver enzyme activity and decreases urea-cycle function. Ammonia levels correlate very well with the level of consciousness and with patient survival.

4. Hepatic cirrhosis

4. Hepatic architecture is deranged and allows blood to be shunted past the liver. This may also occur after surgical portal-caval shunt procedure.

5. Liver failure

5. The excessive number of damaged liver cells decreases liver uptake and conversion of ammonia.

6. GI bleeding associated with hepatic cirrhosis

6. The liver, already diseased by cirrhosis, is unable to convert the excessive ammonia load to urea effectively.

7. Exercise

7. Plasma ammonia levels may be elevated immediately after exercise because of increased tissue catabolism.

8. Protein ingestion

8. Recent protein ingestion will result in a significant increase in plasma ammonia.

9. Alkalosis
   Distal renal tubular damage

9. In both metabolic and respiratory alkalosis, blood ammonia increases. The increase is due to renal retention of ammonia. Urinary ammonia decreases (34).

Conditions Related to Decreases

Rationale
(Urine)

1. Renal damage

1. Because of damage to renal tubules, the area of the kidneys that deaminates glutamic acid to ammonia, urinary excretion is decreased.

Drug Influences: The following drugs may influence test results. The drugs are listed alphabetically by generic name and divided into columns according to the effect of the drug. Examples of trade names are in parentheses.

The following drugs may cause an increase in test results:

Serum

Hypokalemia and alkalosis
   chlorothiazide (Aldoclor)
   chlorthalidone (Hygroton)
   ethacrynic acid (Edecrin)
   furosemide (Lasix)

Hepatic impairment
   ammonium salts (in cough preparations)
   asparaginase (Elspar)
   barbiturates
   ethanol (grain alcohol)
   glucose (Hydra-Lyte)
   hydroflumethiazide (Diucardin)
   morphine
   thiopental (pentothal sodium)
Potential ammonia source
   acetazolamide (Diamox)
   isoniazid (Laniazid)
   levoglutamide (Nature's Bounty)
Miscellaneous
   tetracycline (Achromycin); large IV dose

Urine

Miscellaneous
   methenamine (Hiprex)

The following drugs may cause a decrease in test results:

Serum

Urease inhibition
   acetohydroxamic acid
Capacity of reacting with ammonia
   arginine
   glutamic acid (Acidulin)
Exogenous ammonia toxicity effect
   diphenhydramine (Benadryl)
   isocarboxazid (Marplan)
   MAO inhibitors (Eutonyl)
Hepatic encephalophy
   lactobacillus acidophilus (Lactinex)
   lactulose (Cephulac)
Reduction of ammonia-producing bacteria
   kanamycin (Kantrex)
   neomycin
   tetracycline (Achromycin)
Miscellaneous
   potassium salts (Slow-K)
   sodium salts (sodium chloride, IV)

Urine

Starvation
   glucose (Hydra-Lyte)

Increased alkalinity
  acetazolamide (Diamox)
  secretin

Carbonic anhydrase inhibition
  mafenide (Sulfamylon)

Related Lab Studies: Monitor response to treatment or progress of disease and adjust nursing care accordingly. See individual tests for information.

Liver function tests
  bilirubin, serum
    direct
    indirect
  bilirubin, urine
  urobilinogen
  alkaline phosphatase
  AST (SGOT)
  ALT (SGPT)
  LDH
  serum protein electrophoresis
  prothrombin time
  cholesterol
  serum immunoglobulin

Reye's syndrome; admission lab work
  ammonia, serum
  ALT (SGPT)
  bilirubin, total
  prothrombin time
  glucose, blood
  BUN
  creatinine
  osmolality, serum
  salicylate level
  blood gases
  lumbar puncture

IMPLICATIONS FOR NURSING CARE
PRETEST: Factors related to the test
Nursing Diagnosis: Potential for injury related to changes in biochemical balance

Guide to assessment	Guide to planning and intervention	Guide to evaluation
Assess patient factors that may influence test results:		

1. NPO 8–12 hours	1. Reduce dietary protein effect on ammonia levels:
	  a. Place patient NPO.
	  b. Explain need of NPO status to patient.
		1. The patient is NPO 8–12 hours.

Guide to assessment	Guide to planning and intervention	Guide to evaluation
2. Comprehensive drug history (See Drug Influences)	2. Identify drugs that may influence test results. Note on lab slip. Consult with physician.	2. Patient's medications do not interfere with accurate lab results.
3. Preexisting conditions (See Increases)	3. Identify preexisting conditions that may influence test results.	3. Patient's preexisting conditions are identified and noted on lab slip.
4. Nonlaboratory personnel drawing blood	4. Inform lab prior to blood drawing. Pack specimen in ice and send to lab stat.	4. Patient's blood ammonia sample does not deteriorate.
5. Hemolysis	5. Prevent hemolysis by: a. Not saturating the skin with antiseptic. b. Not probing venipuncture site or leaving the tourniquet on too long. c. Not forcefully withdrawing specimen. d. Not withdrawing specimen too slowly. e. Not agitating or handling specimen too roughly.	5. Patient's values are not influenced by hemolysis.
6. Knowledge deficit	6. Explain test to patient (family): a. Define ammonia (See Description). b. Explain procedure (See Procedure).	6. The patient demonstrates knowledge by defining test and explaining procedure.

Patient Preparation Checklist

1. √ NPO for 8–12 hours.
2. √ Comprehensive drug history; note pertinent drugs on lab slip.
3. √ Preexisting conditions noted on lab slip (See Increases).
4. √ Lab is aware of when blood is being drawn.
5. √ Prevention of hemolysis of specimen.
6. √ Patient knowledge; explain test to patient.

CONSIDERATIONS FOR NURSING CARE RELATED TO ABNORMAL TEST RESULTS
POSTTEST: Factors related to the results of the test
Nursing Diagnosis: Alteration in biochemical balance

Guide to assessment	Guide to planning and intervention	Guide to evaluation
Assess patient factors that may be influencing test results. Nursing history and/or physical exam that is suggestive of:		

1. Possible increased ammonia level
  a. Those with
    Newborn hemolytic disease
    Severe congestive heart failure
    Reye's syndrome severe liver disease
    Cirrhosis and GI bleeding or electrolyte imbalances
	1. Discourage increased ammonia levels:
	  a. Recognize patients at risk for increased blood ammonia levels.
	  b. Promote liver health:
	    (1) Encourage nutritious diet.
	    (2) Inform patients of the relationship of excessive alcohol intake and liver damage.
	    (3) Refer patients with jaundice for medical evaluation.
		1. Patient's ammonia levels remain within normal limits.

2. Reye's syndrome
 	
  a. Stage I, signs and symptoms:
    Child—
    Prodromal viral illness
    Persistent vomiting
    Lethargy
    Listlessness
    Disinterest in environment
  Stage II, signs and symptoms:
    Hyperventilation
    Delirium
    Hepatic dysfunction
    Hyperactive reflexes
  b. Hepatic dysfunction
    ↑ Ammonia
    ↑ ALT (SGPT)
    ↑ Prothrombin time
	2. Control the progression of Reye's syndrome:
	  a. Recognize early signs and symptoms of disease. Refer to physician immediately for emergency care.
	
	b. Protect mitochondrial metabolism:
	  (1) Administer 10–15% glucose solution as prescribed.
		2. Patient recovers without sequela.
		
		b. Patient's liver function studies return to normal.

Guide to assessment	Guide to planning and intervention	Guide to evaluation
	(2) Measure intake and output.	
	(3) Control fever through cool environment or by sponging.	
3. Hepatic encephalopathy, signs and symptoms: Liver flap (asterixis) Slight confusion Untidiness Daytime sleepiness General inappropriate behavior Deterioration of simple thought processes and problem-solving skills	3. Control ammonia levels:	3. Patient's ammonia levels return to normal.
	a. Recognize early signs of hepatic encephalopathy.	
	b. Eliminate, as possible, sources of protein breakdown:	b. Patient's ammonia levels return to normal.
	(1) Give no protein diet.	
	(2) Give IV glucose or total parenteral nutrition to meet nutrient needs.	
	(3) Insert nasogastric tube for patient with GI bleeding.	
	(4) Sterilize bowel with Neomycin (or bowel preparation antibiotic): (a) Do not exceed 3 g for total daily dose. (b) Take vital signs. (c) Measure intake and output.	
(d) Signs of nephrotoxicity: Oliguria or anuria Flank pain Monitor urinalysis Monitor BUN	(d) Be alert to signs of nephrotoxicity. (e) Consult with physician about concurrent administration of diuretics, because in this situation they should not be given together.	
(5) Sorbitol	(5) Give high, large water volume cathartic enemas to induce osmotic diarrhea.	

Guide to assessment	Guide to planning and intervention	Guide to evaluation
(6) Lactulose	(6) Decrease bacterial colonic action by giving lactulose.	
	(7) Resume protein diet cautiously after ammonia levels return to normal. Detect any signs of returning encephalopathy. Consult physician immediately.	
c. Transfusions of stored blood Potassium loss Thiazide diuretics Alkalosis	c. Be aware of factors that may cause an increase in blood ammonia levels in person with compromised liver.	

Test:	Amylase
Abbreviation:	AMS
Reference Values:	*Serum*

Adults   60–180 Somogyi U/dl (11)
              5–81 IU/L
Children   45–200 dye U/dl
              80–180 Somogyi U/dl (23)
Urine
35–260 Somogyi U/hr

Specimen: Serum, urine

Description: Amylase (AMS) is an enzyme produced principally in the pancreas but also in the salivary glands, liver, fallopian tubes, and skeletal muscle. Because it is a small molecule, it is filtered through kidney glomeruli and excreted in the urine. Amylase is responsible for breaking down starch into its component sugars. Serum and urine amylase is used as a diagnostic test for pancreatic disease.

Procedure: (red top tube)

Serum
1. Order blood to be drawn prior to medications or Hypaque dye.
2. 2–7 ml of venous blood is drawn from the patient.

Urine
1. A timed specimen is usually collected (2, 12, or 24 hr).
2. No special container is needed, but urine should be refrigerated.
3. Collect and discard urine specimen; begin timing.
4. Be sure to note exact collection time period.
5. Save *all* urine during collection time period as measurement is quantitative. If a specimen is discarded, start collection over.
6. See Patient Preparation Checklist.

Conditions Related to Increases

1. Acute pancreatitis

Rationale

1. The increase results from the enzyme escaping into the interstitial tissue and peritoneal cavity with increased reabsorption of AMS through the lymphatic and venous systems (11). In acute pancreatitis, high levels of serum AMS usually last 48–72 hours. The return to normal values is due to renal clearance. Levels are rarely elevated in chronic pancreatitis (See Decreases 2).

Urine AMS shows elevation several hours after serum levels begin to rise; urine levels remain elevated longer. For this reason, urine levels are useful diagnostically.

2. Common bile duct calculi or obstruction

2. Obstruction of the pancreatic duct causes subsequent backup of AMS into the bloodstream.

3. Perforated peptic ulcer

3. Ulcer may perforate pancreas, causing a secondary pancreatitis.

4. Intestinal obstruction

4. Secondary obstruction of pancreatic duct from intestinal distention causes a backup of AMS in the bloodstream.

5. Peritonitis

5. There is a natural secretion of AMS into the intestine. Rupture of the intestine releases free AMS into peritoneal cavity with increased absorption through the lymphatic and venous systems.

6. Spasms of sphincter of Oddi

6. Spasms of the sphincter between the common bile duct and duodenum prevents normal secretion of AMS.

7. Trauma
   Post-op gastric resection
   Ruptured ectopic pregnancy

7. Increase is due to the enzyme in the peritoneal cavity, which is absorbed into the bloodstream.

8. Cholecystitis
   Peptic ulcer

8. Inflammation causes a transient pancreatitis.

9. Macroamylasemia

9. In this condition, amylase molecules bind to protein molecules that become too big to pass through glomeruli. The increase in serum AMS is sometimes misinterpreted as serious disease. This is most often seen in patients with malabsorption and/or alcoholism. There is no correlation with any particular disease state (11).

10. Alcoholic intoxication

10. Causes stimulation of pancreatic secretion.

11. Parotid gland disease
    Diabetic ketoacidosis
    Acute respiratory insufficiency

11. There is increased absorption of salivary AMS into the bloodstream from increased salivary gland AMS secretion.

Conditions Related to Decreases

1. Hepatitis, severe
   Cirrhosis of liver
   Carcinoma of liver
   Poisoning
2. Advanced chronic
   pancreatitis
   Advanced cystic fibrosis
3. Hyperglycemia

Rationale

1. There is marked destruction of the liver, which is an AMS-producing organ (24).

2. Destruction of the pancreas, which is an amylase-producing organ, decreases enzyme production.

3. Inhibits enzyme activity (11).

Drug Influences: The following drugs may cause an increase in serum AMS. The drugs are listed alphabetically by generic name and divided into columns according to the effect of the drug. Examples of trade names are in parentheses.

Drug-induced pancreatitis
   dexamethasone (Dexadron, Dexasone)
   furosemide (Lasix)
   L-Asparaginase
   methanol
   salicylates (aspirin)
   thiazides and related diuretics (Aquapres, Hygroton, Diuril, Hydrodiuril, Enduron, etc.)

Stimulation of pancreatic secretion
   ethyl alcohol (liquor, grain alcohol)

Increased Spasms of Sphincter of Oddi
   bethanechol (Urecholine)
   Hypaque dye
   meperidine hydrochloride (Demerol; causes less spasm than opiates)
   opiates (morphine, codeine)

Increased AMS activity
   chloride salts

The following drug may cause a decrease in serum AMS due to an inhibition of enzyme activity:
   citrate

Related Lab Studies: Monitor response to treatment or progress of disease and adjust nursing care accordingly. See individual tests for information.

Acute pancreatic disease
   urinary amylase ↑
   serum lipase ↑
   blood glucose ↑
   calcium ↓
   potassium ↓

IMPLICATIONS FOR NURSING CARE
PRETEST: Factors related to the test
Nursing Diagnosis: Potential for injury related to changes in biochemical balance

Guide to assessment	Guide to planning and intervention	Guide to evaluation
1. Comprehensive drug history	1. Order serum amylase to be drawn prior to medications or Hypaque dye given to patient: a. Report drugs the patient is receiving that may influence lab results to the patient's physician and to the laboratory.	1. The patient receives no interfering medication prior to blood drawing: a. Drugs the patient is currently receiving that may influence test results are identified and the proper people notified.
2. Preexisting conditions (See Increases/Decreases)	2. Record preexisting conditions on lab slip.	2. Patient's preexisting conditions are noted on lab slip.
3. Lack of patient knowledge	3. Explain test to patient: a. Define test (See Description). b. Record preexisting conditions on lab slip.	3. The patient demonstrates knowledge of test by defining test and explaining procedure.

Patient Preparation Checklist

1. √ Blood drawn prior to medications or diagnostic dyes given.
2. √ Preexisting conditions and drugs noted on lab slip.
3. √ Procedure for urine collection.
4. √ Explain test to patient (See Description and Procedure).

CONSIDERATIONS FOR NURSING CARE RELATED TO ABNORMAL TEST RESULTS
POSTTEST: Factors related to the results of the test
Nursing Diagnosis: Alterations in biochemical balance

Guide to assessment	Guide to planning and intervention	Guide to evaluation
1. Nursing history and/or physical exam suggestive of acute pancreatic disease a. Increase in peritoneal fluid	1. Reduce stimulation of pancreatic secretions by: a. Giving prescribed anticholinergic drugs and maintaining NPO, gastric suction, fluid intake treatment plan.	1. The patient demonstrates reduced pancreatic stimulation by: a. Reduced intestinal distention.

Guide to assessment	Guide to planning and intervention	Guide to evaluation
b. Pain that is in abdomen and back and is boring, bandlike, and constant	b. Give pain medication as needed (See Drug Influences) and help the patient assume position of comfort.	b. Diminished verbal and nonverbal communication of pain.
2. Spasms of sphincter of Oddi Acute, severe, deep, cramping pain	2. Reduce spasms by: a. Giving nonopiate pain medication. b. Encouraging low-fat diet. c. Discouraging use of alcoholic beverages.	2. The patient is free of pain due to spasms of sphincter of Oddi.
3. Diabetic ketoacidosis	3. Be alert to signs/symptoms of complications of acute pancreatitis that affect amylase secretion.	3. The patient is free of complications of pancreatitis.
4. History of alcohol abuse	4. Discourage use of alcoholic beverages by explaining relationship to pancreatitis (See Increases 10).	4. The patient explains relationship of alcohol consumption to acute pancreatitis.

Test:	Antinuclear Antibodies Fluorescent Screening Procedure
Abbreviation:	ANA, FANA
Reference Value:	Negative (titer below 1:20; may vary lab to lab)
Specimen:	Serum
Description:	Antinuclear antibodies are antibodies formed against the nucleus of body cells. They are, by themselves, noninvasive and do not destroy cells. When the antinuclear antibody reacts with a portion of a cellular nucleus as the antigen, it causes an antigen-antibody reaction that results in tissue damage.

Antinuclear antibodies can be identified with a fluorescent screening procedure. The procedure demonstrates the antibody attachment to cells. Four characteristic patterns have been demonstrated in the way ANA attaches to the nucleus. The diffuse or homogeneous pattern is the most frequently seen pattern and is characteristic of systemic lupus erythematosus (SLE), although it may also be seen in rheumatoid arthritis. The peripheral or shaggy pattern is the strongest pattern seen in SLE. It is also seen in drug-induced SLE-like syndromes, but the titer is about 1:20–1:50 compared to 1:250 in SLE. Other patterns are the speckled pattern, seen in other connective tissue diseases, and the nucleolar pattern, seen in scleroderma and Sjögren's disease. It is seen rarely in SLE.

Fluorescent ANA procedure is done to aid in the diagnosis of, and follow immunosuppressive therapy in, SLE.

Procedure:	(red top tube)
	1. No food or fluid restrictions.
	2. 2–10 ml of blood is drawn from the patient.
	3. Observe puncture site for bleeding, evidence of hematoma, or infection.

Conditions Related to Increases

1. Systemic lupus
     erythematosus
   Rheumatoid arthritis
   Felty's syndrome
   Progressive systemic sclerosis
   Dermatomyositis/polymyositis
   Infectious mononucleosis
   Viral hepatitis
   Atypical pneumonia

Rationale

1. In autoimmune diseases and occasionally in response to an infection, in certain drugs, and in apparently healthy people, the body may respond to portions of the cell nucleus as foreign and produce antibodies to it.

Drug Influences: The following drugs may influence test results. The drugs are listed alphabetically by generic name and divided into columns according to the effect of the drug. Examples of trade names are in parentheses.

The following drugs may cause an increase of false positive test result.

Prolonged use-related (higher in women)
   anticonvulsants (Dilantin, Mesantoin)
   ethosuximide (Zarontin)
   hydralazine (Apresoline)
   methyldopa (Aldomet)
   procainamide (Pronestyl)
   trimethadione (Tridione)

Hypersensitivity reaction
   oxyphenisatin

TB patient-related
   isoniazid (INH)

Miscellaneous
   aminosalicylic acid (PAS)
   chlorpromazine (Thorazine)
   clofibrate (Atromid-S)
   gold salts (Myochrysine)
   griseofulvin (Fulvicin)
   methysergide (Sansert)
   oral contraceptives
   penicillin
   phenylbutazone (Azolid)
   propylthiouracil
   quinidine
   reserpine
   streptomycin
   sulfonamides
   tetracyclines

Related Lab Studies: Monitor response to therapy or progression of disease and adjust nursing care accordingly. See individual lab tests for specific information.

SLE
   CBC
   platelet count
   sedimentation rate
   protein electrophoresis
   urinalysis
   creatinine clearance
   *serum complement studies
   radioimmunoassay, LE factor
   *serology (false positive)
   indirect immunofluorescent antibody
   LE prep

---

*Not discussed in this book.

IMPLICATIONS FOR NURSING CARE
PRETEST: Factors related to the test
Nursing Diagnosis: Potential for injury related to changes in immune-autoimmune factors

Guide to assessment	Guide to planning and intervention	Guide to evaluation
Assess patient factors that may influence test results: 1. Comprehensive drug history (See Drug Influences), especially Hydralazine Procainamide Isoniazid Oral contraceptives	1. Note interfering drugs on lab slip.	1. Patient's medications do not interfere with test results.
2. Knowledge deficit	2. Explain test to patient: a. Define antinuclear antibodies (See Description). b. Explain procedure (See Description and Procedure).	2. The patient demonstrates knowledge of test by defining test and explaining procedure.

Patient Preparation Checklist

1. √ Interfering drugs noted on lab slip (See Drug Influences).
2. √ Patient knowledge; explain test to patient (See Description/Procedure).

CONSIDERATIONS FOR NURSING CARE RELATED TO ABNORMAL TEST RESULTS
POSTTEST: Factors related to the results of the test
Nursing Diagnosis: Alterations in immune-autoimmune factors

Guide to assessment	Guide to planning and intervention	Guide to evaluation
Assess patient factors that may be influencing test results. Nursing history and/or physical exam suggestive of: 1. Positive ANA test Drug therapy that causes SLE-like syndrome (See Drug Influences)	1. Recognize drugs that cause SLE-like syndrome and consult with physician.	1. Patient's lab values are normal.

Guide to assessment	Guide to planning and intervention	Guide to evaluation
2. Systemic lupus erythematosus	2. Promote disease remission: a. Prevent precipitation of disease by: (1) Initiating nursing measures to prevent infection. (2) Advising patient to use sunscreen if in the sun. (3) Advising patient to consult with physician before using over-the-counter drugs. (4) Exploring positive ways of responding to stress. (5) Seeking mental health help as needed. (6) Advising patient to keep well rested and eat a well-balanced diet. (7) Administering antibiotics as prescribed.	2. Patient achieves remission.
b. Drug therapy: Corticosteroids Salicylates Nonsteroidal antiinflammatory agents Antimalarial drugs Immunosuppressive drugs	b. Decrease inflammation: (1) Administer drugs as prescribed. (2) Educate patient to side effects and precautions of steroids. (3) See a, 1–7 above.	
c. Lupus Foundation of America, Inc. Arthritis Foundation	c. Encourage participation in support groups.	

Test:	Antistreptolysin O Test
Abbreviation:	ASO, ASL
Reference Values:	For ASO titers

Age	Normal Upper Limits
Under 5 years	85 Todd U
School age	170 Todd U
Adults	125 Todd U

Check specific method and values with local lab.

Specimen:	Serum
Description:	In response to infection by group A beta-hemolytic streptococci, the body develops antibodies to the antigens produced by the bacteria. The antigens are called streptolysin O, the antibodies are called antistreptolysin O antibodies (ASO). These antibodies do not offer protection against future infection. The antibodies can be measured and are useful as a diagnostic tool.

The purpose for testing is as an aid in diagnosing poststreptococcal glomerulonephritis or rheumatic fever and as confirmation of recent infection.

Procedure:
1. No food or fluid restrictions.
2. Up to 5 ml of blood is drawn from the patient. Capillary tubes may be used.
3. Observe site for bleeding or evidence of hematoma or infection.
4. Serial tests may be done to observe response to therapy.

Conditions Related to Increases

1. Recent group A beta-hemolytic streptococcal infection, especially streptococcal pharyngitis
   ASO test
2. Streptococcal pharyngitis
   Streptococcal pyoderma
   Streptodornase method

Rationale

1. In response to streptolysin O antigen.

2. ASO test often misses this infection. Streptodornase is the test most helpful in diagnosing this disease. The antibodies detected are to the antigen streptococcal desoxyribonuclease (DNAse B) produced by all group A streptococci.

Conditions Related to Decreases

1. Streptococcal pyoderma

2. Antibiotic therapy
   Corticosteroid therapy

Rationale

1. If ASO test is used, there is a 75% chance of a false-negative result.
2. These drugs may suppress antibody activity.

Drug Influences: See 2, Decreases.

Related Lab Studies

  throat culture
  WBC
  erythrocyte sedimentation rate
  C-reactive protein (CRP)
  Urinalysis
  *serum complement level
  BUN
  creatinine clearance
  skin lesion culture

IMPLICATIONS FOR NURSING CARE
PRETEST: Factors related to the test
Nursing Diagnosis: Potential for injury related to streptococcal infection

Guide to assessment	Guide to planning and intervention	Guide to evaluation
Assess patient factors that may influence test results: 1. Antibiotic or corticosteroid	1. Recognize interfering drugs: a. Schedule test *before* therapy is begun. b. Consult with physician. c. Note on lab slip if the patient is already on medication.	1. Patient's lab values are not falsely low because of interfering drug therapy.
2. Known history of recent streptococcal infection	2. Note preexisting infection on lab slip.	2. The patient's recent streptococcal infection is noted on lab slip.
3. Prevent hemolysis	3. Prevent hemolysis by: a. Not probing venipuncture site or leaving tourniquet on too long. b. Not forcefully withdrawing specimen. c. Not withdrawing the specimen too slowly. d. Not handling the specimen roughly. e. Not oversaturating skin with antiseptic.	3. Patient's values are not influenced by hemolysis.

*Not discussed in this book.

Guide to assessment	Guide to planning and intervention	Guide to evaluation

4. Knowledge deficit about test	4. Explain test to patient:
	  a. Define ASO or DNAse B (See Description and 2 Increases).
	  b. Explain procedure (See Procedure).
		4. The patient demonstrates knowledge of test by defining test and stating procedure.

5. Knowledge deficit about streptococcal infections	5. Initiate specific preventive teaching of streptococcal infections:
	
	  a. Teach that sore throats should be cultured and those positive for streptococcus should be treated.
	
	  b. Explain that family members should have throat cultures and positive cultures should be treated.
	
	  c. Initiate treatment for impetigo lesions.
	
	  d. Consult with physician for systemic antimicrobial therapy as needed for impetigo lesions.
	
	  e. Emphasize the need to complete antimicrobial treatment.
		5. The patient states an understanding of the need for early detection and treatment of streptococcal infections.

Patient Preparation Checklist

1. √ Drug history (See 1 above).
2. √ Known streptococcal infection noted on lab slip.
3. √ Patient knowledge; explain test to patient (See Description/Procedure).
4. √ Patient knowledge of streptococcal infections (See 5 above).

CONSIDERATIONS FOR NURSING CARE RELATED TO ABNORMAL TEST RESULTS
POSTTEST: Factors related to the results of the test
Nursing Diagnosis: Potential for injury related to streptococcal infection

Guide to assessment	Guide to planning and intervention	Guide to evaluation
Assess patient factors that may be influencing test results. Nursing history and/or physical exam suggestive of: 1. Sore throat Impetigo	1. Eradicate streptococcal infection by: a. Administering antimicrobial therapy. (Penicillin is drug of choice.) b. Encouraging family members with suggestive symptoms to seek diagnosis and treatment. c. Teaching patients to take entire course of therapy, and why.	1. Patient's ASO titer returns to normal limits.

Test:	Arterial Blood Gases	
Abbreviation:	ABGs	
Reference Values:	*Arteriopuncture*	*Skin-Puncture (Arterialized)*
	pH 7.35–7.45	*Newborn* 7.33–7.49
		2 days–1 month 7.32–7.43
		1 month 7.34–7.43
		2 months–1 year 7.34–7.46
		Child and adult
		M 7.35–7.45
		F 7.36–7.44
	pCO_2 35–45 mm Hg	*Newborn* 26.8–40.4
		2 months–2 years 26.4–41.2
		Child and adult
		M 36.2–46.2
		F 33.1–43.1
	pO_2 75–100 mm Hg	*Newborn*
		Unreliable (35)
		Child and adult
		80–105 (34)
		Transcutaneous pO_2
		monitoring in infants
		Reference value: 50–110 mm
		Hg (106)

HCO_3 *Premature*   18–26
  mmol/L

Full-term infant
to 2 years   20–26 mmol/L
2 years–adult   22–26 mmol/L

Base excess/deficit
 −2mEq to + 2mEq
CO_2 content
cord blood   15.0–
20.2 mmol/L
  (venus blood)
child   18.27 mmol/L
  (venous blood)
adult   24–35 mmol/L
  (venous blood)

Specimen:	Arterial or arterialized blood (venous blood for CO_2 content).
Description:	Arterial blood gas analysis is one measurement of respiratory function. It is also a valuable tool in diagnosing acid-base imbalance. Acid-base imbalances are frequently complex and require a series of measurements. The nurse must pay close attention to the patient's past medical history as well as present condition.

pH, the abbreviation for potential for hydrogen, measures acidity or alkalinity. An increase in pH reflects a decrease in the hydrogen ion concentration (H^+) and is called alkalinity. Conversely, a decrease in pH shows an increase in the hydrogen ion concentration and is called acidity. The three systems in the body that control hydrogen ion concentration, and therefore, the pH, are the buffer, respiratory, and renal systems. Respiratory-controlled alterations in pH can take place in a matter of minutes. Kidney-controlled alterations in pH take several hours. It takes only seconds for the chemical cellular buffer systems to make adjustments.

pCO_2 (partial pressure of carbon dioxide) indicates alveolar ventilation. The arterial pCO_2 and pH measurements are reflective of ventilatory and acid-base balance. In response to stimulation of a change in pH due to a change in hydrogen ion concentration, respirations change depth and then rate to adjust CO_2 exchange to preserve carbonic acid balance. A pCO_2 above 46 mm Hg indicates hypercarbia or hypoventilation. A pCO_2 below 35 mm Hg indicates hypocarbia or hyperventilation.

pO_2 (partial pressure of oxygen) measures oxygen delivery from inspired air into the blood. Anything that disrupts the diffusion of gases (pO_2/pCO_2) between pulmonary and capillaries influences pO_2 levels. Accurate interpretation of pO_2 levels is in combination with pH, pCO_2, and physical assessment.

HCO_3 (bicarbonate) measures the carbonic acid-bicarbonate buffer system. This system is controlled by the kidneys; carbonic acid is controlled by respiration. A method of reporting all the buffer ions in the serum is designated base excess/base deficit. A decrease in buffer ions is called base deficit; an increase is called base excess.

CO_2 content is a general measurement of total blood carbon dioxide. It is a measurement of carbon dioxide from combined forms and is very close to the actual level of bicarbonate. Because of this, it is a good indicator of the bicarbonate-carbonic acid buffer system. This test is a way of looking at the chemical-cellular buffer system and determining what kind of acid-base disturbance is taking place.

Procedure:

(heparinized syringe or capillary tubes)

Arterial Puncture

1. The patient's temperature and respiratory rate are taken.
2. The most accurate results are obtained if the patient rests quietly at least 15 minutes prior to blood drawing.
3. The radial artery is usually chosen because it is easily accessible and has available collateral circulation. Other arteries that might be chosen are the brachial or femoral.
4. The wrist is extended over a rolled towel to place the radial artery close to the surface of the skin.

5. The skin is sterilized with an antiseptic agent such as beta-dine.

6. A heparinized syringe or Vacutainer is used.

7. The artery is stabilized with two fingers of one hand.

8. Blood is withdrawn (2–5 ml); air is removed; the blood is placed on ice and taken immediately to the lab for analysis.

9. Results are most accurate if determinations of pCO_2 and pO_2 are done 5–10 minutes after drawing the blood.

Skin-Puncture Method (34)

For infants

1. Follow numbers 1 and 2 above.

2. The puncture area is warmed 3–10 minutes to increase the rate of arterial blood flow.

3. The heel is the preferred site on neonates. On older infants the fleshy part of the middle finger is preferred. No edema should be present at the puncture site.

4. The site is cleansed with 70% isopropyl alcohol and wiped dry with a sterile sponge. Betadine is not recommended as a disinfectant for skin-puncture sites.

5. The skin is lanced and the first drop of blood wiped away.

6. Heparinized glass capillary tubes are filled with bubble-free blood and one end sealed.

7. The site is covered with a sterile sponge and gentle pressure is exerted until the bleeding stops. The limb should be held above the heart after blood is drawn. Adhesive bandages should not be used, as the infant may suck them off and aspirate them.

8. The sealed specimens are transported in ice water. Results are most accurate if determinations are made immediately after the sample is drawn.

Conditions Related to Increases in pH	Rationale

1. Metabolic alkalosis
  pH ↑ 7.45
  HCO_3 ↑ 29 mEq/L
  CO_2 ↑ 27 mEq/L
  pCO_2 ↑ 40 mm Hg if compensating
  pO_2 normal
  Base excess
	In this condition there is a deficit of hydrogen, potassium, or chloride ions and an excess of base (HCO_3).

*Caused by:
  Gastric losses from N/G tube, vomiting, lavage
  Diuretic therapy
  Adrenal cortical hyperfunction
  Aldosteronism
  Steroid therapy
	The loss of large amounts of hydrogen, potassium, and chloride stimulates retention of bicarbonate by the kidneys. This upsets the bicarbonate-carbonic acid system in favor of bicarbonate, and the pH increases.

*May not be listed according to frequency of occurrence.

Excessive intake of alkalies; IV fluids high in $NaHCO_3$
Excessive intake of acid-stomach alkalizing agents with poor renal function

A large alkali intake will raise the serum base level and so increase the serum pH. The body tries to realign the bicarbonate-carbonic acid balance. The major compensatory mechanism is hypoventilation to increase pCO_2 and conserve carbonic acid.
The kidneys conserve H^+ by excreting large amounts of potassium. The chemical-cellular buffer system causes intracellular H^+ to change place with extracellular potassium, increasing serum H^+. These last two compensatory mechanisms can cause a dangerous potassium deficit.

2. Respiratory alkalosis
   pH ↑ 7.45
   HCO_3 ↓ 24 mEq/L
   CO_2 ↓ 22 mEq/L
   pCO_2 ↓ 40 mm Hg
   pO_2 normal
   Base deficit
*Caused by:
   Hyperventilation due to
     Hysteria
     Anxiety
     Exercise
     Fever
     Mechanical ventilation
   Stimulates increased respiratory rate
     CNS disease
     High altitude
     Intracranial surgery
     Early salicylate poisoning

   Medical conditions
     Hyperthyroidism
     Carcinoid syndrome
     Thiamine deficiency
     Delirium tremens
     Acute myocarditis
     Resolving pneumonia
     Asthma (intrinsic, severe)
     Pulmonary congestion and hypostasis
     Shock

2. Rapid, deep breathing (hyperventilation) blows off excessive amounts of CO_2. This CO_2 deficit due to pulmonary loss disrupts the ratio of bicarbonate to carbonic acid and causes the pH to rise.

The causes of respiratory alkalosis are usually psychogenic or from environmental factors or diseases that are not necessarily respiratory in origin. In order to compensate, the body decreases respiration until CO_2 levels become high enough to stimulate breathing. Also, the body uses the chemical-cellular buffer system; hydrogen ions come out of the cells in exchange for potassium ions, and potassium deficit may become a problem. Finally, the third mechanism, the kidneys, restricts tubular acid losses and bicarbonate reabsorption. These are medical conditions in which respiratory alkalosis may occur from hyperventilation, overstimulation of the respiratory center, or greatly increased metabolism.

---

*May not be listed according to frequency of occurrence.

Conditions Related to Decreases in pH

1. Metabolic acidosis
   pH ↓ 7.35
   HCO_3 ↓ 25 mEq/L
   CO_2 ↓ 22 mEq/L
   pCO_2 ↓ 40 mm Hg
   pO_2 usually normal
   Base deficit
   *Caused by:
   Accumulation of organic acids, for ex-
   ample, ingestion of
     Ammonium chloride
     Paraldehyde
     Salicylates
     Methanol
     Boric acid
   Diabetic ketoacidosis
   Lactic acidosis
   Shock
   Hypothermia
   Hypokalemia
   Renal failure
   Ketogenic diets
   Loss of HCO_3
     Renal tubular acidosis
     Diarrhea, severe
     Carbonic anhydrase inhibition from
       drugs such as Diamox, Ethamide,
       Cardase

2. Respiratory acidosis
   ph ↓ 7.36
   HCO_3 ↑ 29 mEq/L
   CO_2 ↑ 27 mEq/L
   pCO_2 ↑ 40 mm Hg
   pO_2 normal or low
   Base excess
   **Caused by:
   Congestive heart failure
   Chronic bronchitis
   Pulmonary emphysema
   Asthma
   Respiratory tract damage
   Chronic obstructive lung disease
   Pulmonary edema
   Pulmonary collapse

Rationale

1. An excess of organic acids and a deficit of bicarbonate, which decreases
   serum pH, describes this condition.
   This condition is primarily renal in
   nature.

   Metabolic acidosis may occur due to
   an accumulation of organic acids in
   the blood or from loss of HCO_3 (as in
   inherited or acquired renal tubular
   acidosis). These variables tilt the acid-
   base balance in favor of acid and the
   serum pH falls. Compensation consists of increased rate and depth of
   respirations (Kussmaul respirations)
   to blow off excess carbonic acid, increased excretion of H^+ by the kidney; and the chemical-cellular buffer
   system moving potassium out of the
   cells in exchange for H^+ to decrease
   extracellular acid.

2. This is a condition caused by hypoventilation leading to retention of
   CO_2 and resulting in carbonic acid excess. This excess upsets the carbonic
   acid-bicarbonate ratio in favor of acid
   and lower serum pH. Respiratory acidosis can be caused by any condition
   that causes hypoventilation and CO_2
   retention. To compensate, the kidneys work to lower H^+ concentration
   by H^+ excretion and sodium retention and to form $NaHCO_3$ to increase
   the base side of the acid-base balance.

---

*Not listed according to frequency of occurrence.
**May not be listed by frequency of occurrence.

Respiratory distress syndrome
Respiratory center depression, e.g.
  Surgical anesthesia
  Prolonged CO_2 overbreathing
  Oversedation
  Head trauma with respiratory center
    damage
Paralysis/weakness of respiratory muscles, e.g.
  Guillain-Barré syndrome
  Acute poliomyelitis
  Myasthenia gravis

Conditions Related to Increases in	**Rationale**
HCO_3 CO_2 pCO_2	See metabolic alkalosis (pH ↑) or respiratory acidosis (pH ↓).

Conditions Related to Decreases in	**Rationale**
HCO_3 CO_2 pCO_2	See metabolic acidosis (pH ↓) or respiratory alkalosis (pH ↑).

Conditions Related to an Increase in pO_2

Rationale

1. Oxygen administration

1. Room air is only 21% oxygen. If a patient has no ventilatory problem, oxygen administration can greatly increase the pO_2. This should be taken into account when evaluating arterial blood gas studies. If the patient's pO_2 is in the normal range of 80–100% and he is receiving oxygen therapy, some amount of respiratory insufficiency is present.

Conditions Related to a Decrease in pO_2   **Rationale**

*Fat embolism
Sickle-cell anemia
Polycythemia, secondary lung disorder/
  disease, e.g., chest trauma, COPD,
  pneumonia, etc.
Congenital heart defects
Respiratory acidosis

A decrease of pO_2 indicates a defect in gas exchange at the pulmonary alveoli/capillary level. The defect in gas exchange may be due to reduced diffusing capacity or shunting of blood that has not been ventilated (oxygenated) or to alveolar-capillary block. Usually the lowered pO_2 is due to a combination of these factors.

---

*May not be listed according to frequency of occurrence.

Drug Influences: Many drugs affect ABGs. The drugs are listed alphabetically by generic name and divided into columns according to the effect of the drug. Examples of trade names are in parentheses.

The following drugs may increase test results:

Metabolic acidosis treatment
  lactate
  tromethamine (THAM)

Metabolic alkalosis
  acetates
  antacids
  carbenicillin (Geocillin)
  carbenoxolone (carbenoxolone sodium)
  laxatives, chronic abuse
  phenylbutazone (Butazolidin)

Respiratory alkalosis
  aspirin
  mafenide (Sulfamylon)
  tubocurarine (Tubocurarine Chloride)

Hypochloremic alkalosis
  mercurial diuretics

Hypokalemic alkalosis
  adrenal steroid therapy

Effect of massive diuresis
  meralluride (Meralluride Sodium)

Alteration of acid-base balance
  sodium bicarbonate

Respiratory depression
  narcotics
  propoxyphene (Darvon)

Miscellaneous
  althesin
  glutamic acid (Magacin)
  silver compounds
  urokinase (Abbokinase), effect in pulmonary embolism patients

The following drugs may cause a decrease in test results:

Metabolic acidosis
  aminosalicylic acid
  aspirin, after prolonged use
  cyclopropane (Trimethylene)
  dimercaprol (BAL in oil)
  ether
  ethoxzolamide (Cardrase)
  fluorides
  xylitol

Respiratory acidosis
   acetone
   methanol (wood alcohol)
   methylenedioxyamphetamine (Methylenedioxyamphetamine HCl)

Lactic acidosis
   ethanol (grain alcohol)
   ethylene glycol
   fructose

Acid-base imbalance
   aminobenzoic acid (Pabirin)
   ammonium chloride (Triaminicol)
   arginine
   calcium chloride (calcium chloride, injection)
   citrates

Effect of acidosis in presence of renal impairment
   minocycline (Minocin)
   tetracycline (Achromycin)

Extracellular acidosis
   dimethadione (Dimethadione)

Inhibition of carbonic anhydrase
   acetazolamide (Diamox)
   mafenide (Sulfamylon)

Respiratory acidosis treatment
   tromethamine (THAM)

Effect of increased respiration and pulmonary ventilation
   aspirin, in toxic doses
   ethamivan (Ethamivan)

Anesthesia effect
   ether

Reduction in arterial oxygen pressure (respiratory effect)
   meperidine (Demerol)

Miscellaneous
   acetazolamide (Diamox); in bronchitis
   althesin
   barbiturates
   heroin
   isoniazid (INH)
   isoproterenol (Isuprel), in chronic lung disease
   neuromuscular relaxants (Flaxedil)
   paraldehyde (Paraldehyde, Sterile), decomposes to acetic acid
   spironolactone (Aldactone)
   trimethadione (Tridione)

Related Lab Studies: Monitor response to treatment or progress of disease and adjust nursing care accordingly. See individual tests for information.

O$_2$ Saturation
Hct
Hgb
potassium
chloride
sodium
osmolality
urinalysis
calcium, serum

IMPLICATIONS FOR NURSING CARE
PRETEST: Factors related to the test
Nursing Diagnosis: Potential for injury related to changes in biochemical balance

Guide to assessment	Guide to planning and intervention	Guide to evaluation
Assess patient factors that may influence test results:		
1. Nutritional status Is patient NPO?	1. Record nutritional status on lab slip.	1. The patient's nutritional influences are noted on lab slip.
2. Comprehensive drug history (See Drug Influences)	2. Identify drugs that may influence test results and note on lab slip.	2. The patient's pertinent drug history is noted on lab slip.
3. Respiratory rate Temperature Receiving O$_2$?	3. Record recent temperature and respiratory rate on lab slip. Record if patient is receiving O$_2$.	3. The patient's metabolic requirements for oxygen (temperature) and ventilatory activity are noted.
4. Skin-puncture procedure	4. Encourage arterial blood flow to area by applying warm compresses 3–10 minutes prior to blood drawing. Laboratory will make request.	4. The patient's skin-puncture site is arterialized sufficiently to achieve accurate test results.
5. Activity	5. Encourage rest 15 minutes prior to blood drawing if possible.	5. The patient is at rest or activity is noted on lab slip.
6. Knowledge deficit	6. Explain test: a. Define ABGs (See Description). b. Explain procedure (See Procedure).	6. The patient/parent demonstrates knowledge by defining ABGs and stating procedure.

Patient Preparation Checklist

1. √ Patient dietary status.
2. √ Influencing drugs and note on lab slip (See Drug Influences).
3. √ Record recent temperature and respiratory rate on lab slip. If receiving O_2, note on lab slip.
4. √ Skin-puncture area warmed.
5. √ Note patient activity.
6. √ Patient knowledge; define and explain procedure (See Definition/Procedure).

CONSIDERATIONS FOR NURSING CARE RELATED TO ABNORMAL TEST RESULTS
POSTTEST: Factors related to the results of the test
Nursing Diagnosis: Alterations in biochemical balance

Guide to assessment	Guide to planning and intervention	Guide to evaluation
Assess patient factors that may be influencing test results. Nursing history and/or physical exam suggestive of: 1. Metabolic alkalosis	1. Promote correction of metabolic alkalosis by:	1. The patient's laboratory findings return to appropriate levels:

a. Symptoms
pH ↑ 7.45
HCO_3 ↑ 29 mEq/L
CO_2 ↑ 27 mEq/L
pCO_2 ↑ 40 mm Hg if compensating
pO_2 normal
Base excess
   Potassium ↓
   Calcium ↓
Respiratory rate ↓
Neuromuscular irritability, fidgeting, twitching, picking at sheets, tingling
Atrial tachycardia
	a. Detecting, reporting, and recording early signs of metabolic alkalosis:
	(1) Evaluating without delay drug and nursing/medical history.
	(2) Evaluating recent lab values if known.
	(3) Checking respiratory rate for rate and depth.
	(4) Checking neuromuscular status.
		a. The patient's symptoms are reported without delay and further complications are prevented.

b. Loss of acids:	b. Preventing loss of acids:	b. The patient is protected from base excess by preventing loss of acids as shown by laboratory results and physical status.

Guide to assessment	Guide to planning and intervention	Guide to evaluation
(1) Nasogastric tubes Potassium/chloride replacement	(1) Replacing, by IV, gastric losses through N/G tube as ordered.	
(2) Vomiting	(2) Initiating nursing measures to control or stop vomiting.	
(3) Diuretic therapy Symptoms of potassium loss	(3) Initiating nursing measures to maintain potassium and chloride balance.	
(4) Steroid therapy Aldosteronism	(4) Detecting, reporting, and correcting early signs of potassium/hydrogen ion loss.	
c. Excessive alkali intake	c. Preventing excessive alkali intake: (1) Detecting early signs of base excess. (2) Knowing what IV solution the patient is receiving. (3) Determining excessive antacid intake. (4) Teaching relationship between alkalosis and alkalizing agents.	c. The patient is protected from base excess due to excessive intake of alkalizing agents.
d. History of potassium loss Diuretic therapy Vomiting Diarrhea	d. Teaching the patient how to replace lost ions by dietary choices: Some high-potassium foods: citrus fruits, bananas, prunes, raisins, watermelon, asparagus, beans, brussels sprouts, cabbage, potatoes, squash.	d. The patient is able to name some foods high in potassium and when/why they should be eaten.
e. Hyperkalemia	e. Being aware of possible complications to treatment.	e. The patient does not experience complications to treatment.
2. Respiratory alkalosis	2. Promote correction of respiratory alkalosis by:	2. Patient laboratory findings return to appropriate levels:
a. Signs/symptoms pH $\uparrow$ 7.45 HCO_3 $\downarrow$ 24 mEq/L CO_2 $\uparrow$ 22 mEq/L pCO_2 $\uparrow$ 40 mm Hg pO_2 normal Serum potassium $\downarrow$ Serum calcium $\downarrow$	a. Detecting, reporting, and recording early signs of respiratory alkalosis by: (1) Evaluating without delay drug and medical/nursing history. (2) Evaluating recent lab values, if known.	a. The patient's symptoms are reported without delay and further complications are prevented.

Guide to assessment	Guide to planning and intervention	Guide to evaluation
Deep, rapid breathing Numbness/tingling of hands and face Headache Tetany Convulsions Arrythmias (from K^+ deficit)	(3) Checking respiratory rate. (4) Checking neuromuscular status. (5) Monitoring cardiac rhythm.	
b. Anxiety Hysteria Exercise	b. Initiating nursing measures to correct hyperventilation: (1) CO_2 rebreathing (breathing into paper bag). (2) Providing calm, quiet, nonthreatening environment.	b. Hyperventilation is resolved.
c. Fever	c. Using nursing measures to reduce fever and maintain normal body temperature.	c. The patient's temperature is normal.
d. Mechanical ventilator set too fast/too deep. Ventilation-assisted patient complains of dizziness; signs of muscletwitching observed	d. Adjusting mechanical respirator properly.	d. The patient's mechanical ventilator is adjusted so respirations are neither too deep nor too fast.
e. Respiratory center stimulation (See Increases 2)	e. Implementing medical/nursing plan to treat underlying cause.	e. The patient is relieved of underlying cause of overstimulated respiratory center and respiration, and ABGs are normal.
3. Metabolic acidosis	3. Promote correction of metabolic acidosis by:	3. The patient's laboratory findings return to appropriate levels:
a. Symptoms pH ↓ 7.35 HCO_3 ↓ 25 mEq/L CO_2 ↓ 22 mEq/L pCO_2 ↓ 40 mm/Hg pO_2 usually normal Base deficit Urinary pH ↓ 4.5 Potassium ↑ Respirations ↑ Rate and depth Neuromuscular: Signs of K^+ excess CNS depression	a. Detecting, reporting, and recording early signs of metabolic acidosis: (1) Evaluating without delay drug and nursing/medical history. (2) Evaluating recent lab values, if known. (4) Checking for signs of potassium excess. (5) Checking for CNS depression.	a. The patient's symptoms are reported without delay and further complications are prevented.

Guide to assessment	Guide to planning and intervention	Guide to evaluation
b. See Decreases 1	b. Implementing medical plan to eliminate underlying cause of metabolic acidosis.	b. The patient's lab results return to normal.
c. Hypothermia, especially newborn and elderly Shock Renal failure Severe dehydration Cardiac arrest Hypoxia Ingestion of certain drugs (See Decreases 1)	c. Initiating nursing measures to prevent accumulation of organic acids: (1) Promoting fluid and electrolyte status with precise I&O and daily weights. (2) Detecting first signs of acidosis and reporting them immediately. (3) Implementing medical plan of treatment as ordered. (4) Administering blood transfusions and intravenous fluids as ordered. (5) Preparing for dialysis as necessary. (6) Keeping patients at risk for hypothermia warm and fed. (7) Patients requiring insulin receive proper medication. (8) Providing O_2 to hypoxic patients. (9) Encouraging nutritionally adequate diet. (10) Teaching drug safety to patients/parents.	c. The patient is prevented from experiencing organic acid buildup.
d. Diabetes mellitus Starvation diets	d. Teaching the patient the relationship of ketone bodies, plasma bicarbonate, and metabolic acidosis.	d. The patient states the process of ketoacidosis.
e. Loss of HCO_3 (See Decreases 1)	e. Promoting bicarbonate balance by: (1) Initiating nursing measures to decrease diarrhea, and rapid peristalsis. (2) Maintaining fluid and electrolyte balance, precise I&O and daily weights.	e. The patient's bicarbonate balance is normal.

Guide to assessment	Guide to planning and intervention	Guide to evaluation
f. Hypoventilation	f. Being aware of complications to treatment.	f. The patient does not experience complications to treatment.
4. Respiratory acidosis	4. Promote correction of respiratory acidosis by:	4. The patient's laboratory findings return to appropriate levels.
a. Symptoms pH $\downarrow$ 7.36 HCO_3 $\uparrow$ 29 mEq/L CO_2 $\uparrow$ 27 mEq/L pCO_2 $\uparrow$ 40 mm/Hg pO_2 normal Base excess Potassium $\uparrow$ Dyspnea, severe Hyperventilation at rest Headache Visual disturbances Disorientation Tachycardia Arrythmias Coma	a. Detecting, reporting, and recording early signs of respiratory acidosis: (1) Evaluating without delay drug and nursing/medical history. (2) Evaluating recent lab values, if known. (3) Checking apical pulse for rate and rhythm. (4) Checking ventilatory ability. (5) Checking orientation, level of consciousness.	
b. CO_2 narcosis symptoms: Drowsiness Irritability Depression Headache Dizziness Confusion Shallow respiration with poor ventilation Tachycardia Arrhythmias	b. Preventing CO_2 narcosis: (1) Being aware of patient's past history. (2) Giving O_2 to patients with chronic lung disease with extreme caution. (3) Knowing normal pO_2 for specific patient. (4) Recognizing symptoms of CO_2 narcosis early.	
c. Decreased respiratory ventilation COPD $\downarrow$ Serum chloride $\uparrow$ CO_2 See 2 Decreases Sedation	c. Promoting improved ventilation by: (1) Administering antibiotics as ordered. (2) Performing or ordering respiratory hygiene by (32): (a) Good mouth care. (b) Postural drainage. (c) Administering bronchodilators and detergents as ordered. (d) Inhalation therapy with nebulization.	(1) The patient is free of infection. (2) The patient achieves improved pulmonary ventilation.

Guide to assessment	Guide to planning and intervention	Guide to evaluation
	(3) Teaching and encouraging patient to do respiratory exercises. (4) Turning, coughing, and deep breathing patient as appropriate. (5) Administering O_2 as ordered. Checking flow meter frequently. (6) Monitoring mechanical ventilation closely. (7) Giving sedatives with caution and monitoring patient's respiratory status carefully.	(3) The patient demonstrates respiratory exercises. (4) The patient is TCDB as appropriate.
d. Ringer's solution NaHCO$_3$ Sodium lactate Calcium gluconate Gastric suction (loss of gastric acid)	d. Implementing medical plan to correct acidosis.	d. Patient's lab values return to appropriate levels.
e. Electrolyte imbalances	e. Promoting fluid and electrolyte balance by: (1) Detecting signs and symptoms of electrolyte imbalances. (2) Administering the correct IV solution. (3) Monitoring fluid and electrolyte intake precisely. (4) Keeping accurate I&O records.	e. Patient's lab values show normal electrolyte values.
f. Tetany CO$_2$ narcosis Respiratory alkalosis	f. Being aware of possible complications to treatment.	f. The patient does not experience complications to treatment.

Test: Aspartate Aminotransferase, also known as Serum Glutamic Oxaloacetic Transaminase

Abbreviation: AST, SGOT

Reference Values: 1–3 days   16–74 U/L
<6 months   20–43 U/L
6 months–1 year   16–35 U/L
1 year–5 years   6–30 U/L
5 years–adult   19–28 U/L

Adult
M   8–46 U/L
F   7–34 U/L

Specimen: Serum

Description: AST (SGOT) is an enzyme found in the heart, liver, kidney, and skeletal muscles. It is released following injury to cells. It was the first enzyme correlated with a transient rise and myocardial infarction. This test is done in conjunction with CPK and LDH isoenzymes in the diagnosis of myocardial infarction. See CPK for complete discussion. See also ALT (SGPT).

Drug Influences: A great many drugs affect AST (SGOT) values. Listed below are some of the drugs that influence test results. The drugs are listed alphabetically by generic name and divided into columns according to the effect of the drug. Examples of trade names are in parentheses.

The following drugs may increase test results:

Hepatic necrosis
  acetaminophen

Hepatotoxicity
  allopurinol (Zyloprim)
  antifungal agents (Fungizone, Mysteclin-F)
  asparaginase (Elspar)
  aspirin
  azathioprine (Imuran)
  carbenicillin (Geocillin)
  clofibrate (Atromid-S)
  colchicine
  cycloserine (Seromycin)
  erythromycin
  flurazepam (Dalmane)
  gentamicin (Garamycin)
  kanamycin (Kantrex)
  lincomycin
  oral contraceptives
  procainamide (Pronestyl)
  pyrazinamide (Tebrazid)
  rifampin (Rimactane)

tetracycline, especially pregnant women
thiothixene (Navane)

Intrahepatic cholestasis
acetohexamide (Dymelor)
anabolic steroids (Anavar, Testryl, Drolban)
desipramine (Norpramin, Pertofrane)
indomethacin (Indocin)
isoniazid (INH)
methyldopa (Aldoclor, Aldomet)
nalidixic acid (NegGram)
phenothiazines (Thorazine, Compazine, Prolixin)
phenytoin (Dilantin)

Miscellaneous
aminosalicylic acid
barbiturates
clindamycin
codeine
ethionamide (Trecator-SC)
guanethidine (Ismelin)
meperidine (Demerol, Meperagan)
mithramycin (Mithracin)
morphine
mushroom poisoning
spectinomycin (Trobicin)
Refer to CPK and ALT for more information.

Test:	Barbiturate Screen
Abbreviation:	None
Reference Values:	Negative

Toxic levels associated with coma and shock

Short-acting barbiturates	3 mg/dl
Hexobarbital	
Pentobarbital	
Secobarbital	
Intermediate-acting barbiturates	4 mg/dl
Amobarbital	
Butabarbital	
Long-acting barbiturates	8–10 mg/dl
Barbital	
Mephobarbital	
Phenobarbital sodium	
Phenobarbital	

Specimen: Serum (gastric contents or urine are also used for screen)

Description: Barbiturates produce sedation and hypnosis by interfering with nerve impulse transmission to the cerebral cortex. Though all the barbiturates have the same physiological effect, there is a great difference in type, absorption rate, and length of action. The most common type, uses, and length of action are:

Type	Uses	Length of Action

Short-Acting:
  hexobarbital (Sombulex)
  pentobarbital
    (Nembutal sodium)
  secobarbital (Seconal,
    Seconal Sodium)
	hypnotic,
	preanesthetic,
	sedation
		4 hours

Intermediate-Acting
  amobarbital (Amytal)
  butabarbital (Butisol
    Sodium)
	hypnotic,
	sedation, acute
	convulsive
	disorders, mild
	sedation for
	anxiety
		4–8 hours

Long-Acting
  barbital
  mephobarbital
    (Mebaral)
  phenobarbital
    (Eskabarb)
  phenobarbital sodium
	mild, prolonged
	sedation,
	anticonvulsant
		6–10 hours

Ultra-Short
  methohexital sodium
    (Brevital Sodium)
	anesthesia	minutes

thiamylal sodium
  (Surital sodium)
thiopental sodium
  (Pentothal sodium)

All but two of the barbiturates are totally metabolized in the liver. Phenobarbital is partially metabolized in the liver, but it is mostly excreted by the kidneys unchanged. Barbital is excreted by the kidneys as a completely unchanged compound.

The purpose of the barbiturate screen is to diagnose toxic barbiturate levels, as an aid in the diagnosis of coma type, or it may be used as a tool in determining therapy for toxic barbiturate levels. The screen may also have medicolegal ramifications because of a connection to suicide or homicide.

Procedure: (red tube top)
1. If for medicolegal purposes, permit must be signed.
2. Approximately 2–10 ml of blood is drawn from the patient.
3. Observe puncture site for bleeding or evidence of hematoma.

Conditions Related to Increases

1. Overdose

2. Drugs (See Drug Influences)

3. Hemolysis

Rationale

1. Barbiturate screen is of greatest value in identifying the specific barbiturate agent ingested. Short-acting, rapidly absorbed barbiturates have more serious implications than the longer-acting types. Ingestion of other drugs or drug addiction will make a difference in the clinical appearance of the patient and in the barbiturate level. Barbiturates cross the placental barrier and appear in breast milk and should be given with caution to pregnant and lactating women.

2. Certain drugs in combination with a barbiturate may potentiate the CNS depressant effect of the drug. The most common combination is barbiturates and alcohol.

3. Hemolysis of the specimen falsely elevates results.

Drug Influences: The following drugs may influence test results. The drugs are listed alphabetically by generic name and divided into columns according to the effect of the drug. Examples of trade names are in parentheses.

The following drugs may cause an increase or false positive test result:

Metabolic conversion in vivo
  antipyrine (Tympagesic)
  disulfiram (Antabuse)
  ethanol
  monoamine-oxidase (MAO) inhibitors (Marplan, Eutonyl, Nardil, etc.)
  primidone (Mysoline)
  Any in vivo barbiturate-containing compound

Miscellaneous
  theophylline

The following drug may cause a decrease or false negative test result:
rifampin (Rifadin, Rimactane)

Related Lab Studies: To monitor condition:

  electrolytes
  urinalysis
  blood gases
  creatinine, creatinine clearance
  BUN
  urinary phenobarbital level

IMPLICATIONS FOR NURSING CARE
PRETEST: Factors related to the test
Nursing Diagnosis: Potential for injury related to poisoning

Guide to assessment	Guide to planning and intervention	Guide to evaluation
Assess patient factors that may influence test results:		
1. Gastric contents Urine	1. Save gastric contents and urine for barbiturate analysis.	1. The barbiturate type is identified.
2. Comprehensive drug history (See Drug Influences) If possible: Name of drug Dosage or number taken Time of ingestion Route Concurrent drug ingestion	2. Take in-depth drug history as possible; put pertinent information on lab slip and in chart.	2. The barbiturate type is identified.
3. Medicolegal involvement	3. Get signed permit from patient or family before test.	3. Permission is obtained.

Guide to assessment	Guide to planning and intervention	Guide to evaluation
4. Hemolysis	4. Prevent hemolysis by: a. Not saturating skin with antiseptic solution. b. Not leaving tourniquet on too long. c. Not probing venipuncture site. d. Not forcefully withdrawing specimen. e. Not withdrawing specimen too slowly. f. Not agitating the specimen roughly.	4. The patient's test values are not falsely elevated due to hemolysis of blood sample.
5. Knowledge deficit	5. Explain test to patient (family): a. Define barbiturate screen (See Description). b. Explain procedure (See Procedure).	5. The patient demonstrates knowledge by defining test and stating procedure.

Patient Preparation Checklist

1. √ Saving gastric contents or urine for analysis.
2. √ Comprehensive drug history and note pertinent information on lab slip.
3. √ Permit signed, as needed.
4. √ Patient knowledge; explain test to patient.

CONSIDERATIONS FOR NURSING CARE RELATED TO ABNORMAL TEST RESULTS
POSTTEST: Factors related to the results of the test
Nursing Diagnosis: Potential for injury related to barbiturate poisoning

Guide to assessment	Guide to planning and intervention	Guide to evaluation

Assess patient factors that may be influencing test results:
1. Patient's condition is worse than patient's history warrants.
   Barbiturate overdose signs/symptoms
   Flushed face
	1. Explore with family or significant companions or patient, if possible, concurrent drug ingestion, especially alcohol. Communicate findings to physician and lab.	1. Concurrent drug ingestion by the patient is identified.

Guide to assessment	Guide to planning and intervention	Guide to evaluation
Pulse ↓ Nystagmus Tendon reflexes ↓ Mental alertness ↓ Speaking difficulty Coordination poor Pupils dilated, nonreactive Coma Death		
2. Barbiturate overdose a. Oral activated charcoal b. Hemodialysis Hemoperfusion	2. Encourage accelerated body clearance of barbiturates by: a. Administering oral activated charcoal as prescribed. b. Preparing patient for hemodialysis. c. Assisting with hemodialysis.	2. The patient's phenobarbital level is decreased and clinical condition is improved.
3. Barbiturate withdrawal Shakiness Anxiety Muscular irritability Orthostatic hypotension Tachycardia Seizures Withdrawal psychosis Hyperpyrexia Death	3. Prevent barbiturate withdrawal syndrome by: a. Being alert to clinical manifestations. b. Recognizing that the barbiturate withdrawal syndrome may occur in a patient recovering from barbiturate overdose. c. Giving gradually tapered doses of phenobarbital until patient is dose-free.	3. The patient does not experience barbiturate withdrawal syndrome.
4. Drug abuse Deliberate overdose	4. Initiate nursing measures to help patient eliminate drug abuse: a. Recognize patient manipulative behavior in trying to get drugs. b. Discourage manipulative behavior; set limits; explore alternative positive behavior. c. Explore methods of coping without the use of drugs.	4. The patient becomes drug-independent.

Guide to assessment	Guide to planning and intervention	Guide to evaluation
	d. Refer, as appropriate, patient to proper facility: (1) Psychiatrist. (2) Mental health-drug abuse clinic. (3) Family therapy. 5. Support community drug abuse programs. 6. Encourage community knowledge about real or potential community drug problems.	

Test: Bence-Jones Protein

Abbreviation: BJP

Reference Value: Negative

Specimen: Urine

Description: The Bence-Jones protein is derived from plasma cell proliferation and abnormal immunoglobulin synthesis due to multiple myeloma. The protein is very small and easily filtered by the glomeruli, but it is also quickly reabsorbed and metabolized (21). It is not until there is more Bence-Jones protein than the tubules can reabsorb that the protein appears in the urine. About 50–80% of patients diagnosed as having multiple myeloma excrete the Bence-Jones protein in their urine.

Procedure:
1. No food or fluid restrictions.
2. Collect first morning voided specimen if possible.
3. Keep urine refrigerated or send to laboratory immediately.

Conditions Related to Increases	Rationale
1. Multiple myeloma	1. Plasma cells are responsible for immunoglobulin synthesis. In this condition, there is synthesis of excessive abnormal immunoglobulins from the proliferation of plasma cells. The excessive production of abnormal Bence-Jones globulins, called myeloma proteins, damages renal tubule cells, increasing the excretion of the Bence-Jones protein.

2. Urine contaminants
   Blood
   Semen
	2. May interfere with electrophoretic field.

3. Leukemia Macroglobulinemia	3. Possible false positive results with these conditions.
4. Old, unrefrigerated urine	4. Due to decomposition of protein at room temperature (11).

Drug Influences: The following drugs may influence test results.
The following drug may cause an increase in or false positive test results:

Nephrotoxic effect
tetracycline (Achromycin)

No in vivo decrease or false negatives found.

Related Lab Studies: Diagnosis of multiple myeloma:
ESR
CBC
urinalysis
RBC indices

calcium, urinary
phosphorus, urinary
*Immunoglobulins, IgG/IgA/IgM
bone marrow aspiration

IMPLICATIONS FOR NURSING CARE
PRETEST: Factors related to the test
Nursing Diagnosis: Potential for injury related to changes in biochemical balance

Guide to assessment	Guide to planning and intervention	Guide to evaluation
Assess patient factors that may influence test results: 1. First A.M. voiding	1. Collect first A.M. voiding, at least 50 ml, from patient. Send to lab immediately (or refrigerate specimen immediately).	1. Patient's specimen is concentrated morning specimen of sufficient quantity. The specimen arrives at lab fresh or is refrigerated immediately.
2. Nephrotoxic drugs	2. Note on lab slip if patient is receiving nephrotoxic drugs.	2. Patient's test values are not influenced by medications.

3. Knowledge deficit	3. Explain test to patient:
	  a. Define test.
	  b. Explain procedure.
		3. The patient demonstrates knowledge by defining test and explaining procedure.

Patient Preparation Checklist

1. √ First A.M. voided specimen or concentrated urine. Urine must be fresh or refrigerated immediately.
2. √ Medication history for nephrotoxic drugs. Note on lab slip.
3. √ Patient knowledge; explain test to patient.

---

*Not discussed in this book.

CONSIDERATIONS FOR NURSING CARE RELATED TO ABNORMAL TEST RESULTS
POSTTEST: Factors related to the results of the test
Nursing Diagnosis: Alterations in biochemical balance

Guide to assessment	Guide to planning and intervention	Guide to evaluation

Assess patient factors that may be influencing test results.
Nursing history and/or physical exam that is suggestive of:
1. Clinical diagnosis of multiple myeloma
Bence-Jones protein in urine
	1. Promote reduction of malignant plasma cells:
	  a. Support patient through radiation experience.
	  b. Administer chemotherapy as prescribed.
	  c. Initiate nursing measures for satisfactory completion of chemotherapy.
		1. The patient's tumor mass decreases in size.

2. Bence-Jones protein in urine	2. Initiate nursing measures to protect kidney function:
	  a. Keep patient well hydrated.
	  b. Encourage mobility.
	  c. Protect patient from infection.
		2. The patient's kidney function is maintained as evidenced by urinalysis.

d. Signs of kidney failure:
    ↓ Urine output
    ↑ Weight gain
    Edema
    ↑ B/P
	d. Be alert to signs of decreasing kidney function.	

Test:	Bilirubin		
Abbreviation:	None		
Reference Values:	Total	Cord	<1.8 mg/dl
		24 hours	Premature 1–6 mg/dl
			Full-term 2–6 mg/dl
		48 hours	Premature 6–8 mg/dl
			Full-term 6–7 mg/dl
		3–5 days	Premature 10–15 mg/dl
			Full-term 4–12 mg/dl
		1 month–Adult	1 mg/dl
	(Direct)	Conjugated	<0.4 mg/dl

Specimen: Serum, urine

Description: Bilirubin is formed in large part from heme of destroyed erythrocytes or from the breakdown of developing red blood cells in the bone marrow or other hemoproteins. Heme is converted to biliverdin in the spleen, kidney, and liver, and unconjugated bilirubin is formed from biliverdin. Unconjugated bilirubin is not water-soluble and is not excreted in the urine. It has a high affinity for brain tissue. The unconjugated or indirect bilirubin is bound to albumin and transported to liver cells. In the liver it is taken up and, with the help of the enzyme glucuronyl transferase, bilirubin is conjugated with glucuronic acid. Conjugated bilirubin is water-soluble, not protein-bound, and is excreted in the urine. Conjugated bilirubin has a low affinity for brain tissue (11).

Bilirubin determinations are useful in evaluating jaundice and in diagnosing liver and hemolytic diseases.

Procedure: (red top tube)
1. The patient should restrict food and fluid at least 4 hours prior to testing. Newborn infants do not need feeding restrictions.
2. Collect 10 μl (0.1 ml) to 5 ml of blood from patient. (Heel stick on newborn.)
3. *Protect blood specimen from light.*
4. Observe puncture site for bleeding or evidence of hematoma.

Conditions Related to Increases

1. Unconjugated hyperbilirubinemia
   Hemolytic jaundice

Rationale

1. In hemolysis, when red blood cell destruction is so excessive that the production of bilirubin is more than the liver can handle, the unconjugated serum bilirubin rises.
   Direct bilirubin is less than 20% of total bilirubin.

2. Hemolytic disease of the newborn

2. Also an unconjugated hyperbilirubinemia. In the newborn infant, the enzyme glucuronidase, needed for conjugating bilirubin, is low, and the protein (and possibly glucose and oxygen) needed for binding unconjugated bilirubin are limited, creating excess indirect or unconjugated bilirubin. Unconjugated bilirubin has an affinity for brain tissue, and this condition puts the infant in great danger if the bilirubin is allowed to rise too high. Infants are given exchange transfusions usually when the total bilirubin is between 16 and 20 mg/dl, depending on infant's general condition.
   Direct bilirubin is less than 20% of total.

3. Unconjugated hepatic jaundice, e.g.
   Gilbert syndrome
   Crigler-Najjar syndrome

3. Genetic defects may cause hyperbilirubinemia. The defects discourage conjugation of bilirubin either from lack of enzymes in the case of Crigler-Najjar syndrome or in intracellular bilirubin transport.
   Direct bilirubin is less than 20% of total.

4. Conjugated hepatocellular jaundice, e.g.
   Hepatitis
   Cirrhosis

4. This jaundice is a result of damage to the parenchyma. The exact mechanism is not understood. Direct bilirubin is 20–40% of total. It may be as high as 60%.

5. Intrahepatic cholestasis, e.g.
   Hepatic drug reactions
   Alcoholic hepatitis
   Primary biliary cirrhosis
   Gram-negative septicemia

5. Bile flow to the duodenum is inhibited, and backup of bilirubin into the bloodstream results in jaundice. Bilirubin is mostly conjugated.
   Direct bilirubin may be 20–50% of total.

6. Posthepatic jaundice

6. The flow of conjugated bilirubin is prevented from flowing into the duodenum. Direct bilirubin is above 50%. Indirect bilirubin is normal because the obstruction is after conjugation has taken place.

Drug Influences: The following drugs may influence test results. The drugs are listed alphabetically by generic name and divided into columns according to the effect of the drug. Examples of trade names are in parentheses.

The following drugs may cause an increase in test results:

Serum

Hepatotoxicity

acetaminophen (Tylenol)
aminobenzoic acid (Pabirin)
amphotericin B (Fungizone)
antifungal agents (Mycostatin)
antimony compounds
arsenicals
azathioprine (Imuran)
bismuth salts (Pepto-Bismol)
boric acid (Blinx)
chlorambucil (Leukeran)
chloramphenicol (Chloromycetin)
chloroform
chlorprothixene (Taractan)
chlortetracycline (Aureomycin)
chlorzoxazone (Paraflex)
clofibrate (Atromid-S)
clonidine (Catapres)
colchicine (Colchicine)
coumarin (Coumadin)
cyclophosphamide (Cytoxan)
cycloserine (Seromycin)
diazepam (Valium)
diethylstilbestrol (Stilbestrol)
ethanol (grain alcohol)
ethionamide (Trecator-SC)
ethoxazene (Serenium)
ethyl chloride (Ethyl chloride spray)
floxuridine (FUDR)
flucytosine (Ancobon)
flurazepam (Dalmane)
gentamicin (Garamycin)

glycopyrrolate (Robinul)
halothane (Fluothane)
iopanoic acid (Telepaque)
kanamycin (Kantrex)
lincomycin (Lincocin)
mesoridazine (Serentil)
metaxalone (Skelaxin)
methanol (wood alcohol)
methotrexate (Mexate)
methoxsalen (Oxsoralen)
methoxyflurane (Penthrane)
methsuximide (Celontin)
methyldopa (Aldomet)
morphine
niacin (Nicotinex)
nitrofurantoin (Furadantin)
organophosphorus insecticides
  (Parathion)
paraldehyde (Paral)
paramethadione (Paradione)
phenacemide (Phenurone)
probenecid (Benemid)
procainamide (Sub-Quin)
progesterone (Progestin)
pyrazinamide (Tebrazid)
sulfonamides
testosterone (Android-T)
tetracycline (Achromycin)
thiothixene (Navane)
thorium dioxide
trimethadione (Tridione)
trioxsalen (Trisoralen)

Cholestatic effect

acetazolamide (Diamox)
acetohexamide (Dymelor)
acetophenazine (Tindal)
aminosalicyclic acid
amitriptyline (Elavil)
butaperazine (Repoise)
carbarsone (Carbarsone)
carphenazine (Proketazine)

methimazole (Tapazole)
methyltestosterone (Android-5)
nalidixic acid (NegGram)
norethindrone (Norlutin)
oxazepam (Serax)
oxymetholone (Adroyd)
oxyphenbutazone (Oxalid)
prochlorperazine (Compazine)

chlorothiazide (Diuril)
chlorpropamide (Diabinese)
dienestrol (Dienestrol Cream)
erythromycin (Ilosone)
estradiol (Estrace)
estrogens (Premarin)
ethacrynic acid (Edecrin)
fluoxymesterone (Android-F)
hydroflumethiazide (Diucardin)
imipramine (Antipress)
indomethacin (Indocin)
isocarboxazid (Marplan)
isoniazid (Laniazid)
meprobamate (Miltown)
methandrostenolone (Dianabol)

promazine (Sparine)
promethazine (Phenergan)
propoxyphene (Darvon)
protriptyline (Vivactil)
quinethazone (Hydromox)
stanozolol (Winstrol)
sulfadiazine (Microsulfon)
sulfamethizole (Bursul)
sulfamethoxazole (Gantanol)
sulfisoxazole (Gantrisin)
thioguanine (Lanvis)
tolazamide (Tolinase)
tolbutamide (Orinase)
trifluoperazine (Stelazine)
trimeprazine (Temaril)

Hemolysis with g-6-PD deficiency
antipyrine (Auralgan)
chloroquine (Roquine)
dimercaprol (BAL in oil)
furazolidone (Furoxone)
nitrofurazone (Furacin)
phytonadione (Aqua Mephyton)

primaquine (Primaquine Phosphate)
sulfacetamide (Cetamide Ophthalmic)
sulfanilamide (Vagitrol Cream)
sulfapyridine (Dagenan)
sulfoxone (Diasone Sodium)

Hemolytic anemia effect
amyl nitrate
antimalarials (Camoquin)
antipruritics (Nupercainal)
busulfan (Myleran)
cephalothin (Keflin)
diphenhydramine (Benadryl)
insecticides (Parathion)

mefenamic acid (Ponstel)
melphalan (Alkeran)
mephenytoin (Mesantoin)
piperazine (Antepar)
pipobroman (Vercyte)
quinidine (Duraquin)
streptomycin (Streptomycin Sulfate)

Urine

Cholestatic effect
acetohexamide (Dymelor)
acetophenazine (Tindal)

imipramine (Antipress)
phenothiazines (Compazine)

Hepatotoxic effect
chorprothixene (Taractan)
ethoxazene (Serenium)
methyldopa (Aldomet)

The following drugs may cause a decrease in test results:

Serum

Bilirubin metabolism
barbiturates
thioridazine (Mellaril)

Combination effect
penicillin
sulfisoxazole (Gantrisin)

Miscellaneous

ethanol, in pregnant women (grain alcohol)
phenazopyridine (Azodine)
sulfonamides

Urine

No in vivo decreases in urine results found.

Related Lab Studies:

  AST (SGOT)
  ALT (SGPT)
  alkaline phosphatase
  serum protein electrophoresis
  Prothrombin time
  urobilinogen, urine and feces
  *thymol turbidity
  Coombs'
  ammonia, plasma
  BUN
  reticulocytes
  amylase, serum
  lipase, serum
  cholesterol, serum

IMPLICATIONS FOR NURSING CARE
PRETEST: Factors related to the test
Nursing Diagnosis: Potential for injury related to changes in biochemical balance

Guide to assessment	Guide to planning and intervention	Guide to evaluation
Assess patient factors that may influence test results:		
1. Food and fluid restrictions, especially fatty food	1. Restrict food and fluids at least 4 hours prior to test. Infants have no fluid restrictions.	1. The patient's values are not influenced by food, especially fatty foods.
2. Comprehensive drug history (See Drug Influences)	2. Identify drugs that may influence test results. Consult with physician. Note influencing drugs on lab slip.	2. The patient's test values are not influenced by medication.
3. Preexisting conditions (See Increases)	3. Note pertinent information on lab slip.	3. Patient's preexisting conditions that are pertinent are noted on lab slip.

4. Lack of patient/parent knowledge	4. Explain test to patient:
	  a. Define test (See Description).
	  b. Explain procedure (See Procedure).
		4. The patient demonstrates knowledge by defining test and stating procedure.

*Not discussed in this book.

Patient Preparation Checklist

1. √ Food and fluids restricted at least 4 hours. Not in infant.
2. √ Interfering drugs noted on lab slip.
3. √ Pertinent preexisting conditions noted on lab slip.
4. √ Patient knowledge; explained test to patient/parents.

CONSIDERATIONS FOR NURSING CARE RELATED TO ABNORMAL TEST RESULTS
POSTTEST: Factors related to the results of the test
Nursing Diagnosis: Potential for injury related to alterations in biochemical balance

Guide to assessment	Guide to planning and intervention	Guide to evaluation
Assess patient factors that may be influencing test results. Nursing history and/or physical exam that is suggestive of:		
1. Hemolytic disease of the newborn	1. Control or prevent hyperbilirubinemia in the infant by:	1. The patient's bilirubin level returns to normal.
a. Mother-fetal history Mother RH negative and Father RH positive or Mother O positive and/or Previous pregnancies	a. Identifying positive history. Consult with physician.	
b. Newborn assessment Skin color: reddish-yellow tinge on blanching Pallor Cyanosis Urine color Edema Activity level Vital signs CNS signs: lethargy, irritability, excitability, convulsions, ↑ or rising bilirubin	b. Being alert to signs of increasing bilirubin. Consulting with physician about findings. c. Maintaining adequate hydration to encourage excretion of bilirubin. d. Administering phototherapy to reduce tissue bilirubin: (1) Expose entire skin surface. Cover eyes, scrotum. Do not occlude nose. (2) Turn infant systematically so all skin surface is exposed. (3) Check that ordered lab work is done.	

Guide to assessment	Guide to planning and intervention	Guide to evaluation
	(4) Follow bilirubin levels and consult with physician as arranged. (5) Turn off bililights during blood drawing. (6) Keep light bulb wavelength effective by routine changing. e. Assisting as necessary with exchange transfusion.	
2. Jaundice ↑ Bilirubin	2. Provide supportive care to encourage return to health: a. Encourage nutritious meals. b. Encourage adequate rest. c. Remove offending drug if intrahepatic cholestasis is suspected. d. Implement plan of care to treat underlying cause of jaundice. e. Administer cholestyramine as prescribed. f. Refer to general nursing care text for nursing care of jaundiced patient.	2. The patient's bilirubin level returns to normal.

Test: Bleeding Time

Abbreviation: None

Reference Values: Template method, below 8 minutes; values vary with laboratories and method used

Specimen: Whole blood

Description: The bleeding test is a test for platelet function and vascular abnormality in hemostasis. The test evaluates platelet aggregation (platelet clot) and the ability of the blood vessel to constrict. Several different methods are in use, but the template method is the most sensitive as it has been standardized.* The test consists of a blood pressure cuff wrapped around the upper arm (supported at level of heart) and inflated to 40 mm Hg. Two small incisions are made in the forearm by a lancet. At timed intervals, filter paper is used to blot blood drops until bleeding stops. The incision is not touched with the filter paper as clot formation would be disturbed. Bleeding time test is done as a screen preoperatively and to identify platelet disorders. For a complete discussion on platelets, refer to Platelet Count.

Procedure: 1. No food or fluid restriction.
2. Check patient history for aspirin ingestion within the past 5 days.
3. See Description for test procedure.
4. Observe incisions carefully for evidence of bleeding or hematoma.
5. Apply direct pressure for 10 minutes or until bleeding stops, or apply pressure dressing for 24 hours in patient with prolonged bleeding time.

Conditions Related to Increases

1. Von Willebrand's disease

2. Thrombocytopenia

3. Deficiency factors
    I (Fibrinogen)
    II (Prothrombin)
    V (Plasma accelerator globulin)
    VII (Serum prothrombin conversion factor)

Rationale

1. An inherited complex bleeding disorder of primary hemostasis and blood coagulation. The prolonged bleeding time is due to defective factor VIII (antihemophilic globulin) and platelet aggregation.

2. Diminished platelets available for adequate platelet functioning.

3. A defect in any of these plasma-clotting factors may increase bleeding time. Also, all factors listed are synthesized in the liver, so liver disease may cause factor deficiencies.

---

*The lancet is standardized in the Simplate® method.

Guide to assessment	Guide to planning and intervention	Guide to evaluation
IX (Christmas factor) XI (Plasma thromboplastin antecedent) Liver disease		
4. Disseminated intravascular coagulation	4. Due to decreased platelet count and abnormal platelet aggregation.	

Drug Influences: The following drugs may influence test results. The drugs are listed alphabetically by generic name and divided into columns according to the effect of the drug. Examples of trade names are in parentheses. Also see drugs under Platelet Count.

The following drugs may cause an increase in test results:

Miscellaneous
aspirin;* inhibits platelet glycolysis
dextran (Macrodex)
ethanol (grain alcohol)
mithramycin (Mithracin); reversible effect
streptokinase (Streptase); dissolves blood clots
trifluoroethylvinyl ether (Fluroxene); during anesthesia
warfarin (Coumadin)

The following drugs may cause a decrease in test results: None reported.

Related Lab Studies: Basic hemostatic screening profile:

bleeding time
platelet count
prothrombin time
activated partial thromboplastin time
thrombin time

IMPLICATIONS FOR NURSING CARE
PRETEST: Factors related to the test
Nursing Diagnosis: Potential for injury related to changes in biochemical balance

Guide to assessment	Guide to planning and intervention	Guide to evaluation
Assess patient factors that may influence test results: 1. Comprehensive drug history (See Drug Influences) Careful aspirin history	1. Identify drugs the patient is currently receiving that may influence test results. Consult	1. Patient's drugs do not interfere with test results.

*Many drugs contain aspirin even though the trade name does not make it obvious. Check patient history carefully.

Guide to assessment	Guide to planning and intervention	Guide to evaluation
	with physician; note drugs on lab slip. Aspirin should be withheld 5 days prior to test.	
2. Preexisting conditions History suggestive of bleeding disorder (See Increases)	2. Identify and note on lab slip pertinent information about preexisting conditions.	2. Patient's pertinent preexisting conditions are noted on lab slip.
3. Lack of patient knowledge	3. Explain test to patient.	3. The patient demonstrates knowledge of test by defining bleeding time and explaining procedure.

Patient Preparation Checklist

1. √ Drug history, especially for aspirin ingestion (See Drug Influences). See 1 above.
2. √ Note pertinent preexisting conditions on lab slip.
3. √ Patient knowledge; explain test to patient (See Description).

CONSIDERATIONS FOR NURSING CARE RELATED TO ABNORMAL TEST RESULTS
POSTTEST: Factors related to the results of the test
Nursing Diagnosis: Alterations in clotting factors

Guide to assessment	Guide to planning and intervention	Guide to evaluation
Assess patient factors that may be influencing test results. Nursing history and/or physical exam suggestive of: 1. Preoperative patient with: ↑ Bleeding time Normal PT Normal APTT Normal platelet count	1. Explore with the patient recent medication history. Look for hidden aspirin in over-the-counter drugs.	1. Patient identifies aspirin-containing medication ingested within the past week and does not require further platelet function workup.

Guide to assessment	Guide to planning and intervention	Guide to evaluation
2. Von Willebrand's disease	2. Replace deficient factor VIII: a. Administer antihemophilic factor (AHF) as prescribed. b. Be alert to signs of possible sensitivity reaction after frequent infusions with a commercial AHF. Give immunosuppressive therapy as ordered.	2. Patient's factor VIII is replaced as needed. The patient does not experience sensitivity to commercial AHF.

Refer to Platelet Count for more information.

Test:	Blood Urea Nitrogen
Abbreviation:	BUN
Reference Values:	Adult 6–20 mg/dl Premature (1 week) 3–25 mg/dl Newborn 4–18 mg/dl Infant-child 5–18 mg/dl
Specimen:	Serum
Description:	Urea is an end product of protein metabolism. As proteins are digested and catabolized, ammonia is formed and then detoxified in the liver as urea. Inadequate excretion of urea due to kidney disease or obstruction is the most common cause of increased BUN. Consequently, BUN is usually used as a screening test for renal disease rather than as a liver function test.
Procedure:	(red top tube) 1. Food and fluids are restricted for 8 hours. 2. 0.5–5 ml of blood is drawn from the patient. 3. Observe puncture site for bleeding or evidence of hematoma.

Conditions Related to Increases

1. Prerenal azotemia
   Congestive heart failure
   Dehydration
   Shock
   Diminished blood volume
2. Postrenal azotemia
   Prostatic hypertrophy
   Renal calculi
   Bilateral ureteral stricture
   Pregnancy
   Scarring of urinary tract
3. Renal disease

4. Catabolic conditions
   Starvation
   Sepsis
   Stress
   Myocardial infarction (24)
   Fever
   Diabetes mellitus
   Tumor necrosis
   Burns
5. Excessive protein intake

Rationale

1. Any cause of decreased renal blood flow decreases the free flow of urine and glomerular filtration and therefore the excretion of urea.

2. Obstruction of urinary flow causes a rise in blood urea due to diminished renal clearance.

3. Decrease in glomerular filtration leads to decreased ability of the kidney to excrete urea.

4. Increase in protein tissue breakdown results in the increase.

5. BUN rises with excessive exogenous protein intake. This is especially true if there is accompanying depressed renal function.

6. GI bleeding

6. Hypovolemia and the collection of blood in the small intestine and the breakdown of blood protein cause BUN to rise (12).

7. Exercise

7. Increase in protein tissue breakdown results in an increase in BUN. Moderate amounts of exercise do not affect BUN if there are sufficient calories available to meet energy demands (18).

8. Infancy
   Late Pregnancy

8. The increase is caused by increased utilization of protein during infancy and late pregnancy.

9. Male, adult

9. Because of larger muscle mass there is an increased amount of protein catabolism.

10. Poison ivy
    X-ray therapy
    Insecticides

10. Increase may occur due to nephrotoxic effect.

Conditions Related to Decreases

Rationale

1. Overhydration

1. Causes dilutional decrease due to absence of tubular absorption of urea. One glass of water will reduce BUN by 1 mg/dl. Frequently, dilutional decrease is 6–8 mg/100 dl or less (24, 27).

2. Early pregnancy

2. Due to physiologic hydremia of early pregnancy.

3. Diminished protein intake

3. Causes a negative nitrogen balance due to diminished or eliminated exogenous protein breakdown.

4. Repeated peritoneal dialysis

4. Due to protein losses into dialysis fluid.

5. Liver failure

5. Due to decreased ability to convert ammonia to urea.

6. Smoking

6. Mechanism not stated (27).

Drug Influences (15, 27): The following drugs may cause an increase in blood urea nitrogen (BUN). The drugs are listed alphabetically by generic name and divided into columns according to effect of drug. Examples of trade names are in parentheses.

Tubular necrosis
   acetaminophen (Tylenol)
   cis-platinum
   hydroxyurea (Hydrea)
   methotrexate

Nephrotoxicity
  amphotericin B (Fungizone)
  capreomycin (Capastat)
  cephaloridine (Loridine, Cephoran)
  chlorthalidone (Hygroton)
  corn oil (Lipomul)
  doxapram (Dopram)
  furosemide (Lasix)
  gentamicin (Garamycin)
  indomethacin (Indocin)
  kanamycin (Kantrex)
  methicillin (Staphcillin)
  mithramycin (Mithracin)
  mitomycin (Mutamycin)
  neomycin (Neobiotic, Mycifradin)
  opiates (morphine, codeine)
  polymixin B (Aerosporin)
  salicylic acid (aspirin)
  sodium bicarbonate
  sulfonamides
  tetracycline
  thiazides (Hydro-Diuril, Aquapres, Diuril)
  triamterene (Dyrenium)
  vancomycin (Vancomycin)

Decreased renal blood flow
  guanethidine (Ismelin)
  methyldopa (Aldomet)
  pargyline (Eutonyl)
  propranolol (Inderal)

Miscellaneous
  spectinomycin (Trobicin)
  radiographic agents

The following drugs may cause a decrease in BUN:

Drug	*Effect*
glucose	protein-sparing effect
paramethasone (Haldrone)	negative nitrogen balance
phenothiazines	decreased urea production if hepatic cirrhosis occurs

Related Lab Studies: Monitor response to treatment or progress of disease and adjust nursing care accordingly. See individual lab tests for information.

  serial BUN
  Hct, Hgb
  creatinine levels
  electrolytes (Na, K, Cl, CO_2)
  urine osmolality

IMPLICATIONS FOR NURSING CARE
PRETEST: Factors related to the test
Nursing Diagnosis: Potential for injury related to changes in biochemical balance

Guide to assessment	Guide to planning and intervention	Guide to evaluation
1. NPO	1. Restrict food and fluids the prescribed amount of time prior to collecting specimen because dietary protein and fluid intake directly affect BUN (See 4, 5 Increases; 1, 3 Decreases).	1. The patient is NPO prior to blood drawing.
2. Preexisting conditions (See Increases/Decreases)	2. Record preexisting conditions on lab slip.	2. Patient's preexisting conditions are listed on lab slip.
3. Comprehensive drug history	3. Consult with physician about and inform lab of drugs the patient is receiving that may influence BUN.	3. The patient's pertinent drug history is discussed with the physician and the lab.
4. Knowledge deficit	4. Explain test to patient. a. Define BUN (See Description). b. Explain procedure (See Procedure).	4. The patient demonstrates knowledge of test by defining BUN and stating procedure.

Patient Preparation Checklist

1. √ NPO as ordered.
2. √ Patient drug history (See Drug Influences); note pertinent information on lab slip.
3. √ Preexisting conditions and note on lab slip.
4. √ Patient knowledge, explain test to patient (See Description, Procedure).

CONSIDERATIONS FOR NURSING CARE RELATED TO ABNORMAL TEST RESULTS
POSTTEST: Factors related to the results of the test
Nursing Diagnosis: Alterations in biochemical balance

Guide to assessment	Guide to planning and intervention	Guide to evaluation
1. Fluid and electrolyte balance Type and amount of IV therapy	1. Demonstrate fluid and electrolyte balance by:	1. The patient's BUN is not influenced by fluid and electrolyte imbalance:

Guide to assessment	Guide to planning and intervention	Guide to evaluation
Water/salt balance I&O VS Skin turgor Mucous membrane Weight gain or loss Headache, flushed skin	a. Recording accurate intake and output. b. Checking VS frequently. c. Weighing patient daily. d. Recording assessment data. e. Comparing BUN to Hct and Hgb.	a. The patient's daily fluid intake is equal to daily fluid output. b. The patient's VS do not show evidence of overhydration or hypovolemia. c. Daily weight is stabilized. e. The patient's lab work is within normal limits.
2. Nutritional status a. Amount of protein intake b. Intake of foods producing alkaline urine (milk, vegetables, some fruits)	2. Teach dietary principles of: a. Protein intake, absorption, and elimination. b. Acid urine-producing foods such as meat, bread, cranberry juice, plums, prunes, and protein foods.	2. The patient demonstrates understanding of dietary principles by dietary choices and correct response to questioning.
3. Obstruction to urinary flow (See 2 Increases) Decreased urine output Severe, spasmodic pain in flank and/or abdomen Hematuria Hydration status Distended bladder	3. Encourage urinary flow by: a. Assisting to position of comfort. b. Using comfort measures such as sitz baths, warm towels, warm fluids, etc. c. Giving analgesics and antispasmodics as ordered. d. Determining intake and encouraging hydration.	3. The patient is free from urinary obstruction as noted by BUN.
4. Decreased renal blood flow and glomerulofiltration Recent medical, surgical, obstetrical, chemical history Diminished urine output	4. Restore renal function by: a. Promoting fluid and electrolyte status with precise I&O and daily weights. b. Administering blood transfusions and intravenous fluids as ordered. c. Preparing patient for dialysis as necessary.	4. The patient's renal function is restored by: a. Balancing hydration and electrolyte status. b. Corrected circulatory insufficiency. c. Hemodialysis.

Test:	Body Fluid Analysis
	Gastric Fluid
	Pleural Fluid
	Semen
	Synovial Fluid
Abbreviation:	None
Reference Values:	(9):

Gastric Fluid
Abnormal is either marked hypersecretion or anacidity
Fasting residual volume   20–100 ml
pH   <3.5
Basal acid output (BAO)   0–6 mEq/hr
Maximum acid output (MAO)   5–40 mEq/hr
  after histamine stimulation
    BAO/MAO ratio   <0.4

Pleural Fluid Analysis
Less than 20 ml

Seminal fluid
Liquefaction   within 20 minutes
Sperm morphology   >70% normal, mature spermatozoa
Sperm motility   >60%
pH   >7.0 (average 7.7)
Sperm count   60–150 million
Volume   1.5–5.0 ml

Synovial Fluid
Glucose   70–100 mg/dl
WBC   0–200 μl
Neutrophiles   <25%
Fibrin clot   absent
Mucin clot   abundant
Viscosity   high
Volume   <3.5 ml

Specimen:	Gastric fluid, pleural fluid, semen, synovial fluid
Description:	Evaluation of specific body fluids can provide valuable information in support of a diagnosis. Gastric analysis is a relatively uncommon procedure. The test is generally done for one of the following reasons: (1) to determine anacidity, which refers to a lack of gastric acidity; (2) to measure gastric acid production; (3) to reveal hypersecretory states; or (4) to evaluate the effectiveness of vagotomy for peptic ulcer disease.

Aspiration of pleural fluid is by thoracentesis. The usual indication for pleural fluid analysis is pleural effusion of unknown etiology.

The seminal fluid analysis is done as part of an infertility workup, and in an abbreviated form postvasectomy, or to confirm alleged rape and rapist identity.

The examination of synovial fluid may be of help in diagnosis of arthritis or septic-arthritis. Fluid may be obtained if effusion is present; the tap is usually dry if there is no effusion because even large joints have very little synovial fluid in them.

Procedures:

Gastric Analysis

1. Food and fluids are restricted for 12 hours prior to test.
2. The patient may need to sign a consent form. Check local institutional policy.
3. A nasogastric tube is inserted either by the nurse or physician.
4. Continuous gentle suction is applied for 1 hour. See Increases/Basal acid output and maximum acid output.
5. All gastric secretion is collected and sent to laboratory.
6. The nasogastric tube is removed.

Pleural Fluid

1. No food or fluid restrictions are necessary.
2. The patient should sign a consent form. Check local institutional policy.
3. The patient either straddles a chair, leans on over-bed table, or is seated in bed with thorax exposed. The patient should be comfortable.
4. The skin is prepared with an antiseptic.
5. The puncture site is determined by examination of chest X-ray and percussion of chest.
6. A local anesthetic is injected.
7. The thoracentesis needle is slowly advanced until the pleural space is reached.
8. After fluid is removed the needle is withdrawn.
9. Pressure is applied over puncture site and a small dressing is applied.
10. Fluid is sent to the laboratory immediately.

Semen Collection

1. A period of abstinence from sexual activity is usual. Check with local laboratory for preferred period of abstinence.
2. The patient masturbates into a collection container.
3. If collection is in other than the physician's office or clinical laboratory, the specimen should be kept warm and arrive at the laboratory within 2 hours.

Synovial Fluid

1. Food and fluids are restricted for 8–12 hours prior to test.
2. The patient should sign a consent form.
3. The patient is positioned with the affected joint fully extended.

4. A local anesthetic is usually given.

5. The patient will feel discomfort as the needle is inserted into the joint.

6. Fluid from the joint is aspirated.

7. If medication is to be injected into site, it is given after synovial fluid is aspirated.

8. The needle is removed and pressure is applied to puncture site for several minutes.

Conditions Related to Increases:	Rationale
1. Gastric analysis Food in stomach after fasting Bile, large amounts Blood Basal acid output Maximum acid output	1. After fasting any food in the stomach is abnormal. Result of obstruction to ampulla of Vater. Flecks of blood are from minor trauma from nasogastric intubation. More than flecks of blood is abnormal. The color may be red or coffee-ground color. Bleeding may occur from ulceration, malignancy, gastritis, or from swallowing nasopharyngeal blood. Increased dramatically in Zollinger-Ellison syndrome. Increased in peptic ulcer. During the hour of collection, samples are divided into 15-minute samples and the acid output is calculated.
2. Pleural fluid	2. Pleural fluid amounts are very small in normal circumstances. Infection, trauma, neoplasms of the pleural cavity, congestive heart failure, etc., cause an increase in pleural fluid. A *transudate* is an effusion from failure to reabsorb fluid or the formation of fluid. An *exudate* is caused by damage to the epithelial cells that line the serous membrane.
3. Seminal fluid High viscosity	3. Highly viscous semen may decrease spermatozoa invasion of cervical mucous.
4. Synovial fluid Appearance Turbidity	4. Synovial fluid is normally crystal clear and pale yellow. Increased turbidity is indicative of increased leukocytes.

Milky	Seen in chronic rheumatoid arthritis, SLE, gout.
Purulent	Increased in septic arthritis; sometimes it is absent in early stages.
Greenish	May be seen in hemophilus influenza arthritis, gout, rheumatoid arthritis.
Bloody	Bleeding into joint.
Leukocytes	Increased leukocytes may indicate bacterial invasion, active gout, or rheumatoid arthritis.
Volume	The normal joint has only 0.1–2.0 ml of fluid. An increase in fluid indicates effusion (9).

Conditions Related to Decreases

Rationale

1. Seminal fluid sperm count

1. A sperm count of less than 20 million/ml is considered abnormal. Impregnation may still take place.

Drug Influences: The following drugs may cause an increase in test values. The drugs are listed alphabetically by generic name and divided into columns according to effect of drug. Examples of trade names are in parentheses.

Gastric analysis
  adrenergic blocking agents
  adrenocorticosteroids
  alcohol
  antacids
  anticholinergics

IMPLICATIONS FOR NURSING CARE
PRETEST: Factors related to the test
Nursing Diagnosis: Potential for injury related to people-provider factors

Guide to assessment	Guide to planning and intervention	Guide to evaluation
Assess patient factors that may influence test results: 1. Gastric analysis Synovial fluid analysis	1. Restrict food and fluids for 12 hours prior to test.	1. Patient's food ingestion does not influence test results.
2. Comprehensive drug history For gastric analysis, see Drug Influences	2. Identify interfering drugs and consult with physician. Hold interfering drugs for 24 hours prior to testing. Note interfering drugs patient is receiving on lab slip.	2. Patient's values are not influenced by patient medication.

Guide to assessment	Guide to planning and intervention	Guide to evaluation
3. Preexisting conditions	3. Fill out lab slip completely.	
4. Lack of patient knowledge	4. Explain test to patient: a. Define test. b. Explain procedure. c. Obtain signed consent as necessary.	4. Patient demonstrates knowledge of test by defining test and stating procedure. Consent form is signed.

Patient Preparation Checklist

1. √ NPO for proper test. See 1.
2. √ Interfering drugs for gastric analysis.
3. √ Lab slip filled out completely.
4. √ Patient knowledge: explain test to patient.
   Obtain Signed Consent as Necessary

CONSIDERATIONS FOR NURSING CARE RELATED TO ABNORMAL TEST RESULTS
POSTTEST: Factors related to the results of the test
Nursing Diagnosis: Alterations in biochemical balance

Guide to assessment	Guide to planning and intervention	Guide to evaluation
Assess patient factors influencing test results. Nursing history or physical exam suggestive of: 1. Positive body fluid analysis results.	1. Implement medical plan of care to treat underlying condition.	1. Patient's lab results return to normal.

Test:	Bone Marrow Aspiration Biopsy
Abbreviation:	None

Reference Values:

	Normal
Cellularity	normal
Megakaryocytes and platelet formation	normal
Granulocytic cells	normal
Neutrophilic ⌐	⌐ any
Eosinophilic ⎬	abnormality is
Basophilic ⌐	⌐ specified
Erythroid cells	
Maturation	normoblastic
Activity	normal
M:E ratio	
Birth	1.85:1
2 weeks	11:1
1–20 months	5.5:1
1–20 years	2.95:1
Adult	4:1

Other cells	*Children*	*Adults*
Lymphocytes	3.0–17.0%	2.7–24%
Plasma cells	0 – 2.0%	0.1– 1.5%
Reticulum cells	0.2– 2.0%	0.1– 2.0%

Specimen: Bone marrow aspirate, bone marrow biopsy

Description: Bone marrow is made up of fat and hematopoietic cells and connective tissue. It is soft and friable and fills the spaces between the fibrous cords of bone in the marrow cavity. After birth, the bone marrow is wholly responsible for the production of erythrocytes, granulocytes, monocytes, and platelets. A small sample of bone marrow is fairly representative of total hematopoietic bone marrow activity.

A bone marrow exam may be done to diagnose hematological diseases, to isolate marrow for bacterial culture, follow disease therapies, or diagnose parasitic infections. Bone marrow aspiration is done in conjunction with peripheral blood studies. Interpretation of results is complex and should be done by a qualified professional.

The bone marrow examination report includes peripheral blood studies and details of the marrow aspirate. Marrow cellularity is observed for hypercellular, hypocellular, or normal activity. Cellularity depends on the place of aspiration and age of the patient and is an overview of the cells. Changes in marrow cell distribution are also noted. The number of megakaryocytes, maturity, and the presence of platelets is observed. The granulocyte series is studied for number of cells. Younger forms such as myeloblasts or progranulocytes are noted. Erythropoiesis is observed for number and maturity of cells and for erythrocyte precursors. The number of plasma cells, lymphocytes, and reticulum cells are studied. The M:E ratio (myeloid to erythroid ratio)—that is, the total number of granulocytes to the total number of normoblasts—is determined. A normal M:E ratio does not necessarily mean that the bone marrow is normal. The exam also includes a search for malignant or unusual cells.

Procedure:

1. The patient/parent signs a consent form.
2. There are no food or fluid restrictions.
3. Patients may be premedicated.
4. The patient is placed in position:
   a. Iliac crest aspiration (most recommended for adults and children after infancy). Patient on side.
   b. Sternal aspiration (not recommended on children before adolescence). Patient on back with arms at side.
   c. Anterior iliac crest aspiration. Patient on back with arms at side.
   d. Vertebral spinous process aspiration. Patient is in sitting position leaning forward, on side, or prone.
   e. Tibial aspiration (used in infants under 1 year of age). A sandbag is placed under the infant's thigh. The infant must be held securely.
5. The skin is prepared with antiseptic and draped.
6. A local anesthetic is injected; usually not in children.
7. A small incision is made for biopsy only.
8. The bone marrow needle with stylet in place is advanced and rotated through the skin (incision) and into the bone marrow cavity.
9. When the needle is in place the stylet is removed and the syringe attached.
10. The syringe is aspirated slowly until a small amount of blood and marrow is aspirated. The aspiration may cause a brief sharp pain.
11. The needle and syringe are removed.
12. Pressure is applied to the area and it is observed for bleeding or evidence of hematoma.
13. A small pressure dressing is applied.
14. The procedure lasts 5–10 minutes.
15. The patient should rest for 30 minutes before resuming activity.
16. The site may be tender for 3–4 days after the test.

Conditions Related to Increases	Rationale
1. Myeloproliferative syndromes Pancytopenia of unknown cause Sideroblastic anemia	1. The increase is due to erythroid hyperplasia. The M:E ratio may be decreased.

Hereditary
Acquired
  Lead poisoning
  Alcoholism

2. Myelocytic leukemia

2. Bone marrow granulocyte (neutrophiles, basophiles, eosinophiles) production is increased.

3. Infections

3. Bone marrow elevations may include
increased lymphocytes, granulocytes, and/or megakaryocytes. The
M:E ratio is also increased.

4. Anemias
Hemolytic
Iron deficiency
Megaloblastic
Chronic blood loss

4. Bone marrow normoblasts are elevated. The M:E ratio may be normal.

5. Aplastic anemia caused by
Chemicals
Radiation
Drugs
Idiopathic

5. Elevated lymphocytes make up 60–
100% of the nucleated cells. Plasma
cells may also be elevated. Generally, the marrow is hypocellular.

6. Myelofibrosis

6. In this condition megakaryocytes
and lymphocytes are elevated,
though there is general bone marrow hypoplasia.

7. Cellular decreases

7. In response to decreases of a bone
marrow cell type, lymphocytes,
granulocytes, plasma cells, and normoblasts may increase production.

8. Lymphocytic leukemia
Leukemoid reaction, lymphocytes
Lymphoma
Infectious lymphocytosis
Viral infections
Infectious mononucleosis

8. In these conditions bone marrow
lymphocytes may be elevated. The
M:E ratio may also be elevated.

9. Macroglobulinemia

9. In this disease there is bone marrow
increase in granulocytes, lymphocytes, and plasma cells. Plasma cells
are important to immunoglobulin
production; plasma cell proliferation
may produce immunodeficiency disease.

10. Radiation

10. May cause an increase in plasma cell
production. Also, may be general
bone marrow hypoplasia with decreased granulocytes and megakaryocytes.

11. Polycythemia vera
    Splenic enlargement
    Idiopathic thrombocytosis
    Chronic myelogenous leukemia
    Posthemorrhage
    Sickle-cell anemia

11. Megakaryocyte production is increased in these conditions. There is erythroid hyperplasia.

12. Agranulocytosis
    Hepatic cirrhosis
    Hodgkin's disease
    Carcinomas
    Multiple myeloma
    Serum sickness
    Ulcerative colitis

12. All of these conditions may show elevated bone marrow plasma cells. In the case of Hodgkin's disease, the exam will give information about the stage of the disease.

Conditions Related to Decreases

Rationale

1. Aplastic (hypoplastic) anemia
   Etiology
     Chemical agents
     Congenital aplasia
     Antineoplastic agents
     Antimetabolites
     Radiation
     Antimicrobials
     Anticonvulsants
     Analgesics
     Antihistamines
     Insecticides
     Idiopathic
     Viral

1. There is general bone marrow hypoplasia with diminished granulocytic and megakaryocyte production. Lymphocytes, plasma cells, and fatty particles are seen on marrow section. The M:E ratio may be normal.

2. Hepatic cirrhosis
   Carcinomas

2. These conditions may show diminished megakaryocyte and increased plasma cell production.

3. Old age (65 years +)
   Osteoporosis

3. Cellularity decreases at a fairly even rate until age 65. Cellularity decreases rapidly in the next 10 years, by about 30 percent.

4. Agranulocytosis

4. Decreased granulocyte activity that shows WBC of 200–3000. Granulocyte cell types are neutrophiles, basophiles, and eosinophiles.

5. Myelofibrosis

5. There is general bone marrow hypoplasia. Megakaryocytes and lymphocytes are elevated. If bone marrow aspiration is done, it may result in a "dry tap" and require bone marrow biopsy.

6. Viral infections

6. There may be hematopoietic depression following viral infections such as rubella. These rarely develop into aplastic anemia.

7. Anemias
   Iron deficiency
   Pernicious
   Posthemolytic
   Posthemorrhagic
   Liver disease
   Polycythemia

7. Decreased M:E ratio is seen in conditions of erythroid hyperplasia.

8. Alcoholism

8. Alcoholism causes bone marrow depression of normoblasts, leukocytes, monocytes, and thrombocytes.

9. Hypothyroidism

9. In about 30 percent of patients with hypothyroidism there is decreased erythroid bone marrow activity with a macrocytic anemia.

Drug Influences: Many drugs may interfere with bone marrow function. Listed below are some of the types of drugs that may influence test results.

The following drugs may cause an increase in bone marrow activity:

folic acid
glucocorticoids
iron preparations
vitamin B_{12}

The following types of drugs may cause a decrease in bone marrow activity:

alkylating agents
analgesics
anticonvulsants
antihistamines
antimetabolites
antimicrobials
antineoplastic agents
antithyroid drugs
chemical agents (benzene, carbon tetrachloride, etc.)
diuretics (thiazide diuretics)
insecticides
phenothiazines
tranquilizers
sulfonamides

Related Lab Studies: Monitor response to therapy or progression of disease and adjust nursing care accordingly. See individual tests for specific information.

CBC
platelet count
reticulocyte count

mono spot test
RBC count with morphology

With chemotherapy
alkaline phosphatase
uric acid
AST (SGOT)
urea nitrogen

IMPLICATIONS FOR NURSING CARE
PRETEST: Factors related to the test
Nursing Diagnosis: Potential for injury related to changes in biochemical balance

Guide to assessment	Guide to planning and intervention	Guide to evaluation
Assess patient factors that may influence test results: 1. Comprehensive drug/ chemical history	1. Report to physician and/or lab drugs the patient is receiving that may influence test results:	1. Drugs or chemicals the patient has ingested or used in the past year that may influence test results are noted. Blood transfusion within the past week is noted.
a. See Drug Influences/ Decreases 1 b. Blood transfusion	a. Be alert to toxic effects of drugs patient is receiving. b. Note cytotoxic agents or blood transfusion within past week on lab slip. c. Recognize decreases in WBC count and report to physician.	

2. Preexisting conditions (See Increases/Decreases)
3. Patient/parent apprehension
   Knowledge deficit
	2. Record preexisting conditions on lab slip.
	3. Explain test:
	a. Define test (See Definition).
	b. Explain procedure (See Procedure).
	c. Support child and reduce fear (as appropriate for age) by:
	  (1) Encouraging child to play with syringe without needle, cotton balls, tape, doll (with supervision).
	  (2) Explaining and illustrating procedure for child.
	  (3) Describing pain/pressure honestly.
		2. Patient's preexisting conditions are noted.
		3. The patient/parent demonstrates knowledge of test by defining the test and stating procedure.

Guide to assessment	Guide to planning and intervention	Guide to evaluation
	(4) Encouraging parent to remain with child if at all possible. (5) Explaining the need for child to be very still and the need for someone to help hold. (6) Talking to the child quietly, constantly, in a somewhat melodic way during procedure. (7) Giving the child permission to yell, but he *must hold still*. (8) Warning the child right before aspiration.	
4. Public lack of knowledge	4. Prevent disease of bone marrow in the community: a. Advise against use of nontherapeutically prescribed drugs. b. Be alert to toxic effect of drugs. c. Encourage antipollution measures, especially concerning chemicals and nuclear safety.	

Patient Preparation Checklist

1. √ Consent form signed.
2. √ Influencing drugs are noted and reported (See Drug Influences).
3. √ Preexisting conditions noted on lab slip (See Increases/Decreases).
4. √ Patient knowledge, apprehension; explain test and procedure (See Description/Procedure).

CONSIDERATIONS FOR NURSING CARE RELATED TO ABNORMAL TEST RESULTS

POSTTEST: Factors related to the results of the test

Nursing Diagnosis: Alterations in biochemical balance related to abnormal blood profile

Guide to assessment	Guide to planning and intervention	Guide to evaluation
Assess patient factors that may be influencing test results. Nursing history and/or physical exam suggestive of:		
1. Aplastic anemia Patient symptoms Pallor Fatigue Infections Unusual bleeding Lab: bone marrow is fatty with few developing cells Peripheral blood ↓ RBC ↓ Reticulocytes ↓ WBC ↓ Platelets	1. Prevent further bone marrow damage and encourage bone marrow activity by:	1. The patient demonstrates improvement by improved lab findings:
a. Comprehensive drug/chemical history Over-the-counter drugs	a. Removing offending agent, if known, as ordered.	a. The patient is protected against further damage to bone marrow by the offending agent.
b. Androgens Steroids	b. Administering androgens and steroids as ordered.	b. The patient's peripheral blood work shows erythropoietic response to drugs.
c. Decreased leukocyte count	c. Initiating measures to protect patient from infection.	c. The patient is protected from infection and further insult to damaged bone marrow.
d. Platelet count below 50,000	d. Initiating nursing measures to protect the patient from bleeding.	d. The patient is protected from loss of blood and further damage to the bone marrow.
e. Need for bone marrow transplant	e. Initiating nursing measures specific to bone marrow transplant (See local hospital protocol/procedure).	e. Patient receives successful bone marrow transplant.
2. Agranulocytosis Patient symptoms Fatigue Weakness Infection	2. Prevent further bone marrow damage and encourage bone marrow activity:	2. The patient demonstrates improvement by improved lab findings:

Guide to assessment	Guide to planning and intervention	Guide to evaluation

Anemia
Uremia
TB
Lab: Bone marrow
  Absence of granulocytes
  (neutrophiles, baso-
  philes, eosinophiles)
Peripheral blood
  WBC; 500–3000
  ↓ Polymorphoneuclear
  cells		

a. Comprehensive drug and chemical history, especially
  Antibiotics (Chloramphenicol)
  Anticonvulsants
  Antithyroid drugs (Thiouricils)
  Gold
  Sulfonamides
  Tripelennamine (Pyrabenzamine)
	a. Remove offending agent and teach patient to use only currently prescribed drugs.	a. The patient is protected against further damage to bone marrow by the offending agent. Bone marrow activity is increased as evidenced by increased monocytes and immature myeloid forms in peripheral blood.

b. Decreased leukocyte count	b. Initiate nursing measures to protect the patient from infection.	b. The patient is protected from infection and further insult to the damaged bone marrow.
c. Androgen therapy	c. Administer androgen therapy as ordered.	c. The patient's marrow activity is stimulated as noted by increased monocyte count and immature myeloid forms in the peripheral blood.

3. Chemotherapy
  Alkylating agents
  Antimetabolites
  Plant alkaloids
  Antibiotics
  Myelosuppressive therapy
Radiation to bones
	3. Detect toxic effects to bone marrow early; report to physician and record findings.	3. Patient's symptoms of extreme fatigue, sore throat, sore mouth, fever, or drop in WBCs are reported to physician immediately.

4. Alcoholism (See 8 Decreases)	4. Teach patient, as appropriate, relationship of alcohol to bone marrow activity.	4. The patient states understanding of alcohol and bone marrow depression.

Guide to assessment	Guide to planning and intervention	Guide to evaluation
5. Myeloproliferative diseases Leukemias Lymphomas, etc.	5. Promote restoration of normal bone marrow function by:	5. The patient's bone marrow shows improvement by reduction or disappearance of abnormal cells in bone marrow and peripheral blood:
a. Chemotherapy	a. Administering chemotherapeutic agent on time and as ordered.	a. The patient receives therapy to achieve maximum effect on different phases of miotic cycle. Lab findings show improvement.
b. Myelosuppressive therapy Polycythemia vera	b. Administering radioactive phosphorus or other myelosuppressive drugs on time and as ordered.	b. The patient's hyperplastic bone marrow is controlled as evidenced by reduced peripheral blood count, decreased number of precursor cells, and increased iron stores on bone marrow exam.

Test: Calcium

Abbreviation: Ca

Reference Values: Premature <1 week   6–10 mg/dl
Full-term ≤1 week   7–12 mg/dl
Child   8–11 mg/dl
Adult   8.9–10.1 mg/dl

Specimen: Serum

Description: Calcium is found throughout the body in cells, in extracellular fluid, and in bones. It is the most abundant electrolyte in the body. It exists in the body in three forms: it is protein-bound to albumin or globulin; or ionized; or a small portion is complexed with organic compounds such as citrate, bicarbonate, or phosphate. Only the ionized calcium is active. Calcium functions in the body to maintain cellular and skeletal integrity, maintains normal transmission of nerve impulses, and plays a role in blood clotting and enzyme activity.

Calcium levels in the bloodstream are regulated by the parathyroid hormone parathormone, calcitonin, and vitamin D.

Serum calcium levels are measured to assess parathyroid disorders, bone disease, neuromuscular irritability, and after surgery to the thyroid or parathyroid gland.

Procedure: (red top tube)
1. Food and fluids, except water, are restricted for 8 hours.
2. Hold influencing medications before test (See Drug Influences).
3. Approximately 10 ml of blood is withdrawn from the patient. Blood may be drawn by skin puncture in the pediatric patient (about 0.5 ml is needed).
4. Specimen should go to laboratory immediately.
5. Observe puncture site for bleeding or evidence of hematoma.

Conditions Related to Increases

Rationale

1. Hyperparathyroidism

1. The polypeptide hormone parathormone acts on the kidneys to decrease reabsorption and increase excretion of phosphate and increase calcium reabsorption. Hyperparathyroidism results in an excess production of parathormone.

2. Neoplasms

2. It is thought that some neoplasms are capable of synthesizing and releasing a parathormone-like peptide.

3. Alkalosis
Ulcer diet
High calcium content in water

3. Excess dietary calcium intake may result in total serum calcium increase.

4. Vitamin D excess
   Sarcoidosis
   Hyperthyroidism
   Multiple myeloma
   Skeletal metastasis
5. Newborn, exchange transfusion

6. Postdialysis
   Renal transplantation
   Uremia

Conditions Related to Decreases

1. Malabsorption
   Sprue
   Acute pancreatitis
   Diarrhea
   Hypoparathyroidism
   Renal disease
   Rickets, vitamin D deficiency
2. Pregnancy
   Lactation

3. Surgical removal of the parathyroids

4. Idiopathic hypoparathyroidism

5. Newborn that is fed cow's milk

4. Calcium is released from bone and floods the extracellular fluid.

5. Acid-citrate-dextrose–treated blood, and calcium gluconate will increase total plasma calcium (34).
6. Increase in serum calcium is from decreased calcium excretion.

Rationale

1. The deficit is from excessive loss of calcium from the body and an inadequate intake of vitamin D.

2. If dietary intake is insufficient for the increased calcium requirement, total serum calcium will be decreased.
3. When parathyroid glands are removed, the source of parathormone is removed.
4. Due to autoimmune destruction of parathyroid glands.
5. Cow's milk contains less calcium/ phosphorus ratio than human milk and may result in decreased serum calcium levels (34).

Drug Influences: The following drugs may influence test results. The drugs are listed alphabetically by generic name and divided into columns according to the effect of the drug. Examples of trade names are in parentheses.

The following drugs may cause an increase in test results:

Serum

Increased calcium absorption and/or retention
   antacids (Tums)
   calcium gluconate (Calcet)
   calcium salts
   dienestrol (Dienestrol Cream)
   ergocalciferol (Deltalin)
   estradiol (Estrace)
   estrogens (Premarin)
   oral contraceptives

Impaired excretion
   chlorothiazide (Aldoclor)
   hydrochlorothiazide (Esidrix)
   methyclothiazide (Enduron)

Increased with breast cancer
   diethylstilbestrol (Stilbestrol)
   dromostanolone (Drolban)
   fluoxymesterone (Android-F)
   methandrostenolone (Dianabol)
   methyltestosterone (Android-5)
   nandrolone (Anabolin)
   oxymetholone (Adroyd)
   testosterone (Android-T)

Urine

Diuretic effect
   bendroflumethiazide (Naturetin); initial diuretic effect
   corticotropin (Acthar)
   dimercaprol (BAL in oil)
   mannitol (Osmitrol)
   metolazone (Diulo)
   viomycin

Impaired reabsorption
   acetazolamide (Diamox)
   furosemide (Lasix)
   mercaptomerin (Thiomerin Sodium)
   triamterene (Dyrenium)

Metabolic effect
   dexamethasone (Decadron)
   prednisolone (Cordrol)
   triamcinolone (Kenalog)

Miscellaneous
   calcitonin (Calcimar)
   cholestyramine (Questran)
   dihydrotachysterol (Hytakerol)

The following drugs may cause a decrease in test results:

Serum

Calcium complexing effect
   citrates (magnesium citrate)
   fluorides (Flo-Tabs)
   magnesium salts (Milk of Magnesia)
   polystyrene sulfonate (Kayexalate)

Vitamin D and parathyroid antagonists
   cortisone (Cortistan)
   prednisone (SK-Prednisone)

Diuretic effect
   acetazolamide (Diamox)
   furosemide (Lasix)

Metabolic effect
   diphenylhydantoin (Dilantin)
   phenobarbital (Barbipil)

Lowered albumin-binding effect
   asparaginase (Elspar)
   ethinyl estradiol (Estinyl)

Miscellaneous
   laxatives (Colace)
   mithramycin (Mithracin)
   tetracycline (Achromycin)

Urine

Impaired excretion
   bendroflumethiazide (Naturetin)
   chlorothiazide (Aldoclor)
   methyclothiazide (Enduron)
   polythiazide (Renese)
   trichlormethiazide (Diurese)

Increased tubular reabsorption
   parathyroid extract (Paroidin)

Decreased GI absorption
   ethinyl estradiol (Estinyl)
   oral contraceptives

Related Lab Studies: Monitor response to treatment or progress of disease and adjust nursing care accordingly. See individual tests for information.

Hypoparathyroidism
   phosphorus, serum
   24-hour urine calcium
   alkaline phosphatase
   *(skull X-ray)

IMPLICATIONS FOR NURSING CARE
PRETEST: Factors related to the test
Nursing Diagnosis: Potential for injury related to changes in biochemical balance

Guide to assessment	Guide to planning and intervention	Guide to evaluation
Assess patient factors that may influence test results: 1. Food and fluids	1. Restrict food and fluids for 12 hours prior to testing. Infants are usually not placed	1. Patient's values are not increased due to dietary calcium.

_____
*Not discussed in this book.

Guide to assessment	Guide to planning and intervention	Guide to evaluation
	NPO, but serum calcium is drawn before feeding.	
2. Comprehensive drug history (See Drug Influences)	2. Identify influencing drugs on test values. Consult with physician. Note medications that must be continued but may interfere with test values on lab slip.	2. Patient's medications do not interfere with test values.
3. Preexisting conditions (See Increases/Decreases) Age	3. Identify pertinent preexisting conditions and note them on lab slip.	3. Patient's preexisting conditions do not interfere with test values.
4. Lack of patient knowledge	4. Explain test to patient: a. Define calcium/phosphorus (See Description). b. Explain procedure (See Procedure).	4. The patient demonstrates knowledge by defining test and stating procedure.
5. Hemolysis	5. Prevent hemolysis by: a. Not saturating skin with antiseptic. b. Not probing venipuncture site or leaving the tourniquet on too long. c. Not forcefully withdrawing specimen. d. Not withdrawing specimen too slowly. e. Not agitating or handling specimen roughly.	5. Patient's values are not influenced by hemolysis.

Patient Preparation Checklist

1. √ Food and fluids restricted 12 hours (not on infants).
2. √ Interfering drugs withheld or noted on lab slip.
3. √ Pertinent preexisting conditions noted on lab slip.
4. √ Patient knowledge; explain test (See Description/Procedure).
5. √ Prevent hemolysis.

CONSIDERATIONS FOR NURSING CARE RELATED TO ABNORMAL TEST RESULTS
POSTTEST: Factors related to the results of the test
Nursing Diagnosis: Alterations in biochemical balance

Guide to assessment	Guide to planning and intervention	Guide to evaluation
Assess patient factors that may be influencing test results. Nursing history and/or physical exam suggestive of: 1. Hypercalcemia	1. Reduce serum calcium by:	1. The patient's serum calcium level is reduced to normal.
a. May be asymptomatic May be rapid and severe Anorexia Nausea Vomiting Weight loss Constipation Polydipsia Polyuria EKG changes Hypertension Deep thigh pain Pathologic fractures Cardiac arrest	a. Recognizing early signs and symptoms of hypercalcemia. Consulting with physician.	
b. Parathyroid tumor	b. Initiating nursing measures to prepare patient for surgery.	
c. PTH-independent hypercalcemia (See 4 Decreases)	c. Implementing medical plan to treat underlying condition.	
d. Isotonic sodium chloride infusion	d. Expanding extracellular fluid volume and promoting renal excretion of excess calcium by administering increased fluids as prescribed.	
e. Diuretics	e. Giving diuretic as prescribed to promote renal excretion of calcium.	
f. Phosphate therapy	f. Promoting phosphate binding with calcium for removal from bloodstream as prescribed.	
g. Mithramycin, calcitonin	g. Inhibiting skeletal reabsorption of calcium by giv-	

Guide to assessment	Guide to planning and intervention	Guide to evaluation
	ing mithramycin and calcitonin as ordered.	

2. Hypocalcemia
  Tetany
  Seizures
  Mental disturbances
  Carpopedal spasms
  Paresthesia
  Laryngeal stridor
  Possibly, respiratory distress
  Chvostek's sign
  Postive Trousseau test
  Emotional complaints
  Dry, coarse, scaly skin
  Alopecia, eyebrows, eyelashes
  Thin nails
  Cataracts
	2. Increase serum calcium by:
	  a. Recognizing signs and symptoms of hypocalcemia. Consulting with a physician.
		2. The patient's serum calcium level returns to normal.

b. Calcium salts Vitamin D	b. Improving intestinal absorption of calcium by giving calcium salts and vitamin D as ordered.	

Test:	Catecholamines
Abbreviation:	None
Reference Values:	Plasma: less than 1 µg/L
	Urine: 0–18 µg/dl per random sample (total catecholamines)
	Below 1 year up to 20 µg/dl/24 hours
	1–5 years up to 40 µg/dl/24 hours
	6–15 years up to 80 µg/dl/24 hours
	Above 15 years up to 100 µg/dl/24 hours
	These are representative of total catecholamine levels
Specimen:	Plasma, urine
Description:	Catecholamines are hormones and amines produced in the brain, sympathetic ganglia, and the adrenal medulla. The major members are epinephrine, norepinephrine, and dopamine. Catecholamine secretion is stimulated by such stimuli as physiologic or psychologic stress, hypoxia, hemorrhage, and a number of drugs (26). Norepinephrine and epinephrine collectively increase the blood pressure and metabolic rate, raise blood sugar, and elevate fatty acid levels. The majority of catecholamines are excreted in the urine as VMA (metabolic end products) with only small amounts excreted as catecholamines or metanephrine (metabolite of epinephrine). Measurement of plasma and urinary catecholamines is most commonly done to diagnose pheochromocytoma, a rare chromaffin tissue tumor (often of the adrenal medulla) secreting excessive amounts of epinephrine and norepinephrine. Since the rate of hormone secretion is not constant, a 24-hour urine collection is usually considered the most significant value.
Procedure:	(lavender top tube)

Plasma

1. Dietary restrictions.
   a. Eliminate amine-rich foods (coffee, tea, cocoa, beer, Chianti, cheese, bananas, avocados) from the diet for 2 days. There may be no dietary restrictions, so check with local laboratory for procedure.
   b. Fast for 10–12 hours prior to test.
2. Venipuncture is performed early morning (usually 6 A.M. to 8 A.M.), or after the patient has been supine in a nonstimulating surrounding for at least 30 minutes.
3. 5 ml of blood is drawn using a special tube. Care is taken to prevent hemolysis.
4. The patient may have a second sample drawn after standing for 10 minutes.
5. If venipuncture will stress the patient, a heparin lock may be used prior to collecting specimen. At least 30 minutes in a non-

stimulating environment is required before collecting sample. (Discard the first 1–2 ml of blood from lock before collecting sample.)

6. Indicate on lab slip whether patient was standing or supine.
7. Observe for bleeding at venipuncture site or for evidence of hematoma.

24-Hour Urine Collection

1. Amine-rich foods may or may not be restricted. Check with local lab. If restricted, see 1 above for list of foods.
2. Collection bottle must be acidified; contact lab. The urine should be refrigerated during the entire collection.
3. Collection.
   a. Discard first voided specimen.
   b. For next 24 hours place all voidings into specimen container immediately after voiding. Keep refrigerated.
   c. Have patient void just prior to completion of the 24 hours and put sample in collection bottle.
4. Record exact start and finish times on lab slip.
5. Send to lab immediately.

Random Urine Sample

1. Collect and place urine into an acidified collection bottle. Obtain collection container from lab.
2. Obtain ordered random urine sample immediately after hypertensive episode, if possible, and send to lab.

Conditions Related to Increases	Rationale
	Plasma and Urine
1. Pheochromocytoma	1. This is a chromaffin tissue tumor that secretes excessive amounts of epinephrine and norepinephrine. Values may be 3–100 times greater than normal.
2. Ganglioneuroma	2. This is a well-differentiated tumor of the sympathetic nervous system that secretes excessive catecholamines.
3. Neuroblastoma	3. One of the most common malignant soft tissue tumors in infancy and childhood, this tumor arises in sympathetic and adrenal medullary tissue and produces increased catecholamines (40).
4. Psychiatric disorders Manic depressive disorders Depressive neurosis	4. These are conditions in which anxiety and depression may cause prolonged stress. Stress is a known cause of elevated catecholamines. If

MAO inhibitors are used for treatment they would contribute to increased levels because MAO is needed to degrade catecholamines (44).

5. Stress
   Normal stressors
      Anxiety, anger
      Vigorous exercise
   Abnormal stressors
      Tetanus
      Widespread burns
      Severe infections
      Severe trauma
      Pancreatitis, peritonitis

5. Stress causes a normal increase in catecholamine output (the fight-or-flight mechanism).

6. Hypoglycemia

6. A compensatory increase in catecholamines occurs because epinephrine increases glycogenolysis and decreases insulin release to increase blood sugar (20). Hypoglycemia is also a stressor.

7. Conditions producing circulatory inadequacy
      Acute myocardial infarct
      Congestive heart failure
      Cor pulmonae

7. When blood volume is inadequate, the baroreceptors try to compensate by stimulating the sympathetic nervous system and the adrenal medulla. This causes an increased release of epinephrine and norepinephrine with a resulting increase in blood pressure.

8. Hypertension, essential and malignant, some cases

8. Elevated catecholamines may be part of the cause of the hypertension.

9. Progressive muscular dystrophy
   Myasthenia gravis

9. Cyclic AMP, a biochemical second messenger, facilitates neuromuscular transmission, and norepinephrine and ephedrine increase cellular levels of AMP. The increased levels may be a compensatory mechanism for the problems with the neuromuscular transmission associated with these diseases. Other studies show that in diseases affecting the integrity of the nerves, there is an increased production of catecholamines from the remaining intact areas (40).

10. Hypothyroidism

10. There is an inverse relationship between catecholamine levels and thy-

roid activity (49). Increased levels may be a compensatory mechanism of the body to maintain normal metabolism since many catecholamine actions mimic thyroid hormone actions.

11. Shock conditions, including electroshock therapy

11. Shock conditions stimulate catecholamine output because they are stressors. In most shock situations, the body is attempting to elevate the blood pressure.

Conditions Related to Decreases

Rationale

Plasma and Urine

1. Diabetes mellitus with existing neuropathy

1. The limited function of the peripheral nerves results in decreased release of norepinephrine.

2. Familial dysautonomia

2. An inherited defect in catecholamine metabolism (1).

3. Transection of cervical spinal cord

3. Results in decreased or absent sympathetic nerve function below level of severance.

4. Malnutrition

4. Decrease may be related to amino acid deficiency. Tyrosine is the amino acid precursor of catecholamines (40).

5. Hyperthyroidism

5. There is an inverse relationship between thyroid activity and catecholamine levels. The decrease levels may be compensatory to keep metabolism balanced.

6. Idiopathic orthostatic hypotension

6. There is either a deficiency or lack of responsiveness to catecholamines (21).

Drug Influences: The following drugs may influence test results. The drugs are listed alphabetically by generic name and divided into columns according to the effect of the drug. Examples of trade names are in parentheses.

The following drugs may cause an increase in test results:

Plasma

Metabolic effect with decreased organ uptake
    chlorpromazine (Thorazine)
    diazoxide (Hyperstat)
    perphenazine (Trilafon)
    phentolamine (Regitine)
    promethazine (Phenergan)

Epinephrine-like effect
   epinephrine (Adrenalin Chloride)
   levodopa (Bendopa)
   methyldopa (Aldomet)

Miscellaneous
   aminophylline (Aminophyllin)
   ethanol (grain alcohol)
   ether
   MAO inhibitors (Eutonyl)
   nitroglycerin (Corobid)

Urine

Release of stored norepinephrine
   rauwolfia (Raupoid)
   reserpine (Alkarau)

Metabolic effect with decreased organ uptake
   prochlorperazine (Compazine)

Miscellaneous
   ethanol (grain alcohol)
   isoproterenol (Isuprel)

   The following drugs may cause a decrease in test results:

Plasma

Normal therapy response
   reserpine (Alkarau)

Urine

Output decrease
   clonidine (Catapres)

Norepinephrine inhibition
   guanethidine (Ismelin)

Miscellaneous
   quabain
   methyldopa (Aldomet)
   radiographic agents

Related Lab Studies:

Diagnosis of pheochromocytoma
   *histamine pressor test
   glucose tolerance test (shows diabetic curve)
   *phentolamine pressor test
   *tyramine pressor test
   ↑ vanillylmandelic acid (VMA)

---

*Not discussed in this book.

IMPLICATIONS FOR NURSING CARE
PRETEST: Factors related to the test.
Nursing Diagnosis: Potential for injury related to biochemical imbalance

Guide to assessment	Guide to planning and intervention	Guide to evaluation
Assess patient factors influencing test results:		
1. Food and fluid restrictions	1. Restrict dietary intake prior to test as ordered (See Procedure).	1. Ingestion of food does not influence lab results.
2. Exercise and stress Resting 15 minutes prior to blood drawing Minimal physical activity during urine collection Environment stress-free before and during specimen collection	2. Decrease influence of stress and exercise by: a. Plasma catecholamines: (1) Inserting heparin lock 24 hours prior to test if needle puncture is stressful to patient. (2) Having patient in relaxed, recumbent position 30 minutes prior to withdrawal of blood sample. b. Urinary catecholamines: (1) Avoiding excessive physical activity while 24-hour urine sample is being collected. (2) Avoiding stressful situations during 24-hour urine sample collection.	2. Stress and exercise by the patient do not influence lab results.
3. Position Recumbent or standing	3. Decrease influence of position on catecholamines by: a. Placing patient in recumbent position 30 minutes prior to withdrawal of sample. b. Assisting patient, as necessary, to stand after initial sample is drawn for second sample to be drawn.	3. The patient's lab results are not influenced by incorrect position.
4. Comprehensive drug history (See Drug Influences)	4. Diminish the influence of drugs on: a. Plasma catecholamines by: (1) Scheduling test before, or at least 1 week after, studies using radioactive substances. (2) Omitting nonprescribed medications, especially those for cold or	4. The patient's lab results are not influenced by nonessential drugs:

Guide to assessment	Guide to planning and intervention	Guide to evaluation
	hay fever for 2 weeks prior to exam. (3) Abstaining from smoking for 24 hours prior to exam. b. Plasma or urine samples by:	
	(1) Reporting drugs the patient is currently receiving to the patient's physician and to the laboratory. (Drugs may be withheld as long as 2 weeks prior to the exam.)	(1) Drugs the patient is currently receiving which may influence test results are identified and the proper department notified.
5. Preexisting conditions (See Increases/Decreases)	5. Record preexisting conditions on lab slip.	5. The patient's preexisting conditions are noted on lab slip.
6. Patient knowledge level	6. Explain test to patient: a. Define catecholamines (See Description). b. Explain procedure (See Procedure).	6. The patient demonstrates knowledge of test by defining test and stating procedure.

Patient Preparation Checklist

1. √ Amine-rich foods are omitted from diet as ordered.
2. √ NPO for 10–12 hours, or as ordered, for plasma catecholamines.
3. √ Decrease exercise and stress during 24-hour urine collection.
4. √ Influencing drugs noted and reported (See Drug Influences).
5. √ Preexisting conditions noted on lab slip (See Increases/Decreases).
6. √ Patient knowledge; explain test and procedure (See Description/Procedure).

CONSIDERATIONS FOR NURSING CARE RELATED TO ABNORMAL TEST RESULTS
POSTTEST: Factors related to the results of the test
Nursing Diagnosis: Alterations in biochemical balance

Guide to assessment	Guide to planning and intervention	Guide to evaluation
Assess patient factors influencing test results: 1. Nursing history and/or physical exam suggestive of a. Pheochromocytoma	1. Excessive catecholamine secretion is prevented by: a. Protecting patient from excessive palpation of abdominal mass by staff and students.	a. The patient is protected from increased catecholamine secretion caused by palpation of abdomen.
b. Stress	b. Initiating nursing measures to establish a nonstressful environment for the patient.	b. The patient appears and acts calm and relaxed.
c. Inadequate circulation	c. Initiating nursing measures to promote adequate circulation.	c. The patient demonstrates adequate circulation by color, vital signs, no complaints of pain, level of consciousness.
2. Nursing history and/or physical exam suggestive of a. Hypertension b. Myasthenia gravis c. Hypothyroidism	2. Decrease catecholamine secretion by administering as ordered: a. Antihypertensive agents b. Anticholinesterase c. Thyroid medication	2. The patient receives ordered medication as scheduled.
3. Nursing history and/or physical exam suggestive of a. Malnutrition	3. Increase catecholamine secretion by: a. Initiating nursing measures to improve nutritional status.	3. The patient's catecholamine secretion is increased by: a. Improved nutritional status.
b. Hyperthyroidism	b. Promoting decreased metabolism by giving antithyroid medication as ordered.	b. Administering antithyroid medication.
c. Idiopathic orthostatic hypotension	c. Administering vasoconstrictor drugs as ordered.	c. Administering vasoconstrictor drugs as ordered.

Test:	Cerebral Spinal Fluid
Abbreviation:	CSF

Reference Values: *Pressure*

Newborn	80–110 mm H_2O
Infant/child	200 mm H_2O
Adult	50–180 mm H_2O

Appearance   clear, colorless

Protein

Premature	65–150 mg/dl
Newborn	20–170 mg/dl
Child	5– 40 mg/dl
Adult	15– 45 mg/dl

Glucose

Premature	24– 63 mg/dl
Newborn	34–119 mg/dl
Child	40– 80 mg/dl
Adult	50– 80 mg/dl

CSF glucose usually two-thirds of blood glucose

Cell Count

Premature	0–25
Newborn	0–22
All others	0–5

Specimen: Cerebral spinal fluid

Description: Cerebral spinal fluid (CSF) is produced at the choriod plexus found in the four ventricular cavities of the brain. The brain floats in the CSF and this protects the delicate brain from sudden pressure variations. The fluid removes CSF metabolic waste products and maintains a steady chemical environment for cerebral metabolism. The study of CSF gives valuable information for the diagnosis of central nervous system disorders.

Procedure:

1. Food and fluids may be restricted for approximately 4 hours prior to test.

2. The patient is placed in a side-lying position, grasping knees. The infant and child will need to be held by the nurse. An alternative position is for patient to straddle a chair, or sit on side of bed.

3. The skin is prepared with an antiseptic solution.

4. The subcutaneous spaces may be anesthetized with a local anesthetic.

5. A spinal tap needle is inserted between L3 and L4 and advanced until the needle enters the subarachnoid space.

6. The patient slowly relaxes his legs.

7. An initial CSF pressure is taken.

8. CSF fluid is collected in 3 test tubes and labeled serially.

9. A closing CSF pressure is taken.
10. The needle is removed.
11. A bandage or small dressing is applied.
12. The specimens are taken to the lab immediately.
13. The patient is usually kept flat 4–6 hours.
14. Fluids, as appropriate, are encouraged.

Conditions Related to Increases	Rationale
1. Pressure	1. Increased venous pressure will increase CSF pressure, coughing, crying, moving, congestive heart failure, etc. A high opening pressure may indicate cerebral edema, space-occupying lesion, subarachnoid hemorrhage, inflammation, thrombosis of the venous sinuses.
2. Appearance	2. Normal CSF is clear, colorless, and hypocellular.
a. Turbidity	a. Turbidity indicates cells present.
b. Red	b. Hemoglobin is present due to RBC lysis from traumatic tap or subarachnoid hemorrhage.
c. Yellow	c. Result of bleeding. Color is from bilirubin formation from hemoglobin degradation in the subarachnoid space. Xanthochromia may be seen with excessive CSF protein or in patients with serum bilirubin above 6 mg/dl (126).
d. Brown	d. Found in CSF fluid of patients with subdural and intracerebral hematomas. Color is from oxidation of hemoglobin.
3. Protein	3. CSF protein increases because of altered capillary permeability, decreased absorption, and local gamma globulin formulation (126). An increase in total protein indicates disease. CSF protein electrophoresis is an aid in diagnosing multiple sclerosis. An assay for myelin basic protein is a new test to aid in the diagnosis of demyelinating disease.
4. Glucose	4. Increase in CSF glucose parallels blood glucose levels and is not diagnostic of CNS disease. See Decreases.
5. Cell count	5. Cell counts need to be done within 1

hour of collection or counts will be wrong due to cell lysis. Immediate refrigeration may preserve them for a short period of time.

a. RBC count

a. After subarachnoid hemorrhage or traumatic tap. Greater than 500 RBCs/μl gives cloudy pink color (126).

b. Leukocytes

b. Excessive number of any kind of leukocytes in CSF fluid is called pleocytosis. Bacterial meningitis may cause WBC counts to be as high as 1,000–12,000 cells/μl.

c. CSF differential cell count

c. Lymphocytes are increased in infection, multiple sclerosis, drug abuse, Guillain-Barré syndrome, and other noninfectious CNS diseases. Monocytes are increased in meningeal irritation as in viral meningitis. Neutrophiles are present in bacterial meningitis and are up to 90% of CSF cells. Plasma cells present are nonspecific and occur in a variety of CNS diseases. Malignant cells are present in brain tumors, blood malignancies, and metastatic carcinomas (110).

Conditions Related to Decreases

1. Pressure

Rationale

1. A decreased opening pressure may mean a subarachnoid block above the needle. The jugular vein or veins are compressed for 10 seconds. If pressure does not rise quickly, a subarachnoid block is suspected. This is called the Queckenstedt test.

2. Glucose

2. Decreased CSF glucose is a signal of infection. Glucose utilization by bacteria, leukocytes, or brain tissue is the cause of the decrease.

Related Lab Studies: In diagnosis of meningitis:

CBC
blood cultures
glucose, serum
electrolytes
urinalysis

IMPLICATIONS FOR NURSING CARE
PRETEST: Factors related to the test
Nursing diagnosis: Potential for injury related to changes in biochemical or biological balance

Guide to assessment	Guide to planning and intervention	Guide to evaluation
Assess patient factors that may influence test results: 1. Fluid/food restrictions	1. Restrict food and fluids as ordered. If an emergency spinal tap, fluids will not be withheld.	1. Patient does not experience nausea during spinal tap.
2. Preexisting conditions Age of patient Tentative diagnosis	2. Note pertinent information on lab slip.	2. Patient's lap slip contains complete information.
3. Lack of patient/parent knowledge	3. Explain test to patient/family: a. Define spinal tap (See Description). b. Explain procedure (See Procedure). c. Have patient sign permit.	3. Patient demonstrates knowledge by defining test and stating procedure. Permit is signed.
4. Nursing responsibilities Preparation of patient Positioning of patient Preserving sterile field Labeling serial specimen Monitoring patient during procedure Monitoring patient after procedure Informing lab of test Keeping specimen warm Delivering specimen immediately to lab personnel	4. Initiate nursing measures to protect patient and patient's CSF from harm.	4. Patient tolerates procedure well and specimen arrives at lab safely.

Patient Preparation Checklist

1. √ Food/fluids restricted as ordered.
2. √ Lab slip filled out completely.
3. √ Patient knowledge; explain test to patient. *Have Patient Sign Permit.*
4. √ Nursing responsibilities (See 4 above).

CONSIDERATIONS FOR NURSING CARE RELATED TO ABNORMAL TEST RESULTS

POSTTEST: Factors related to the results of the test

Nursing Diagnosis: Potential for injury related to changes in biochemical or biological balance

Guide to assessment	Guide to planning and intervention	Guide to evaluation
Assess patient factors that may be influencing test results:		
1. Need for postspinal tap follow-up	1. Protect cerebral spinal environment.	1. The patient does not experience complications from spinal tap.
a. Fluid replacement	a. Encourage fluids, as appropriate, for CSF fluid replacement.	
b. Infected tapsite	b. Check spinal puncture site for signs of inflammation.	
c. Central nervous system deterioration	c. Detect negative neurological signs and consult with physician immediately.	
2. Medical diagnosis	2. Implement medical plan of care to treat underlying cause of disease.	2. The patient's CSF returns to normal.

Test:	Chloride
Abbreviation:	Cl
Reference Values:	*Serum*
	Newborn 96–106 mEq/L
	Children 96–105 mEq/L
	Adult 95–105 mEq/L
	Urine
	110–254 mEq/L/24° urine
	Sweat
	10–35 mEq/L
	>60 mmol/L considered diagnostic for cystic fibrosis
Specimen:	Serum, urine, sweat

Description: Chloride is the major anion in the extracellular compartment. The highest distribution of chloride is found in gastric juice and the extracellular fluid. A normal diet supplies the body's need for chloride, and it is completely absorbed through the intestines, with only a small amount lost in the feces. It is excreted through the kidneys and a small amount is lost through perspiration. Like sodium, the reabsorption of chloride by the kidneys is promoted by aldosterone, and excretion is regulated by the concentration of electrolytes. The intake and output of chloride are inseparable from those of sodium. Chloride, along with sodium, helps to maintain extracellular osmotic pressure and regulate water balance. Chloride plays a role in the acid-base balance of the body as chloride competes with bicarbonate for sodium ion combination. Hydrogen ion loss occurs with chloride loss in approximately the same amount. Chloride is also essential for the production of hydrochloric acid by the gastric mucosal cells. Serum and urinary chloride levels are done to determine the body's fluid and electrolyte balance and detect acid-base disturbances. Chloride sweat values are done to confirm the diagnosis of cystic fibrosis. Chloride imbalances generally occur with sodium imbalance.

Procedure: (red top tube)

Serum
1. No food or fluid restrictions.
2. 0.5–3 ml of venous blood is withdrawn from the patient. Capillary blood may be drawn.
3. Observe puncture site for bleeding or evidence of hematoma.

Urine
1. Collection container needs no preservative or refrigeration (34).
2. Collection:
   a. Discard first voided specimen.

b. Begin timing.

c. For the next 24 hours place all voidings into specimen container immediately after voiding.

d. Having patient void just prior to completion of 24 hours and put sample in collection bottle.

3. Record exact start and finish times on lab slip.

4. Send to lab.

Sweat

1. This test should be done by well-trained technicians.

2. Questionable results should be repeated.

3. In infants, the right leg is the area of choice. Otherwise, the flexor surface of the right forearm is used. *The chest is never used* (possibility of electrically induced cardiac arrest).

4. Analysis:

a. The area is cleansed.

b. A gauze pad with a measured amount of pilocarpine solution and a gauze pad saturated with normal saline solution cover the electrodes attached to the skin.

c. The area is given minute electrical charges every few seconds for 5 minutes (iontophoresis).

d. The area is cleansed and dried and a weighed dry gauze pad covered by plastic is applied and left in place 30–40 minutes.

e. The gauze is carefully removed and placed in a weighing bottle.

f. The difference in the weight of the gauze pad placed on the patient after iontophoresis gives the weight (concentration) of sweat chloride.

5. Any complaints of burning by the patient need immediate attention:

a. *Stop* the test.

b. Call technician immediately.

Conditions Related to Increases	Rationale
	Serum
1. Hyperparathyroidism	1. Increased loss of bicarbonate causes chloride to be retained by the kidneys. This is due to the effect of parathormone decreasing the reabsorption of bicarbonate in the renal tubules.
2. Renal tubular acidosis	2. In this disease there is decreased hydrogen ion secretion, increased chloride ion concentration, and increased bicarbonate loss.
3. Primary aldosteronism	3. Excessive amounts of aldosterone cause increased reabsorption of chlo-

4. Exercise, vigorous

5. Cushing's disease

6. Severe dehydration
   Diabetes insipidus

7. Hyperventilation
   Salicylate toxicity
   Fever
   Head trauma

8. Acute renal failure
   Uremia
   Urinary obstruction
   Nephritis
9. Jejunoileal bypass

ride along with sodium.

4. If exercise results in larger losses of water through perspiration than sodium and chloride, serum chloride levels will be elevated.

5. In this disease there is an excess production of ACTH, which causes increased levels of adrenocorticoid hormones that lead to increased sodium and chloride retention.

6. In these conditions ions become concentrated in a decreased extracellular fluid volume (94).

7. Rapid deep breathing associated with these conditions causes a respiratory alkalosis that results in large amounts of base being excreted by the kidneys. There is a corresponding increase in chloride and hydrogen ions (91).

8. Diseased kidneys may no longer be able to regulate chloride ion concentration.

9. The exact causes for chloride levels being elevated are unknown, but this phenomenon has occurred in up to one third of the patients with this surgery (87).

Conditions Related to Decreases

1. Vomiting
   Gastric suctioning
2. Addison's disease

3. Salt-losing renal disorders
   Polycystic kidney disease
   Medullary cystic disease
   Interstitial nephritis
4. Heat Stress

5. Diabetic ketosis

6. Burns

Rationale

1. These conditions cause a loss of gastric juices high in chloride content.
2. Lack of aldosterone causes decreased reabsorption of chloride and sodium by the kidneys.
3. Kidney tubules lose their ability to reabsorb sodium and chloride.

4. Increased loss of chloride in perspiration leads to decreased serum levels especially if fluid replacement is by plain water.
5. Ketonic anions replace chloride in the serum (94).
6. There is a loss of sodium and chloride into edema at the burn site due

7. Extracellular fluid excess
   Edema
   Congestive heart failure
8. Metabolic alkalosis

9. Delayed processing of blood sample

10. COPD

to damaged capillaries.

7. A dilution of electrolytes occurs due to the increased extracellular fluid volume (94).
8. As bicarbonate levels increase, serum chloride levels decrease due to increased excretion of chloride by the kidneys.
9. If blood sample is not processed promptly, false low serum levels may be reported due to the shift of chloride from plasma to red blood cells.
10. In the case of COPD there is a low serum chloride and elevated CO_2. To buffer the increased carbonic acid, bicarbonate ions are retained and chloride ions are excreted.

Conditions Related to Increases

1. Salicylate toxicity

2. Dehydration

3. Salt-losing renal disorders
   Polycystic kidney disease
   Medullary cystic disease
   Interstitial nephritis
4. Addison's disease

Rationale

Urine

1. Increased amounts of chloride are excreted along with the hydrogen ion as the body attempts to lower the blood pH.
2. High sodium and chloride losses occur in the urine as the body tries to reduce the osmolality of the extracellular fluid.
3. The kidneys lose their ability to retain sodium and chloride.

4. The lack of corticosteroids leads to increased urinary losses of chloride and sodium.

Conditions Related to Decreases

1. Excessive perspiration

2. Congestive heart failure

3. Prolonged vomiting
   Gastric suctioning

Rationale

Urine

1. The kidneys conserve chloride due to an increased chloride loss through diaphoresis.
2. Increased aldosterone production causes sodium and chloride to be retained by the kidneys.
3. Kidneys conserve chloride due to the low serum chloride resulting from

4. Hypochloremic metabolic acidosis

loss of gastric fluid high in HCl.

4. Loss of chloride from the body leads to an increase in bicarbonate blood levels to maintain equality of total anions in extracellular fluid. This causes a metabolic alkalosis. As the kidneys excrete the bicarbonate to raise the blood pH, chloride is retained by the kidneys.

Conditions Related to Increases

Rationale

Sweat

1. Cystic fibrosis

1. An inherited disease of the exocrine glands that raises chloride levels in sweat.

2. Premenopausal adult women

2. There is a cyclic fluctuation of sweat electrolytes reaching a peak 5–10 days prior to the onset of menses (11).

Conditions Related to Decreases

Rationale

1. Deficient electrolytes

1. Abnormal sweat results will occur if patient is deficient in electrolytes prior to testing (11).

Drug Influences: The following drugs may cause an increase in test results. The drugs are listed alphabetically by generic name and divided into columns according to the effect of the drug. Examples of trade names are in parentheses.

Serum

Added chloride effect
   ammonium chloride (Triaminicol)
   potassium chloride (Slow-K)
   saline

Salt retention effect
   androgens (Android-F)
   corticosteroids (Celestone)
   diazoxide (Hyperstat)
   estrogens (Premarin)

   guanethidine (Isemlin)
   methyldopa (Aldomet)
   oxyphenbutazone (Oxalid)
   phenylbutazone (Butazolidin)

Nephrotoxic effect
   Methoxyflurane (anesthetic agent)
   Triamterene (Dyrenium)

Urine

Diuretic effect
   ammonium chloride (Triaminicol)
   benzthiazide (Aquapres)
   chlorthalidone (Hygroton)

   hydrochlorothiazide, effect 5 hours post
      oral dose (Esidrix)
   hydroflumethiazide (Diucardin)

cyclothiazide (Anhydron)   metolazone (Diulo)
digitalis (Lanoxin)   spironolactone (Aldactone)
furosemide (Lasix)

The following drugs may cause a decrease in test results:

Serum

Hypochloremic alkalosis
  aldosterone   cortisone (Cortistan)
  bicarbonates   hydrocortisone (Cortef)
  corticotropin (Acthar)   prednisolone (Cordrol)

Diuretic effect with inhibited tubular reabsorption
  ethacrynic acid (Edecrin)   metolazone (Diulo)
  furosemide (Lasix)   polythiazide (Renese)
  hydroflumethiazide (Diucardin) triamterene (Dyrenium)

Hypochloremic acidosis
  acetazolamide (Diamox)

Chloride retention
  corticosteroids (Celestone)
  mafenide (Sulfamylon)

Related Lab Studies: Monitor response to therapy and/or progression of disease and adjust nursing care accordingly.

  electrolytes (sodium, potassium, chloride, CO_2 content)
  osmolality, serum/urine
  aldosterone, renin levels
  salicylate levels
  urinalysis
  arterial blood gases (ABGs)
  blood urea nitrogen (BUN)
  creatinine
  Hct/Hgb

IMPLICATIONS FOR NURSING CARE
PRETEST: Factors related to the test
Nursing Diagnosis: Potential for injury related to changes in biochemical balance

Guide to assessment	Guide to planning and intervention	Guide to evaluation
Assess patient factors that may influence test results:		
1. Comprehensive drug history (See Drug Influences)	1. Report to lab and physician drugs the patient is receiving that may influence lab results.	1. Drugs patient is receiving do not interfere with test results.
2. Preexisting conditions	2. Record preexisting conditions on lab slip.	2. Patient's preexisting conditions noted on lab slip.

Guide to assessment	Guide to planning and intervention	Guide to evaluation
3. Lack of patient knowledge	3. Explain test to patient: a. Define chloride (See Description). b. Explain test procedure (See Procedure).	3. Patient demonstrates knowledge of test by defining test and stating procedure.

Patient Preparation Checklist

1. √ Influencing drugs noted and reported (See Drug Influences).
2. √ Preexisting conditions noted on lab slip (See Increases/Decreases).
3. √ Patient knowledge; explain test and procedure (See Description/Procedure).

CONSIDERATIONS FOR NURSING CARE RELATED TO ABNORMAL TEST RESULTS
POSTTEST: Factors related to the results of the test
Nursing Diagnosis: Alterations in biochemical balance

Guide to assessment	Guide to planning and intervention	Guide to evaluation
Assess patient factors influencing test results:		
1. Increased serum chloride	1. Correct or prevent increased serum chloride (hyperchloremia) by:	1. The patient will demonstrate normal electrolyte balance by:
a. Signs and symptoms: Stupor Rapid, deep breathing Weakness Coma Sodium imbalances Potassium imbalance	a. Detecting and reporting signs/symptoms of hyperchloremia.	a. Showing no evidence of increased chloride.
b. Identify patients with potential for hyperchloremia (See Increases)	b. Recording accurately intake/output.	b. Showing adequate hydration.
c. Heat stress Excessive sweating (water loss)	c. Teaching principles of heat stress by: (1) Identifying sodium and chloride increases. (2) Replenishing water losses as they occur.	c. The patient is able to give return explanation of sodium/chloride/water balance and state methods of replacing water loss.

Guide to assessment	Guide to planning and intervention	Guide to evaluation
	(3) Discouraging strenuous activity that produces excessive sweating during hot days.	
d. Salicylate poisoning	d. Teaching prevention of overdosage with salicylates. (1) Child-proof bottle caps. (2) Proper dosage adjustment. (3) Careful monitoring of salicylate levels during long-term treatment for arthritis.	d. The patient is able to state safety measures related to accidental overdose.
2. Signs and symptoms of decreased serum chloride: Hypertonicity of muscles Tetany Depressed respirations Potassium imbalances Sodium imbalances	2. Correct or prevent further decreased serum chloride (hypochloremia) by:	2. The patient will demonstrate normal electrolyte balance by:
	a. Detecting and reporting signs/symptoms of hypochloremia. b. Recording accurate intake/output.	a. Showing no evidence of hypochloremia. b. Showing adequate hydration.
c. Vomiting	c. Providing nursing measures to reduce vomiting.	c. Diminished vomiting.
d. N/G tube	d. Irrigating N/G tubes with normal saline as ordered.	d. Showing no signs of electrolyte imbalance due to gastric chloride losses.
e. Diaphoresis	e. Instituting measures to prevent excessive diaphoresis. Replace fluid loss with bouillon or fruit juices as appropriate.	e. Replacing sodium/chloride/water losses.
f. Hypochloremia	f. Administer ammonium hydrochloride, L-lysine monohydrochloride or arginine hydrochloride as ordered by physician.	f. The patient's chloride levels are within normal limits.

Test:	Cholesterol
Abbreviation:	None
Reference Values:	*Total cholesterol*

Full-term infant   50–120 mg/dl
1–2 years   70–190 mg/dl
2–16 years   135–250 mg/dl
Adult   120–330 mg/dl

HDL-cholesterol
F   Mean 55 mg/dl
M   Mean 45 mg/dl

LDL-cholesterol
F   Mean 131.1 mg/dl
M   Mean 135.5 mg/dl
Values vary with laboratory

Specimen: Serum or plasma

Description: The body lipid cholesterol is a steroid alcohol compound. It is formed chiefly in the reticulum cells of the liver. It is discharged from the liver into the blood and bile. Cholesterol is a precursor for many steroid hormones. Cholesterol is also utilized by the body to form bile acids and is part of all cell membranes. About 500 mg of cholesterol is excreted in the feces daily (7). Cholesterol is transported in the blood by attaching to blood proteins. These cholesterol-containing proteins also have other lipids attached and are called lipoproteins. The lipoproteins are classified into four major groups. The classifications are:

Lipoprotein	*Abbreviation*	*Major Lipid*
1. High density lipoprotein	HDL	Cholesterol
2. Low density lipoprotein	LDL	Cholesterol
3. Very low density lipoprotein	VLDL	Triglyceride
4. Chylomicrons		Triglyceride

In identifying patients at risk for coronary artery disease (CAD), measurements of HDL-cholesterol and total serum cholesterol are beneficial.

Serum cholesterol levels are measured to evaluate the risk of coronary artery disease and as a tool in evaluating nephrotic syndrome, hepatic disease, and thyroid function.

Procedure: 1. The patient should restrict food and fluids for 12–14 hours before the test.
2. The patient should eat a normal diet for 2 days prior to the test and should abstain from alcohol for 24 hours prior to testing.

3. Approximately 10 ml of blood is withdrawn from the patient.

4. Observe puncture site for signs of bleeding or evidence of hematoma.

Conditions Related to Increases

1. Coronary artery disease

Rationale

1. ↑ LDL-cholesterol
   ↓ HDL-cholesterol
   ↑ Triglycerides
   LDL are cholesterol-rich and are absorbed into the smooth muscle cell of the arterial wall. (See 1 Decreases). Excess weight and high saturated fat diets increase LDL-cholesterol.

2. Nephrotic syndrome

2. Because of large protein losses, the liver compensates by increasing synthesis of all plasma proteins, including lipoproteins. The increase is because the lipoproteins are not excreted but accumulate in the blood (7).

3. Starvation
   Diabetes mellitus, poorly controlled

3. If insufficient carbohydrates are available, lipids are mobilized from body stores and increase in the bloodstream as they are carried to the liver (7).

4. Biliary tract obstruction

4. Cholesterol is part of the makeup of bile. With increased bile in the blood, cholesterol levels are also increased.

5. Hypothyroidism

5. Tissue utilization and storage and excretion of cholesterol are decreased in hypothyroidism (7).

6. Excessive lipoprotein levels

6. Certain hereditary disorders have been identified that result from a defect in catabolism of lipids called sphingolipids. The result is an accumulation of lipids in various body organs and the CNS (11).

Conditions Related to Decreases

1. Low risk coronary artery disease

Rationale

1. ↓ LDL-cholesterol
   ↑ HDL-cholesterol
   Normal Triglyceride
   The transporation of cholesterol from body cells to the liver is by HDL transport. The liver either utilizes the cholesterol or excretes it unchanged. This lowers serum cholesterol and protects the body against the devel-

opment of ischemic heart disease. Strenuous exercise, diet low in saturated fats, and about 6 oz. of alcohol a week work to increase HDL-cholesterol and decrease LDL-cholesterol.

2. Malnutrition
   Malabsorption

2. Dietary protein may be insufficient to synthesize lipoproteins, and caloric intake may be high enough to discourage mobilization of lipid stores.

3. Liver disease
   Cirrhosis

3. The damaged liver cells may be unable to synthesize cholesterol.

4. Hyperthyroidism

4. The increased utilization of fat because of the high metabolic rate is the reason why cholesterol levels are decreased in this condition.

Drug Influences: The following drugs may influence test results. The drugs are listed alphabetically by generic name and divided into columns according to the effect of the drug. Examples of trade names are in parentheses.

The following drugs may cause an increase in test results:

Cholestatic Effect
acetohexamide (Dymelor)
acetophenazine (Tindal)
anabolic steroids
chlorpromazine (Thorazine)
gold (Solganal)
meprobamate (Miltown)
methandrostenolone (Dianabol)
methimazole (Tapazole)
methyltestosterone (Virilon)
oxymetholone (Adroyd)
prochlorperazine (Compazine)
promazine (Sparine)
sulfonamides
testosterone (Android-T)
thiabendazole (Mintezol)

Effect of Prolonged Hormone Action
corticosteroids (Celestone)
corticotropin, after initial fall (Acthar)
cortisone (Cortistan)

Hepatotoxic Effect
arsenicals
diphenylhydantoin (Dilantin)
paramethadione (Paradione)

The following drugs may cause a decrease in test results:

Hepatotoxic Effect
allopurinol (Lopurin)
antimony compounds
asparaginase (Elspar)
chloroform
chlortetracycline (Aureomycin)
colchicine (Colchicine)
erythromycin (Ilosone)
isoniazid (Laniazid)
lincomycin (Lincocin)
MAO inhibitors (Eutonyl)
tetracycline (Achromycin)

Therapeutic Intent
androsterone
cholestyramine (Questran)
clofibrate (Atromid-S)
colestipol (Colestid)
dextrothyroxine (Choloxin)

estrogens (Premarin)
insulin
niacin (Nicotinex)
nicotinyl alcohol (Roniacol)

Inhibition of Hepatic Synthesis
chlorpropamide (Diabinese)
clomiphene (Clomid)

haloperidol (Haldol)
tolbutamide (Orinase)

Miscellaneous
aminosalicylic acid
triiodothyronine (Thyrolar)

Related Lab Studies: In diagnosis of coronary artery disease:

HDL-cholesterol fraction
LDL-cholesterol fraction
triglycerides
*lipoprotein electrophoresis
*lipoprotein phenotype

IMPLICATIONS FOR NURSING CARE
PRETEST: Factors related to the test
Nursing Diagnosis: Potential for injury related to changes in biochemical balance

Guide to assessment	Guide to planning and intervention	Guide to evaluation
Assess patient factors that may influence test results:		
1. Food and fluid restrictions Alcohol restrictions	1. Restrict food and fluid, except water, for 12–14 hours prior to test. The patient should eat a normal diet for 2 days prior to test. Instruct patient to abstain from alcohol for 24 hours prior to test.	1. Patient's lab values are not falsely elevated due to recent ingestion of food or alcohol.
2. Comprehensive drug history	2. Identify drugs that may interfere with test values. Consult with physician. Note interfering drugs on lab slip.	2. Patient's lab values are not influenced by medication.

3. Preexisting conditions (See Increases/Decreases)
   Age
   Sex
	3. Identify preexisting conditions that may influence test results. Note on lab slip.	3. Patient's preexisting conditions do not influence test values.

4. Knowledge deficit	4. Explain test to patient: a. Define test (See Definition).	4. The patient demonstrates knowledge by defining test and stating procedure.

*Not discussed in this book.

Guide to assessment	Guide to planning and intervention	Guide to evaluation
	b. Explain procedure (See Procedure).	
5. Preventive health teaching	5. Increase public awareness of LDL-cholesterol and triglyceride levels to coronary artery disease: a. Encourage low saturated fat diet. b. Encourage personal daily exercise program. c. Discourage smoking. d. Discourage high alcohol intake. e. Encourage slow weight loss program.	5. Local statistics show deaths due to preventable heart disease decrease.

Patient Preparation Checklist

1. √ Food and fluids, except water, restricted 12–14 hours.
2. √ Interfering drugs noted on lab slip (See Drug Influences).
3. √ Preexisting conditions, age, and sex noted on lab slip.
4. √ Patient knowledge; explain test to patient.
5. √ Preventive health teaching (See 5 above).

CONSIDERATIONS FOR NURSING CARE RELATED TO ABNORMAL TEST RESULTS
POSTTEST: Factors related to the results of the test
Nursing Diagnosis: Alterations in biochemical balance

Guide to assessment	Guide to planning and intervention	Guide to evaluation
Assess patient factors that may be influencing test results. Nursing history and/or physical exam that is suggestive of: 1. Positive history for coronary artery disease C/o chest pain Cigarette smoking Hypertension High saturated fat diet Obesity	1. Be alert to risk factors in the patient's history.	1. Patient's factors are recognized.

Guide to assessment	Guide to planning and intervention	Guide to evaluation
Hypothyroidism Family history of heart disease Dizziness or fainting		
2. Coronary artery disease ↑ LDL-cholesterol ↓ HDL-cholesterol ↑ Triglycerides Dyspnea Fatigue Palpitations Chest pain Syncope Edema Hepatomegaly Heart murmurs	2. Recognize symptoms of coronary artery disease.	2. Patient's symptoms are recognized.
3. Need for health teaching	3. Promote the decrease of LDL-cholesterol and triglycerides by: a. Teaching patient negative correlation between LDL and heart disease. b. Teaching patient the positive correlation between HDL and decreased risk of heart disease. c. Arranging consultation with dietician for HDL foods and slow weight loss program, as appropriate. d. Exploring with patient ways of developing a personal daily exercise program. Impressing upon patient the need for such a program. e. Emphasizing that no smoking and low alcohol consumption may help to decrease LDL and increase HDL.	3. The patient's LDL-cholesterol and triglyceride levels decrease and HDL-cholesterol increases.

Test:	Clotting Time, Lee-White Coagulation Time, Coagulation Time
Abbreviation:	None
Reference Values:	Clotting time 5–15 minutes
Specimen:	Whole blood
Description:	This is a nonspecific test of blood coagulation. It consists of placing blood in 3 plain glass tubes and tilting the blood gently every 30 minutes. The time it takes for the blood to form a solid clot is the clotting time. This test has generally been replaced by the activated partial prothrombin time (APTT) because the clotting time may not pick up problems of mild to moderate severity. The test may be used to monitor heparin therapy or to evaluate the intrinsic pathway of blood coagulation.

Drug Influences: The following drugs may influence test results. The drugs are listed alphabetically by generic name and divided into columns according to the effect of the drug. Examples of trade names are in parentheses.

The following drugs may cause an increase in test results:

Miscellaneous
   aspirin
   carbenicillin (Geocillin)
   dicumarol (Dicumarol)
   heparin (Panheprin); dose-related
   mithramycin (Mithracin); reversible effect
   phosphorus (thiacide tablets)
   tetracycline (Achromycin)
   warfarin (Coumadin)

The following drugs may cause a decrease in test results:

Miscellaneous
   aminophylline (Mudrane)
   epinephrine (Adrenalin Chloride); increased factor V activity
   oral contraceptives

Refer to APTT (Partial Thromboplastin Time, Activated) for more information.

Test: Cold Agglutinins

Abbreviation: None

Reference Value: Less than 1:16

Specimen: Serum

Description: In response to respiratory infection by Mycoplasma pneumoniae, the body usually develops an antibody that is tested on
acute and convalescent sera. These antibodies demonstrate activity by agglutination temperatures below 37° C and are called
cold agglutinins. Blood is drawn during the acute stage of disease
and again in 4 weeks; if there is a fourfold rise in titer, as well
as positive clinical findings, the diagnosis of M. pneumoniae
pneumonia is made. Cold agglutinins disappear after several
weeks.

Cold agglutination can be reversed upon warming. The cold
agglutination activity can take place in distal portions of the body
upon exposure to cold temperatures and this results in hemolytic
anemia or occlusion of microcirculation causing Raynaud's phenomenon.

Procedure: (Prewarmed red top tube)
1. No food or fluid restrictions.
2. Up to 5 ml of blood is drawn from the patient. Capillary blood
can be used.
3. *Do Not Refrigerate:* Send to the laboratory immediately.
4. Observe puncture site for bleeding or evidence of hematoma.

Conditions Related to Increases	Rationale
1. Mycoplasma pneumoniae pneumonia	1. During acute illness, titers may be above 1:32.
2. Infection other than M. pneumoniae Conditions such as Cirrhosis Hemolytic anemia Pregnancy Aged Healthy individual	2. Slight elevations may occur above 1:16.
3. Prelymphoma idiopathic cold agglutinin disease	3. Extremely high titers of 1:1,000–1:1,000,000 are seen occasionally. These patients may develop hemolytic anemia with occlusion of the microcirculation.
4. Waldenström's macroglobulinemia	4. Described as related to the increased plasma immunoglobulin manifestation of this disease.

Conditions Related to Decreases

1. Antibiotic therapy

Rationale

1. Cold agglutinins may not develop.

Drug Influences: See number 1, Decreases above.

Related Lab Studies: In diagnosis of Mycoplasma pneumoniae pneumonia:

CBC
urinalysis
Coombs', indirect

IMPLICATIONS FOR NURSING CARE
PRETEST: Factors related to the test
Nursing Diagnosis: Potential for injury related to changes in biochemical environment

Guide to assessment	Guide to planning and intervention	Guide to evaluation
Assess patient factors that may influence test results.		
1. Antibiotic therapy	1. Note on lab slip if patient is receiving antibiotic therapy.	1. Patient's antibiotic therapy noted on lab slip.
2. Knowledge deficit	2. Explain test to patient: a. Define test (See Description). b. Explain procedure (See Procedure).	2. Patient demonstrates knowledge by defining test and stating procedure.
3. Hemolysis	3. Prevent hemolysis by: a. Not probing venipuncture site or leaving tourniquet on too long. b. Not withdrawing blood forcefully. c. Not withdrawing blood too slowly. d. Not handling specimen roughly. e. Not saturating skin with anesthetic.	3. Patient's blood does not hemolyze.

Patient Preparation Checklist

1. √ If on antibiotics, it is noted on lab slip.
2. √ Patient knowledge; explain test (See Description/Procedure).

CONSIDERATIONS FOR NURSING CARE RELATED TO ABNORMAL TEST RESULTS
POSTTEST: Factors related to the results of the test
Nursing Diagnosis: Alterations in biochemical environment

Guide to assessment	Guide to planning and intervention	Guide to evaluation
Assess patient factors that may be influencing test results. Nursing history and/or physical exam suggestive of: 1. Intravascular symptoms Pallor Numbness Jaundice Purpura Painful, swollen extremities Cramping, fingers and toes Acrocyanosis Urinalysis shows hemoglobinuria	1. Prevent intravascular agglutination by: a. Keeping patient warm. b. Recognizing signs and symptoms. c. Administering antibiotics as prescribed.	1. The patient does not experience intravascular agglutination.

Test:	Complete blood count
Abbreviation:	CBC

Reference Values:

	Hematocrit (Hct)	Hemoglobin (Hgb)
Newborn	57–68%	17–21 g/dl
1 week	46–62%	15–20 g
1 month	31–41%	11–14 g
3–5 months	30–36%	10–12 g
1 year	29–41%	11–13 g
2–10 years	36–41%	11–13 g
Adult		
Male	40–54%	14–18 g
Female	37–47%	12–16 g

Red blood cell count (RBCs)

Newborn	4.4–5.8 million/µl
2 months	3 –3.8 million/µl
Children	4.6–4.8 million/µl
Adults	
Male	4.5–6.2 million/µl
Female	4.2–5.4 million/µl

White blood cell count and differential (WBC ≤ diff.)

Newborn	7,000–35,000
1 week	4,000–20,000
1 month	6,000–18,000
3–5 months	6,000–17,000
6–11 months	6,000–16,000
1 year	6,000–15,000
2–10 years	7,000–13,000
11–15 years	5,000–12,000
Adult	4,300–10,000
Neutrophiles	55–70%
Lymphocytes	20–40%
Monocytes	2– 8%
Eosinophiles	2– 4%
Basophiles	0.5–1%

Values vary with laboratory.

Specimen:	Whole blood

Description:	The complete blood count is a collective overview of the peripheral blood. The test provides a great deal of information about the hematologic system as well as other organ systems. The CBC consists of hemoglobin and hematocrit measurements, red blood and white blood counts, as well as study of the cell types, forms, and structures. The test is ordered as a screening test. It is usually performed on every patient admitted to the hospital.

Refer to individual tests for more information about:

Increases
Decreases
Drug Influences
Related Lab Studies
Pretest Implications
Posttest Considerations

Test:	Direct Coombs' Test or Direct Antiglobulin Test; Indirect Coombs' Test or Indirect Antiglobulin Test; Coombs' Test
Abbreviation:	Direct Coombs', DAGT Indirect Coombs', IAGT
Reference Values:	Negative—both tests.
Specimen:	Whole blood
Description:	The Coombs' test, or antiglobulin test, gives valuable information concerning immunohemolytic conditions. As red blood cells become sensitized, they are coated with immunoglobulins. By adding antihuman globulin antibodies to patient red blood cells, abnormal antibodies cause the patient RBCs to agglutinate. The direct antiglobulin test (DAGT) concerns the testing directly to the patient's blood. The antihuman serum antibody (Coombs' serum) is mixed with washed patient red cells; if agglutination takes place it is known that abnormal antibodies are on the cells and the test is positive. The indirect antiglobulin test (IAGT) can indirectly identify certain antibodies. This is accomplished by mixing serum with known antigens and allowing the specimen to incubate so suspected immunoglobulins can coat the cells. Then Coombs' serum is added, and if the cells agglutinate the test is positive. These tests are ordered to identify hemolytic processes (blood transfusion reaction, hemolytic disease of the newborn) and as part of the blood screening prior to transfusion.
Procedure:	(red top tube) 1. No food or fluid restrictions. 2. 10 ml of blood is drawn from the patient. Cord blood is used in the newborn. 3. Observe puncture site for bleeding or evidence of hematoma.

Conditions Related to Positive Reactions	Rationale
	Direct
1. Hemolytic disease of the newborn	1. Test performed on neonatal cord blood. If the test is positive, maternal antibodies are present.
2. Acquired autoimmune hemolytic anemia	2. A drug, chemical, or other substance acts as the antigen. Antibodies to the antigen attach to the RBC and ultimately destroy it. Because of the antibodies' presence, the Coombs' test is positive.

Drug Influences: The following drugs may influence test results. The drugs are listed alphabetically by generic name and divided into columns according to the effect of the drug. Examples of trade names are in parentheses.

The following drugs may cause an increase in test results:

Immunological response
  aminopyrine
  cephaloridine (Loridine)
  cephalothin (Keflin sodium)
  chlorpromazine (Thorazine)
  chlorpropamide (Diabinese)
  diphenylhydantoin (Dilantin)
  isoniazid (Laniazid)
  melphalan (Alkeran)
  methyldopa
  penicillin
  phenacetin
  phenylbutazone (Butazolidin)
  quinidine (Duraquin)
  quinine (Quinamm)
  sulfonamides

Immune hemolytic anemia
  sulfonylureas (Orinase)

Miscellaneous (mechanism obscure)
  ethosuximide (Zarontin)
  hydralazine (Apresazide)
  procainamide (Procan S.R.)
  streptomycin
  tetracycline (Achromycin)

The following drug may cause a decrease in test results:

Miscellaneous
  Salicylazosulfapyridine (Azulfidine)

Related Lab Studies: In hemolytic disease of the newborn:

Cord blood for
  Rh typing
  ABO typing
  direct Coombs'
  RBC and morphology
  RBC indices
  glucose
  bilirubin, total and direct

IMPLICATIONS FOR NURSING CARE
PRETEST: Factors related to the test
Nursing Diagnosis: Potential for injury related to changes in biochemical balance

Guide to assessment	Guide to planning and intervention	Guide to evaluation
Assess patient factors that may influence test results.		
1. Comprehensive drug history (See Drug Influences)	1. Identify drugs that may influence test results. Note	1. Patient's medications do not influence patient values.

Guide to assessment	Guide to planning and intervention	Guide to evaluation
Blood products	them on lab slip.	
2. Diagnosis	2. Inform lab of preexisting	2. Patient's pertinent preexist-
Transfusion history	conditions by noting pertinent	ing conditions are noted on
Pregnancy	information on lab slip.	lab slip.
Cord blood		
3. Knowledge deficit	3. Explain test to patient:	3. Patient (parent) demon-
	a. Define Coomb's test.	strates knowledge by defining
	b. Explain procedure.	test and stating procedure.

Patient Preparation Checklist

1. √ Interfering medications and note on lab slip.
2. √ Pertinent information on lab slip. See 2 above.
3. √ Patient knowledge; explain tests to patient.

Test:	Cortisol, ACTH stimulation test, dexamethasone suppression test
Abbreviation:	DST (for dexamethasone suppression test)
Reference Values:*	*Cortisol* 7 A.M.–9 P.M. 5–25 µg/dl 4 P.M.–6 P.M. 2–13 µg/dl *Dexamethasone suppression test* Less than 5 µg/dl any sample *ACTH stimulation test* More than 18 µg/dl or 2–3 × baseline value
Specimen:	Plasma
Description:	As the end product in the glucocorticoid pathway, cortisol is the most important glucorticoid. Cortisol is secreted by the adrenal cortex in response to the influences of adrenocorticotrophic hormone (ACTH), stress, and a diurnal rhythm. The main functions of glucocorticoids are in the metabolism of carbohydrates and proteins, the regulation of the immune system and in the adaptive response mechanism to stress. Cortisol is conjugated in the liver and excreted in the urine. About 5% of cortisol is excreted unchanged in the urine. Cortisol levels are measured to evaluate pituitary-adrenal activity or adrenal-cortical functioning. There are a variety of tests to measure cortisol levels. To measure increased cortisol activity, the dexamethasone suppression test is done; to measure decreased cortisol activity, the ACTH stimulation test is given. Cortisol levels without steroids are done for baseline values.
Procedure:	(green top tube) *Plasma Cortisol or Dexamethasone Suppression Test (DST)* 1. Normal diet for 3 days prior to test. 2. For the DST the patient is given a dose(s) of dexamethasone the day before the test. 3. The patient should engage in only mild physical activity the day before the test. 4. The patient is NPO 10–12 hours prior to the early morning blood drawing. 5. Blood is drawn between 6 A.M. and 9 A.M. before the patient gets out of bed and prior to breakfast. 6. 0.5 ml–5 ml of blood is drawn from the patient. 7. Blood is drawn about 4 P.M. 8. Observe puncture site for bleeding or evidence of hematoma. 9. It is imperative to follow local institutional guidelines for this test.

*Values are adult values within 1 week of life. There is no sex variation.

ACTH Stimulation Test
1. The patient is NPO 10–12 hours prior to the test.
2. The patient should engage in only mild physical activity for 1 day prior to the test.
3. Baseline blood specimen is drawn at peak ACTH secretion level between 6 A.M. and 8 A.M., before the patient is up or has eaten breakfast.
4. The patient is given Cortrosyn, an ACTH analogue (IM or IV).
5. At specified intervals, usually 30 minutes and 60 minutes, blood samples are drawn from the patient.
6. Observe puncture site for bleeding or evidence of hematoma.
7. It is imperative to follow local institutional guidelines for this test.

Conditions Related to Increases   Rationale

Normally, the limbic-hypothalamic-pituitary-adrenal axis uses a negative feedback system in the secretion of cortisol. The hypothalamus and emotion regulating limbic system stimulate the adrenal glands to release cortisol. Cortisol release inhibits further production of ACTH.

Hypothalamus/limbic system → pituitary stimulation → ACTH release → adrenal gland release of cortisol → ACTH inhibition → cortisol inhibition.

1. Melancholia

1. The DST evaluates the response of pituitary adrenal inhibition. In patients with melancholia, there is a lack of pituitary-adrenal inhibition, that is, there is resistance to suppression of plasma cortisol. After dexamethasone is given, if any blood sample has a value of more than 5 μg/dl the patient is considered a nonsuppressor and, along with clinical evaluation, may be diagnosed as positive for melancholia. The normal response to dexamethasone is cortisol suppression for 24 hours. See 6 Increases for medical exclusion list for DST.

2. Cushing's disease

2. In this disease there is a hypothalamic disorder that allows an increased rate of corticotropin-releasing factor (CRF) release that stimulates ACTH release and subsequently increases plasma cortisol levels. The DST in this disease is a useful technique in the differential diagnosis of hypothalamic disorders versus adrenal tumor. Dexamethasone dosage is higher in testing for this disease.

3. Cushing's syndrome

3. Cushing's syndrome, or hypercortisolemia, is caused by an adrenal tumor. Because of the tumor, the cortisol secretion is mostly ACTH-independent and there is no dexamethasone suppression.

4. Stress
   Hospitalization
   Surgery
   Fever
   Hypoglycemia
   Examinations
   Difficult blood drawing episode (especially pediatrics)
   Anesthesia
   Activity, etc.

4. The transient, moderate increases are part of the adaptive response mechanism to stress.

5. Diurnal rhythm

5. There is a circadian pattern to ACTH release and thus cortisol release. Plasma cortisol levels are highest in the early morning (between 6 A.M. and 8 A.M.) and at the lowest level between 9 P.M. and 4 A.M. This rhythm is true for people with normal sleep-wake patterns. People with prolonged changes in sleep patterns may have a different rhythm.

6. *Medical exclusion list for DST:
   Major physical illness
   Trauma, fever, nausea, dehydration
   Temporal lobe disease
   Pregnancy
   High dose estrogen therapy
   Cushing's disease
   Unstable diabetes
   Malnutrition
   Anorexia nervosa
   Heavy alcohol use
   Alcohol withdrawal
   Electroconvulsive therapy
   Other endocrine diseases are questionable

6. All these conditions interfere with the hypothalamic-pituitary-adrenal axis in some way and so are apt to cause false positive results.

Conditions Related to Decreases

Rationale

1. Adrenocorticoid insufficiency
   Addison's disease

1. This is a condition in which there is primary adrenal-cortical insufficiency. The cause may be from an autoim-

---

*Taken from James C. Ritchie and Bernard J. Carroll, "A New Test to Identify Depression," *Lab World*, September 1981.

mune reaction, adrenocortical destruction, or it may be idiopathic. The adrenal gland does not respond to ACTH stimulation and cortisol is not released. The ACTH stimulation test is the test used to demonstrate this problem. The normal response is for the post-Cortrosyn values to be 2–3 times the baseline value. See Procedure. This disease may cause a false negative DST.

2. Anterior pituitary hypofunction
   Hypophysectomy
   Postpartum pituitary necrosis
   Space-occupying tumors
   Starvation
   Severe anemia

2. The decreased cortisol levels are due to the failure of the pituitary gland to produce adequate amounts of ACTH either because of gland removal, destruction, obliteration due to tumor, or an inadequately nourished gland. This kind of hypocortisolism is called secondary adrenal insufficiency. This condition may cause a false negative DST.

3. Congenital adrenal enzyme disorders
   (Congenital adrenal hyperplasia)

3. There are five enzymes involved in the synthesis of cortisol. A deficiency in any one of these enzymes results in diminished synthesis of the glucocorticoid.

4. Iatrogenic adrenal insufficiency

4. After high dose prolonged treatment with steroids there may be adrenal suppression. Tapering steroids and testing for adrenal recovery is a way of monitoring this problem.

Drug Influences: The following drugs may influence test results. The drugs are listed alphabetically by generic name and divided into columns according to the effect of the drug. Examples of trade names are in parentheses.

The following drugs may cause an increase in test results:

Plasma

Therapeutic intent
   corticotropin (Acthar)

Hormonal action
   cortisone (Cortistan)   hydrocortisone (Cortef)
   estrogens (Premarin)   oral contraceptives

Miscellaneous
   ethanol (grain alcohol)   methadone (Dolophine HCL)
   lithium (Lithonate-S)   tetracosactrin

Urine

Effect of therapy
  corticotropin (Acthar)

Hormonal effect
  oral contraceptives

The following drugs may cause a decrease in test results:

Plasma

Diminished ACTH secretion
  levodopa (Bendopa)

Miscellaneous
  androgens
  barbiturates
  dexamethasone (Decadron)
  diphenylhydantoin (Dilantin)
  glucose; when serum glucose is increased

Urine

Altered cortisol secretion
  hydrochlorothiazide (Esidrix)
  DST

The following drugs may cause a false positive test result:

Increased hepatic clearance
  barbiturates
  carbamazepine (Tegretol)
  glutethimide (Doriden)
  meprobamate (Equanil, Miltown)
  methaqualone (Quaalude)
  methyprylon (Noludar)
  phenytoin (Dilantin)
  reserpine; questionable

Measured as cortisol
  synthetic steroid therapy; chronic, high doses

The following drugs may cause false negative results:

Inhibition of production of corticotrophin-releasing factor
  benzodiazepines; high doses (Valium)
  cyproheptadine

Hypothalmic-Pituitary-Adrenal Axis Suppression
  synthetic steroid therapy; chronic, high doses

Related Lab Studies: In the diagnosis of Cushing's syndrome or disease:
  Urinalysis
  17-KS
  17-OHCS
  ACTH stimulation test
  dexamethasone suppression test
  *metyrapone test
  electrolytes, serum/urine (Na, K, Cl, CO_2 content)
  glucose tolerance test
  CBC

---

*Not discussed in this book.

IMPLICATIONS FOR NURSING CARE
PRETEST: Factors related to the test
Nursing Diagnosis: Potential for injury related to changes in biochemical balance

Guide to assessment	Guide to planning and intervention	Guide to evaluation
Assess patient factors that may influence test results.		
1. NPO 10–12 hours	1. Prevent increased glucocorticoid activity by: a. Maintaining patient NPO 10–12 hours. b. Allowing patient water to drink.	1. The patient's test values are not influenced by increased glucocorticoid activity due to metabolism of carbohydrates and proteins.
2. Comprehensive drug history (See Drug Influences)	2. Withhold interfering drugs for 2 weeks as prescribed. Note any interfering drugs on lab slip.	2. Patient's test values are not influenced by unnecessary medication.
3. Preexisting conditions (See Increases, especially 6; See Decreases also)	3. Consult with physician about interfering conditions. Note them on lab slip.	3. Patient's test values are not influenced by preexisting interfering conditions.
4. Lack of patient knowledge	4. Explain test to patient: a. Define cortisol (See Description). b. Explain procedure (See Procedure).	4. The patient is able to define test and explain procedure.
5. Possibility of staff error Wrong test Incorrect procedure	5. Prevent test error by: a. Being informed of which test is to be performed. b. Following institutional guidelines carefully.	5. Patient's results are not influenced by staff error.

CONSIDERATIONS FOR NURSING CARE RELATED TO ABNORMAL TEST RESULTS
POSTTEST: Factors related to the results of the test
Nursing Diagnosis: Alterations in biochemical balance

Guide to assessment	Guide to planning and intervention	Guide to evaluation
Assess patient factors that may be influencing test results. Nursing history and/or physical exam suggestive of:		
1. Melancholia Plasma cortisol, ↑ 5 µg/dl Some symptoms of depression: Depressed mood	1. Encourage cortisol inhibition by: a. Giving prescribed somatic medication. b. Encouraging the patient to take the prescribed medi-	1. The patient's DST converts to normal.

Guide to assessment	Guide to planning and intervention	Guide to evaluation
Weight loss/gain Decreased appetite Insomnia Agitation/retardation Lack of pleasure Fatigue Worthlessness Guilt Difficulty concentrating Thoughts of suicide	cations. c. Assisting with DST monitoring for continued therapy. d. Discussing with the patient reasons for testing and medication.	
2. Cushing's disease	2. Promote cortisol suppression by:	2. The patient achieves normal cortisol levels through successful management of cause of disease.
a. Anterior pituitary tumor	a. Supporting patient through *all* of radiation treatments.	
b. Need for hypophysectomy	b. Initiating nursing measures to prepare patient for surgery.	
c. Replacement of hormonal therapy posthypophysectomy or irradiation d. Hormonal replacement Patient education	c. Administering pituitary-dependent hormones as prescribed. d. Teaching patient need to continue hormone replacement.	
e. Hypothalamic disorder Plasma cortisol ↓ 24-hour urine collections 17-OHCS 17-KS DST	e. Administering high dose dexamethasone as prescribed and assist with cortisol level monitoring as necessary.	
3. Cushing's syndrome Adrenal tumor	3. Encourage control of cortisol secretion by: a. Initiating nursing measures to prepare patient for adrenalectomy and specifically: (1) Protect patient from infection; recognize only mild symptoms may be representative of serious infection. (2) Attempt to keep stress to a minimum.	3. The patient's cortisol levels are normal: (1) The patient is protected from infection due to glucocorticoid suppression of immune system and inflammatory reactions.

Guide to assessment	Guide to planning and intervention	Guide to evaluation
	(3) Understand emotional lability and inform patient of positive physical changes after adrenalectomy. (4) Administer preop cortisol preparation as prescribed. b. Administering cortisol replacement postoperatively. c. Teaching patient about cortisol replacement.	
4. Addison's disease	4. Maintain adequate cortisol levels: a. Administer cortisol. Recognize signs of excessive long-term cortisol therapy (Cushinoid signs). b. Attempt to maintain stress-free environment: (1) Consistency of care givers. (2) Protect from infection. (3) Consult with physician about any signs of infection, high-stress situations, etc. (4) Be responsive to patient. c. Plan with patient self-medication with glucocorticoids. Include: (1) Route. (2) Dosage. (3) Action of drug. (4) Signs of overdosage and underdosage. (5) When to call physician for dosage readjustment, e.g., illness, emotional stress, minor surgery. (6) Patient should wear medical alert bracelet.	4. The patient's cortisol level is normal.
5. Acute adrenal insufficiency Severe	5. Initiate nursing measures to correct acute adrenal insufficiency:	5. The patient's severe glucocorticoid deficiency is corrected as evidenced by

Guide to assessment	Guide to planning and intervention	Guide to evaluation
hypotension Hyperkalemia Vascular collapse	a. Administering fluids: (1) Strict I&O, hourly. (2) Hourly infusion check. (3) Plasma as ordered. c. Take vital signs to monitor hypotension. d. Protect the patient from additional stress. (See 4b above.)	cortisol levels and clinical evaluation:
e. Glucocorticoid excess/ overhydration Generalized edema Hypertension Paralysis, flaccid Hypokalemia Psychoses Loss of consciousness	e. Detect signs of overdosage with glucocorticoids and IV fluids.	e. The patient does not demonstrate signs of overhydration/glucocorticoid excess.
6. Congenital adrenal hyperplasia Signs/Symptoms In 21-hydroxylase deficiency Dehydration Shock Pernicious vomiting ↓ sodium, serum ↑ k⁺, serum In 11-beta-hydroxylase and 21 hydroxylase deficiency, virilization of female genitalia	6. Replace insufficient cortisol: a. Instruct family in use of medication and technique needed. b. Teach family about disease and what can be done for treatment. c. Refer for follow-up to community health nurse.	

Test:	C-Reactive Protein
Abbreviation:	CRP
Reference Values:	Negative
Specimen:	Serum

Description

C-reactive protein is an abnormal globulin that rapidly appears in the serum as a response to a variety of inflammatory stimuli (5, 8, 11, 21). It is called an acute phase reactant because it is one of the protein responses that occur in association with an inflammatory stimulus. The C-reactive protein is so named because it forms a precipitate with the somatic C carbohydrate of pneumococci (21, 30, 33). The amount of precipitation determines the degree of inflammation. The reason for measurement is as a diagnostic tool in the workup of rheumatic fever and as an indicator in following the course of the disease. It also is used as an early indicator of inflammation. The absence of CRP rules out rheumatic activity (21).

Procedure:

(red top tube)
1–3 ml of venous blood is drawn from the patient.

Conditions Related to Increases	**Rationale**
1. Acute myocardial infarction	1. CRP appears in serum within 24–48 hours of acute episode. CRP begins to fall in about 72 hours and becomes negative in 1–2 weeks (9). Production is stimulated by products of injured tissue.
2. Bacterial/viral diseases	2. Production is stimulated by bacterial infections and various pyrogenic agents (21).
3. Gangrene	3. CRP appears and disappears within serum before the erythrocyte sedimentation rate shows change. When steroids or salicylates suppress the inflammatory process, CRP will disappear.
4. Malignancies	4. In response to injured tissue, CRP levels appear in the serum. Levels are more likely to be seen in active, widespread disease. In some malignancies, levels may be almost normal during periods of remission.
5. Rhematoid arthritis	5. There is a 70–80% chance of increase (21) and this is sometimes used as an indicator of disease activity.
6. Rheumatic fever	6. Measurement of CRP is a valuable aid in the diagnosis of questionable rheu-

matic fever as CRP is elevated early in the disease. CRP will remain positive in the presence of active carditis (9).

7. Systemic lupus erythematosus

7. CRP is elevated even during apparent remissions (9).

Drug Influences: The following drugs may influence test results. The drugs are listed alphabetically by generic name and divided into columns according to the effect of the drug. Examples of trade names are in parentheses.

The following drugs may cause an increase in test results:

Altered liver metabolism and/or estrogen effect
    estrogens (Premarin)
    oral contraceptives

The following drugs may cause a decrease in test results:

Progesterone effect
    oral contraceptives

Related Lab Studies

In rheumatic fever:
    ↑ erythrocyte sedimentation rate (ESR)
    ↑ leukocytes
    ↑ antistreptolycin O titer (ASO Titer)
    Throat culture; positive for group A streptococci

IMPLICATIONS FOR NURSING CARE
PRETEST: Factors related to test
Nursing Diagnosis: Potential for injury related to changes in biochemical balance

Guide to assessment	Guide to planning and intervention	Guide to evaluation
Assess patient factors that may influence test results:		
1. Comprehensive drug history	1. Consult with physician and indicate on lab slip drugs the patient is receiving that may influence presence of C-reactive protein.	1. The patient's pertinent drug history is discussed with physician and lab.
2. Preexisting conditions a. See Increases b. History of recent streptococcal pharyngitis	2. Record preexisting conditions on lab slip.	2. The patient's preexisting conditions are noted on lab slip.
3. Knowledge deficit	3. Explain test to patient: a. Define CRP (See Description). b. Explain procedure (See Procedure).	3. The patient demonstrates knowledge of test by defining test and stating procedure.
4. Knowledge deficit	4. Initiate specific preventive teaching of streptococcal in-	4. The patient states an understanding of the need for

Guide to assessment	Guide to planning and intervention	Guide to evaluation
	fections: a. Teach that sore throats should be cultured and those positive for streptococcus should be treated. b. Explain that family members should have throat cultures and positive cultures should be treated. c. Emphasize the need to complete antimicrobial treatment of positive streptococcal throats.	early detection and treatment of streptococcal infections.

Patient Preparation Checklist

1. √ Drug history (See Drug Influences).
2. √ Preexisting conditions and note on lab slip (See Increases).
3. √ Patient knowledge; explain test to patient (See Description/Procedure).
4. √ Patient knowledge of streptococcal infections (See 4 above).

CONSIDERATIONS FOR NURSING CARE RELATED TO ABNORMAL TEST RESULTS
POSTTEST: Factors related to the results of the test
Nursing Diagnosis: Alterations in biological balance

Guide to assessment	Guide to planning and intervention	Guide to evaluation
Assess patient factors influencing test results: 1. Recent history of streptococcal pharyngitis of patient, family or close friends. Symptoms: Sudden onset of sore throat Throat reddened with exudate Swollen tender cervical nodes	1. Prevent return of rheumatic fever or additional cases of the disease by: a. Referring family members and those in close association with the patient for throat cultures. b. Teaching that all people with positive streptococcal throat cultures should be treated.	1. The patient is free from the threat of a recurrence of rheumatic fever. a. The patient's family and close associates have throat cultures, b. and those with positive cultures are treated and

Guide to assessment	Guide to planning and intervention	Guide to evaluation
Headache and fever Abdominal pain (children)	c. Explaining the need for antimicrobial therapy to be continued for at least 10 days.	c. remain on antimicrobial therapy for the prescribed amount of time.
2. See above	2. Eradicate streptococcal infection by: a. Giving complete antimicrobial therapy (penicillin is drug of choice). b. Teaching need for long-term antimicrobial prophylaxis to prevent further attacks.	2. The streptococcal organism is eliminated by: a. Giving complete antimicrobial therapy. b. Complying with prophylactic treatment.
3. Observe for signs of carditis: Apical diastolic heart murmur Ventricular diastolic gallop Distant, dull, muffled heart sounds Friction rub present Lengthening of P-R interval Dyspnea Tachycardia (sleeping pulse) Peripheral venous congestion	3. Protect the patient from permanent cardiac damage by: a. Restricting physical activity according to the degree of carditis.	3. The patient is protected from permanent cardiac damage by: a. Reducing cardiac workload by decreasing physical activity.

b. Need for antimicrobial therapy
  Penicillin
  Erythromycin
  Sulfonamides
	b. Administering antimicrobial drugs as ordered.	b. Eliminating any remaining streptococcus and/or preventing recurrence of infection.

c. Need for antiinflammatory drugs
  Salicylates
  Steroids
	c. Administering antiinflammatory drugs.	c. The rheumatic inflammatory process is suppressed.

d. Lack of patient knowledge and/or noncompliance to treatment	d. Teaching why prophylactic medication should be continued; follow-up visits kept; and the affected person protected from close association with those with respiratory diseases or sore throats.	d. The patient demonstrates understanding by correct explanation and compliance to long-term treatment for protection against recurrence of disease.

Test: Creatine phosphokinase, Creatine kinase

Abbreviation: CPK, CK

Reference Values: Newborn 30–100 U/L
Child 15–50 U/L
Adults
  M 23–99 U/L
  W 15–57 U/L

Isoenzymes
CPK-BB None
CPK-MB 0–7 IU/L
CPK-MM 5–70 IU/L

Specimen: Serum

Description: Creatine phosphokinase is an enzyme found principally in heart muscle, skeletal muscle, and the brain. Three isoenzymes have been separated by electrophoresis. They are CPK_1, or BB fraction, found in the CNS tissue; CPK_2, the MB fraction, found almost exclusively in cardiac muscle; and CPK_3, the MM fraction, found in skeletal muscle. Because of CPK's role in energy storage for muscular activity, measuring isoenzymes helps to differentiate elevations.

CPK measurements aid in the diagnosis of acute myocardial infarction and muscular disorders.

Procedure: (red top tube)
1. No food or fluid restrictions.
2. Approximately 5 ml of blood is drawn from the patient.
3. Observe puncture site for bleeding or evidence of hematoma.

Conditions Related to Increases

Rationale

1. Myocardial infarction

1. Enzymes are released from necrotic myocardial cells. CPK-MB elevations appear 2–8 hours after the infarct episode, continue to rise to peak at 18–24 hours. Elevations are gone by about 48 hours after the epidode began.

2. Cerebral thrombosis
Brain infarction
Cerebral embolism
Meningitis

2. Activity of CPK–BB found in CNS tissue.

3. Muscular activity or injury
Hyperthyroidism
Progressive muscular dystrophy
Myotonia atrophica
Exercise
Intramuscular injections

3. Muscular activity increases CPK-MM activity found in skeletal muscle.

Drug Influences: The following drugs may influence test results. The drugs are listed alphabetically by generic name and divided into columns according to the effect of the drug. Examples of trade names are in parentheses.

The following drugs may cause an increase in test results:

Effect of IM injections

ampicillin (Omnipen)
analgesics
carbenicillin (Geocillin)
chlorpromazine (Thorazine)
clindamycin (Cleocin)
digoxin (Lanoxin)
meperidine (Demerol)

narcotics
penicillin
phenothiazines (Compazine)
saline
tubocurarine (Tubocurarine Chloride)

Poisoning (probable muscle origin)

barbiturates
carbromal (Carbrital)
ethchlorvynol (Placidyl)

Effect of administration during anesthesia

halothane (Fluothane)
succinylocholine (Anectine)

Enzyme activator effect

insulin

Miscellaneous

clofibrate (Atromid-S)

The following drugs may cause a decrease in test results:

Miscellaneous

ethanol (grain alcohol)
phenothiazines (Compazine); in schizophrenics with high initial values

Related Lab Studies: Monitor response to treatment or progress of disease and adjust nursing care accordingly. See individual tests for information.

In suspected myocardial infarction

LDH isoenzymes
AST (SGOT)
CBC

IMPLICATIONS FOR NURSING CARE
PRETEST: Factors related to test
Nursing Diagnosis: Potential for injury related to changes in biochemical balance

Guide to assessment	Guide to planning and intervention	Guide to evaluation
Assess patient factors that may influence test results: 1. Comprehensive drug history	1. Identify drugs that may influence test results. Consult with physician. Note on lab slip if patient has had recent	1. Patient's test values are not influenced by medication.

Guide to assessment	Guide to planning and intervention	Guide to evaluation
	IM injection. Note interfering drugs on lab slip.	

2. Knowledge deficit	2. Explain test to patient:
	  a. Define test.
	  b. Explain procedure.
		2. The patient is able to define test.

3. Hemolysis	3. Prevent hemolysis by:
	  a. Not saturating skin with antiseptic.
	  b. Not probing venipuncture site or leaving tourniquet on too long.
	  c. Not forcefully withdrawing specimen.
	  d. Not withdrawing specimen too slowly.
	  e. Not agitating or handling specimen roughly.
		3. Patient's values are not influenced by hemolysis.

Patient Preparation Checklist

1. √ Interfering drugs noted on lab slip. Recent IM injections noted on lab slip.
2. √ Patient knowledge; explain test to patient.
3. √ Prevention of hemolysis.

CONSIDERATIONS FOR NURSING CARE RELATED TO ABNORMAL TEST RESULTS
POSTTEST: Factors related to the results of the test
Nursing Diagnosis: Alterations in biochemical balance

Guide to assessment	Guide to planning and intervention	Guide to evaluation

1. Nursing history and/or physical exam indicative of myocardial infarction:
  Severe, crushing chest pain, possibly radiating into the left arm and/or up the sides of the neck
  Dyspnea
  Cyanosis
	1. Prevent further myocardial damage by:
	  a. Positioning patient in semi-Fowler's position.
	  b. Administering O_2 by cannula at prescribed rate.
	  c. Promoting patient rest by grouping nursing activities to allow rest periods.
		1. The patient's cardiac enzyme studies return to normal and remain normal.

Guide to assessment	Guide to planning and intervention	Guide to evaluation
	d. Placing patient on bed rest, progressing activity slowly as ordered and as tolerated by the patient. e. Eliminating as many environmental stressors as possible. f. Administering coronary vasodilators, beta-adrenergic blocking agents, sedatives and tranquilizers as ordered. g. Administering stool softeners as ordered; allowing patient to use the commode for bowel movement. h. Teaching patient to: (1) Engage in moderate activity that does not produce chest pain. (2) Avoid activities that produce chest pain, dyspnea, or fatigue. (3) Avoid performing valsalva maneuver. (4) Avoid overeating, and rest 1 hour after meals. (5) Lose weight, if necessary, and stop smoking; provide support to help the patient. (6) Avoid caffeine-containing drinks. (7) Develop positive ways of decreasing and/or coping with stress.	

2. Shock
  Decreased blood pressure
  Increased pulse and respirations
  Cold, moist skin
  Decreased temperature
  Pallor
  Slow capillary filling
  Thirst
  Restlessness, apprehension
  Nausea, vomiting
	2. Prevent further myocardial damage resulting from decreased blood flow by:
	a. Administering medications to relieve pain as ordered.
	b. Administering vasopressors as ordered.
	c. Administering IV fluids as ordered.
		2. The patient's cardiac enzyme studies return to normal and remain normal.

Guide to assessment	Guide to planning and intervention	Guide to evaluation
3. Thromboemboli: Severe, crushing chest pain "Indigestion" Dyspnea, sensation of suffocation Hemoptysis Pain in calf of leg Positive Homan's sign	3. Prevent further myocardial damage caused by secondary thromboemboli by: a. Administering anticoagulants as ordered. b. Applying antiembolic stockings. c. Encouraging the patient to do flexion-extension exercises of legs every hour while awake and every 4 hours at night.	3. The patient's cardiac enzyme studies return to normal and remain normal.

Test:	Creatinine, Creatinine Clearance
Abbreviation:	Cr, CrCl
Reference Values:	*Serum*

Serum
1–18 months   0.2–0.5 mg/dl
2–12 years   0.3–0.8 mg/dl
13–20 years   0.5–1.2 mg/dl
Adults   0.8–1.5 mg/dl

Urine
*children   0.7–1.5 g/24 hr
 Adults
 M   1.0–2.0 g/24 hr
 F   0.8–1.8 g/24 hr

Specimen: Serum
Urine, 24-hour specimen

Description: Creatinine (Cr) is a nonprotein end product in the breakdown of creatine phosphate in the skeletal muscle. The concentration in the bloodstream is proportional to the amount of active muscle tissue in the body and is normally maintained at a constant rate. Creatinine is removed from the body by the glomerular filtration action of the kidneys at a rate that is close to the rate of serum creatinine production. A very small amount of creatinine is added to the urine by tubular secretion (17). Because creatinine production is not significantly affected by factors such as protein intake, hydration, urine volume or protein metabolism, it is a valuable measure of kidney function. Generally, if a patient's creatinine level is double that which is normal for that patient, it can be assumed that 50% of the nephrons are nonfunctioning (39).

Creatinine clearance (CrCl) studies are the most practical and effective indicators of renal failure. The CrCl reflects the rate at which the creatinine is taken from the serum and excreted or cleared by the kidney. Done correctly, they are more sensitive than single serum creatinine values, which are elevated only when at least 50% of the kidney parenchyma is not functioning (38).

Procedure: (red top tube)

Serum

1. Food and fluid may be restricted; check with local lab.
2. 0.5–2 ml of blood is drawn from the patient.
3. Observe for bleeding at venipuncture site or for evidence of hematoma.

---

*Not discussed in this book.

Urine

1. Encourage fluid intake for adequate urine flow; discourage excessive protein intake.
2. Urine collection may be either a 24-hour urine collection or timed urine specimen collection for a shorter time period.
3. Check with local lab as special collection container may be used.
4. Save all urine during collection time; refrigerate.
5. Indicate on lab slip exact time of start and finish.
6. Blood specimen is drawn during 24-hour urine collection so lab must be notified.
7. Send entire specimen to lab.
8. Note on lab slip patient's height and weight.

Conditions Related to Increases

Rationale

Serum

1. Prerenal origin
   Congestive heart failure
   Bilateral renal artery thrombosis
   Hypovolemic shock
   Cardiogenic shock
   Dehydration (all causes)
   Hypovolemia
   Toxic conditions of pregnancy
   Hypertension

1. The increase in serum creatinine is caused by a decrease in the volume of blood to the kidneys, which results in a decreased glomerular filtration rate. The creatinine cannot be excreted in normal amounts and the serum level rises.

2. Postrenal origin
   Prostatic hypertrophy
   Renal calculi
   Bilateral ureteral stricture

2. Any obstruction of the urinary flow results in a rise in serum creatinine due to diminished renal clearance. Obstruction is usually bilateral and severe to result in this increase (7).

3. Renal origin
   Chronic glomerulonephritis
   Diabetic nephropathy
   Polycystic kidney disease
   Chronic pyelonephritis
   Nephrosclerosis
   Nephritis

3. Decrease in glomerular filtration leads to decreased ability of the kidney to excrete creatinine. The creatinine remains in the serum.

4. Excessive exercise

4. An excessive increase in muscle use over an extended length of time means that more energy is expended and there is an increase in the amount of creatine being converted to creatinine.

5. Extra large muscle mass

5. With increased muscle mass there is more creatine present, which results in increased production of serum creatinine.

Conditions Related to Decreases

1. Muscular origin
   Muscular dystrophies
   Myasthenia gravis
   Amyotonia congenita
   Muscle weakness
2. Catabolic states
   Starvation
   Acromegaly (in late stages)

3. Hyperthyroidism

4. Pregnancy

Rationale

1. With these conditions there is a decrease in the total muscle mass so there is less creatine available to be converted to creatinine.

2. There is a decrease in total muscle mass because of muscle weakness and muscle atrophy. As a result of this, there is less creatine available to be converted to creatinine.

3. In addition to the rationale in 2 above, it is believed that excess thyroid hormone may inhibit the conversion of creatine to creatinine (7).

4. It is believed that the kidneys increase in size during pregnancy. This leads to an increase in glomerular filtration rate and renal plasma flow, which results in a decrease in serum creatinine (37).

Conditions Related to Increases

1. Excessive exercise

2. Extra large muscle mass
3. Fever
   Sepsis
   Excessive trauma

Rationale

Urine

1. Assuming that kidney function is normal, the increase in serum creatinine results in more creatinine in the glomerular filtrate and an elevated excretion of urine creatinine.

2. See rationale in 1 above.
3. In these conditions, the urine creatinine increases as more creatine is released from the muscle and converted to creatinine.

Conditions Related to Decreases

1. Prerenal origin
   Congestive heart failure
   Bilateral renal artery thrombosis
   Hypovolemic shock
   Cardiogenic shock
   Dehydration (all causes)
   Hypovolemia
   Toxic conditions of pregnancy
   Hypertension
2. Postrenal origin
   Prostatic hypertrophy
   Renal calculi

Rationale

1. Urine creatinine decreases because there is a decrease in the volume of blood flow through the kidneys. Creatinine is excreted by glomerular filtration so decreased blood volume means decreased urine creatinine.

2. The flow of urine is obstructed in these conditions. If the obstruction is severe, there is diminished renal

Bilateral ureteral stricture

3. Renal origin
   Chronic glomerulonephritis
   Diabetic nephropathy
   Polycystic kidney disease
   Chronic pyelonephritis
   Nephrosclerosis
   Nephritis

4. Muscular origin
   Muscular dystrophies
   Myasthenia gravis
   Amyotonia congenita

5. Hyperthyroidism

6. Age

clearance and a decrease in urine creatinine.

3. Decrease in glomerular filtration leads to decreased ability of the kidney to excrete creatinine.

4. In these conditions, the decreased muscle mass results in a decrease in the serum creatinine produced. Because there is less creatinine in the blood, there is a resultant decrease in the excretion of creatinine in the urine.

5. As in 4 above. This decrease may also be due in part to the excess thyroid hormone blockage of serum creatine to creatinine (7).

6. After age 20, the creatinine clearance concentrations decrease 6 ml/min/decade because of the decreasing numbers of functioning nephrons (38).

Drug Influences: The following drugs may influence test results. The drugs are listed alphabetically by generic name and divided into columns according to the effect of the drug. Examples of trade names are in parentheses.

The following drugs may cause an increase in test results:

Serum Creatinine

Nephrotoxic effect
   acetaminophen (Tylenol)
   amphotericin B (Fungizone)
   arsenicals
   barbiturates
   capreomycin (Capastat Sulfate)
   cephaloridine (Loridine)
   chlorthalidone (Hygroton)
   colistimethate (Coly-Mycin M)
   colistin (Coly-Mycin S)
   co-trimoxazole (Bactrim)
   demeclocycline (Declomycin)
   doxycycline (Vibramycin)
   gentamicin (Garamycin)
   ipodate (Oragrafin)
   kanamycin (Kantrex)

   lipomul (corn oil)
   methicillin (Staphcillin)
   mithramycin (Mithracin)
   mitomycin (Mutamycin)
   neomycin
   nitrofurantoin (Macrodantin)
   penicillin
   phosphorus (thiacide tablets)
   polymyxin (Aerosporin)
   streptokinase (Streptase)
   streptomycin
   tetracycline (Achromycin)
   triamterene (Dyrenium)
   viomycin

Transient azotemia effect
  oxacillin (Prostaphlin)
  phenacetin

Miscellaneous
  clofibrate (Atromid-S), possibly derived from muscle damage

Urine

Anabolic effect
  oxymetholone (Anadrol-50)

Miscellaneous
  corticosteroids (Celestone); associated with negative nitrogen balance
  fluoxymesterone (Halotestin)

Urine Clearance

Decreased tubular reabsorption
  isosorbide (Isordil)

Miscellaneous
  furosemide (Lasix)
  methylprednisolone (Medrol)

The following drugs may cause a decrease in test results:

Serum

Miscellaneous
  cannabis (marijuana)

Urine

Anabolic effect
  anabolic steroids
  androgens (Android-F)
  nandrolone (Anabolin)

Urine Clearance

Nephrotoxic effect
  amphotericin B (Fungizone)
  mitomycin (Mutamycin)

Renal damage and/or failure
  iopanoic acid (Telepaque)
  paromomycin (Humatin)
  vancomycin
  viomycin

Decreased renal blood flow
  triamterene (Dyrenium)

Related Lab Studies: Monitor response to treatment and/or progression of disease and adjust nursing care accordingly. See individual tests for information.

In renal failure:
  ↑ BUN
  electrolytes (↑ K, ↓ Na, ↓ CO_2, Cl ↑ or ↓)
  ↓ total protein

↓ serum osmolality
↓ hematocrit and hemoglobin
*retrograde pyelography

In muscular dystrophies:
↑ serum creatine
↑ urine creatine
*muscle biopsy
*electromyography
↑ aldolase
↑ AST (SGOT)
↑ creatine kinase (CK/CPK)

IMPLICATIONS FOR NURSING CARE
PRETEST: Factors related to the test
Nursing Diagnosis: Potential for injury related to changes in biochemical balance

Guide to assessment	Guide to planning and intervention	Guide to evaluation
Assess patient factors influencing test results:		
1. Food and fluids	1. Restrict food and fluid for 8 hours before a serum creatinine test. This restriction does not apply to a serum creatinine sample drawn during a creatinine clearance study. Instruct the patient to avoid eating *excessive* amounts of meat prior to the test. Maintain proper hydration during creatinine clearance to insure a good urine flow.	1. Ingestion of food or fluids does not influence test results.
2. Vigorous exercise	2. Instruct patient to avoid vigorous exercise prior to a creatinine test or during a creatinine clearance test.	2. Patient avoids excessive exercise prior to and during the testing.
3. Comprehensive drug history (See Drug Influences)	3. Remind physician and inform lab of drugs the patient is receiving which may influence creatinine level.	3. Patient's pertinent drug history is discussed with physician and lab.
4. Preexisting conditions (See Increases/Decreases)	4. Record preexisting conditions on lab slip.	4. Patient's preexisting conditions are noted on lab slip.
5. Knowledge deficit	5. Explain tests to patient: a. Define tests (see Description). b. Explain procedure (see Procedure).	5. Patient demonstrates knowledge of tests by defining tests and explaining procedure.
6. Nursing staff factors influencing test results:	6. Control staff factors influencing test results.	6. Patient's lab results are accurate.

*Very age dependent, check with local lab.

Guide to assessment	Guide to planning and intervention	Guide to evaluation
a. Knowledge deficit	a. (1) Urine specimens are timed accurately. (2) Proper preservatives are present in the urine collection bottle. (3) Urine is stored correctly. (4) Laboratory technician is notified to obtain a serum creatinine during the time the urine is being collected.	

Patient Preparation Checklist

1. √ Correct test procedure and patient preparation for creatinine and creatinine clearance test.
2. √ Patient drug history (see Drug Influences).
3. √ Preexisting conditions and note on lab slip (see Increases/Decreases).
4. √ Patient knowledge; explain test to patient (see Description/Procedure).

CONSIDERATIONS FOR NURSING CARE RELATED TO ABNORMAL TEST RESULTS
POSTTEST: Factors related to the results of the test
Nursing Diagnosis: Alterations in biochemical balance

Guide to assessment	Guide to planning and intervention	Guide to evaluation
Assess patient factors that may be influencing test results:		
1. Obstruction of urinary flow (See serum increases 2, and urine decreases 2) Decreased urine output Severe, spasmodic pain in flank and/or abdomen Hematuria Hydration status Distended bladder	1. Encourage urinary flow by: a. Assisting to position of comfort. b. Using comfort measures such as sitz baths, warm towels, warm fluids, etc. c. Giving analgesics and antispasmodics as ordered. d. Determining intake and encouraging hydration.	1. Patient is free from urinary obstruction as noted by an adequate output and a normal urine and serum creatinine.

Guide to assessment	Guide to planning and intervention	Guide to evaluation
	e. Checking to be sure that urinary drainage systems are functioning properly.	
2. Decreased renal blood flow and glomerulofiltration	2. Restore renal function by	2. Patient's renal function is restored by:
	a. Promoting fluid and electrolyte status with precise I&O and daily weights.	a. Balancing hydration and electrolyte status.
Recent medical, surgical, obstetrical, chemical history	b. Administering blood transfusions and intravenous fluids as ordered.	b. Corrected circulatory insufficiency.
Diminished urine output	c. Preparing patient for dialysis as necessary.	c. Hemodialysis.
3. Uncontrolled disease conditions (e.g., diabetes, hyperthyroidism, hypertension) that can lead to increases or decreases in creatinine (see Increases/ Decreases)	3. Promote control of disease conditions that influence creatinine levels by: a. Reinforcing patient teaching regarding disease processes and appropriate methods of control. b. Administering medications and treatments which help to control those conditions (e.g., thyroid inhibitors, insulin, diuretics, stress management).	3. The patient will not develop increases or decreases in creatinine as a result of uncontrolled disease conditions.

Test:	Cultures
Abbreviation:	None
Reference Value:	Normal flora or no growth
Description:	Cultures identify the presence and type of microorganisms. A culture medium is an environment that encourages organism growth. The right medium must be present. Organisms grow at different rates. It may take only 12–24 hours for some organisms to grow, while others may take 6–8 weeks.

Aerobic organisms are those that live in the presence of oxygen. Anaerobic organisms live without oxygen. The anaerobic organisms are most numerous but it is the aerobic organisms that cause most infections.

IMPLICATIONS FOR NURSING CARE
Nursing Diagnosis: Potential for injury related to changes in biological environment

Guide to assessment	Guide to planning and intervention	Guide to evaluation

Assess patient factors that may influence test results:
1. General signs of infection
  Fever
  C/o increasing pain 3 days postsurgery
  Fatigue
  Malaise
  C/o pain
  Red, sore, swollen wound
  Exudate
  ↑ WBC
	1. Detect signs of infection. Consult with physician as necessary.	1. Patient's signs of infection are identified.

2. Antibiotics
  Name
  Route
  Duration received
	2. Collect specimen before giving antibiotics. Note on lab slip if patient is taking antibiotics.	2. The patient's lab results are not influenced by antibiotics.

3. Immunosuppressant drugs	3. Initiate measures to protect patient on immunosuppressant drugs from infection.	3. The patient does not experience an infection.
4. Possible isolation	4. Place patient with potentially infectious condition in isolation until bacteriology reports are confirmed.	4. Patient's infection is isolated.

5. Hospitalization	5. Prevent nosocomial infection by:
	  a. Using proper aseptic technique.
	  b. Checking patients on antibiotic therapy for suprainfection.
		5. The patient is free of nosocomial infection.

Guide to assessment	Guide to planning and intervention	Guide to evaluation
6. Specimen collection	6. Collect specimen correctly: a. Use correct container. b. Collect correct amount. c. Fill lab slip out completely. d. Label specimen. e. Take to lab immediately. f. Consult with lab if in doubt.	6. The patient's results are not influenced by collection procedure.
7. Prevent infection	7. Encourage patient to practice good health measures by: a. Eating a nutritious diet. b. Getting sufficient rest. c. Planning daily exercise program.	7. The patient is free of infection.

Patient Preparation Checklist

1. √ Culture obtained prior to antibiotic therapy.
2. √ Note if on antibiotic therapy (name, route, duration).
3. √ Identification of culture.
4. √ Collection procedure (see 6 above).
5. √ Patient knowledge; explain test to patient (parent).

Test:	Digoxin level
Abbreviation:	None
Reference Values:	Therapeutic level 0.8–2 ng/ml Toxic level over 2 ng/ml
Specimen:	Serum

Description: Digoxin, a substance not normally present in the blood, is a cardiac glycoside derived from the plant *Digitalis lanta*. Digoxin increases the force of myocardial contractions, lengthens the refractory period, and reduces the heart rate. Digoxin is 75–80% absorbed through the gastrointestinal tract and excreted largely unchanged through the kidneys (40). A small amount is excreted in the stool but this means of excretion is of little significance except in cases of renal failure. The expected half-life of digoxin in the adult is 35 hours, with shorter times found in infants and longer times found in premature infants. The onset of action is approximately 30 minutes after oral ingestion and peaks in 1.5–5 hours. Serum blood levels are helpful when the specimen is obtained during the plateau phase, which occurs 6 hours after oral ingestion. Serum digoxin levels are currently used as a guide to establish therapeutic dosages and confirm suspected toxicities. A change in the level for an individual patient is generally more useful than an isolated reading. Disease state and body condition may predispose an individual to digoxin toxicity even though blood levels reflect a therapeutic range. Such conditions include hypokalemia, hypothyroidism, hypomagnesemia, acid-base disturbances, hypoxia, and diffuse heart disease. Do not confuse the cardiac glycosides digoxin and digitoxin. Although they have similar effects in the body, serum levels and body half-life differ.

Procedure: (red top tube)
1. Order digoxin level to be drawn at least 6–8 hours after last oral dose of digoxin.
2. No food or fluid restrictions.
3. 0.5–3 ml of blood is drawn from the patient.
4. Observe puncture site for bleeding or evidence of hematoma.

Conditions Related to Increases	**Rationale**
1. Renal disease	1. With renal impairment the amount of digoxin eliminated from the body decreases, leading to an increase in digoxin level.
2. Digoxin overdose	2. Increase in amount of digoxin ingested leads to increased blood levels. This may be a result of dosage alteration by patients.

3. Specimen drawn after administration of digoxin but before plateau phase.

3. If the specimen is obtained before the plateau phase, very high values may be obtained due to the distribution in the body. These high levels do not result in toxicity because they do not reflect myocardial drug levels (11, p. 483).

4. Jaundice

4. False increases in digoxin levels have been reported (24).

Conditions Related to Decreases

Rationale

1. Impaired gastrointestinal motility and/or malabsorption

1. 75–80% of digoxin is absorbed after oral ingestion. Impaired function of gastrointestinal tract will reduce the amount of digoxin absorbed.

2. Uremia

2. False decreased levels have been reported (24).

Drug Influences: The following drugs may cause an increased chance of digoxin toxicity. The drugs are listed alphabetically by generic name and divided into columns according to effect of the drug. Examples of trade names are in parentheses.

Increases K$^+$ depletion
   amphotericin B
   diuretics, potassium-losing (Lasix, Hygroton, Edecrin, thiazides)
   glucose infusions

Causes cardiac arrhythmias
   calcium preparations
   reserpine (Serpasil)
   succinylcholine (muscle relaxant used during surgery, manipulative procedures, and electroshock therapy)
   sympathomimetics (adrenergic drugs, such as theophylline derivatives, epinephrine, ephedrine, isoproterenol, etc.)

Bradycardia
   propranolol (Inderal)

Increased absorption
   propantheline (Pro-Banthine Bromide)

The following drugs may cause a decrease in the absorption of digoxin or digoxin availability:

Decreases absorption
   antacids
   Kaopectate
   metoclopramide

Increases breakdown in the liver
   barbiturates

Decreases half-life
  chlolestyramine (Cuemid, Questran)

Decreases effectiveness
  spironolactone (Aldactone)

Related Lab Studies: Monitor response to digoxin and observe for signs and symptoms of toxicity.

  electrolytes (Na, K, Cl, CO_2 content)
  *EKG for potassium and digoxin effect
  BUN
  creatinine

IMPLICATIONS FOR NURSING CARE
PRETEST: Factors related to the test
Nursing Diagnosis: Potential for injury related to changes in chemical balance

Guide to assessment	Guide to planning and intervention	Guide to evaluation

Assess patient factors that may influence test results:
1. Comprehensive drug history
  See Drug Influences
  Note date, time, route, and amount of last dose of digoxin
  Check for ingestion of *digitoxin* during last 6–8 weeks
	1. Report drugs the patient is receiving that may influence lab results to the patient's physician and to the laboratory:
	  a. Order digoxin level to be drawn at least 6–8 hours after last oral dose of digoxin (11).
	  b. Report *digitoxin* ingestion that has occurred during last 6–8 weeks to the laboratory.
	  c. Clarify the cardiac glycoside ordered since testing for wrong glycosides results in errors.
	  d. Administer the correct cardiac glycoside.
		1. The patient's digoxin level is not negatively influenced by staff error in ordering the test, giving the correct drug, or filling out lab slip.

2. Preexisting conditions (See Increases/Decreases)
3. Knowledge deficit
	2. Record preexisting conditions on lab slip.
	3. Explain test to patient:
	  a. Define digoxin (See Description).
	  b. Describe procedure (See Procedure).
		2. Patient's preexisting conditions are noted on lab slip.
		3. The patient demonstrates knowledge of test by defining test and stating procedure.

*Not discussed in this book.

```
┌─────────────────────────────────────────────────────────────────┐
│                    Patient Preparation Checklist                  │
│  1. √ Date, time, route, and amount of last digoxin dose recorded │
│       on lab slip.                                                │
│  2. √ Blood drawn 6–8 hours after last dose of oral digoxin; and  │
│       time specimen was drawn recorded on slip.                   │
│  3. √ Influencing drugs noted and reported (See Drug Influences). │
│  4. √ Explain test to patient (See Description and Procedure).    │
│  5. √ Type of glycoside ordered.                                  │
└─────────────────────────────────────────────────────────────────┘
```

CONSIDERATIONS FOR NURSING CARE RELATED TO ABNORMAL TEST RESULTS

POSTTEST: Factors related to the results of the test
Nursing Diagnosis: Alterations in chemical balance related to digoxin level

Guide to assessment	Guide to planning and intervention	Guide to evaluation
Assess patient factors that may be influencing test results:		
1. Therapeutic effects of digoxin:	1. Recognize therapeutic effects of digoxin by:	1. The patient demonstrates therapeutic dioxin levels by:
a. Heart rate Adults 60–120 Infants/children 90–160	a. Checking apical heartbeat for rate and rhythm before each dose for 1 full minute.	a. Heart rate regular and rate within normal limits.
	b. Auscultating chest and recording chest sounds every 4 hours or as needed.	b. The patient's breath sounds upon auscultation are normal.
	c. Measuring and recording intake and output.	c. The patient demonstrates balanced intake and output.
	d. Observing for signs of edema; check sacral area and buttocks of patients on bed rest.	d. The patient does not demonstrate signs of edema.

2. Digitalis toxicity
History of digoxin intake
Serum digoxin:
  level over 2 mg/ml
Signs/symptoms of digitalis toxicity
  Anorexia
  Nausea
  Vomiting
  Headache
  Fatigue
  Visual disturbances
  Pulse below 60/min. in adults; below 90–110/min. in children
  EKG changes
	2. Correct digitalis toxicity by:
	
	a. Discontinuing digoxin as ordered by physician.
	b. Placing the patient on cardiac monitor.
	
	c. Administering potassium for low serum K^+ levels as ordered by physician.
	d. Monitoring and controlling life-threatening arrhythmias until excess digoxin is excreted.
		2. The patient's digoxin toxicity is corrected:
		
		a. Digoxin is discontinued as ordered.
		b. The patient demonstrates normal sinus rhythm on EKG.
		c. The patient's serum K^+ level is normal.
		
		d. The patient does not demonstrate physical signs of digoxin toxicity. Serum digoxin levels are normal.

Guide to assessment	Guide to planning and intervention	Guide to evaluation
Identify patients with increased sensitivity to digoxin (See Description)		
3. Lack of patient education related to digoxin therapy	3. Implement teaching plan regarding digoxin therapy to include:	3. The patient states understanding of digoxin therapy:
	a. Teaching name and desired effect of digoxin and amount of medication to be taken.	a. The patient states name, dosage, and desired effect of digoxin.
	b. Stressing not to change dosage unless ordered by physician.	
	c. Stressing importance of following the physician's *most recent* instructions.	
	d. Teaching symptoms of toxicity to be reported to physician.	d. The patient states symptoms of toxicity to be reported.
	e. Teaching pulse-taking and recording.	e. The patient demonstrates pulse-taking and regular/irregular rhythms by tapping a finger (47).
	f. Teaching the relationship between potassium and digoxin if taking diuretics.	f. The patient is able to state the potassium/digoxin/diuretic relationship to digoxin toxicity.
	g. Teaching dietary potassium supplements.	g. The patient is able to list dietary sources of potassium.

Test:	Dilantin (Phenytoin)
Abbreviation:	None
Reference Values:	Therapeutic levels 10–20 µg/ml Toxic levels over 20 µg/ml
Specimen:	Serum

Description: Dilantin is a drug currently used to treat seizure disorders and cardiac arrhythmias. It acts in the body by altering ion movement across cell membranes. Absorption from the gastrointestinal tract is slow, sometimes variable, and occasionally incomplete (41, p. 454). About 90% of Dilantin is bound to plasma protein. Metabolism takes place in the liver by hepatic microsomal enzymes, it is excreted into the bile, then the urine. Five to 20% is excreted unchanged in the urine. It takes several hours to reach peak plasma levels after an oral dose. The half-life of Dilantin is 10–45 hours, depending on the patient's age. After beginning or increasing Dilantin dosage, about 5 days are required before new plasma concentrations achieve a steady state (21). Once the therapeutic range is obtained, small increases in the Dilantin metabolism dosage may greatly alter the serum level. This is because the metabolism of Dilantin becomes independent of serum concentrations. The purpose of the test is to monitor plasma levels to determine toxicities and evaluate dosage regimes.

Procedure: (check tube color with testing lab)
1. No food or fluid restrictions.
2. 0.5–3 ml of venous blood is drawn from the patient.
3. Observe puncture site for bleeding or evidence of hematoma.

Conditions Related to Increases

1. Uremia

2. Liver disease

3. Dosage increase

Rationale

1. Dilantin is 70–95% bound to plasma protein. In uremia, serum protein binding is decreased, causing an increased percentage of free drug.
2. Decreased functioning of the liver interferes in the metabolism of Dilantin.
3. Once a therapeutic range is achieved, small increases in the dose cause greater serum levels than the increased dosage would have caused at subtherapeutic levels. This is because serum concentrations are not linearly related to daily dose (96, p.235).

Conditions Related to Decreases

1. Infectious mononucleosis

2. Pregnancy

Rationale

1. Increased clearance of drug has been described (34).
2. Due to decreased absorption.

Drug Influences: The following drugs may influence test results. The drugs are listed alphabetically by generic name and divided into columns according to the effect of the drug. Examples of trade names are in parentheses.

The following drugs may cause an increase in test results:

Plasma protein displacement
aspirin
sulfisoxazole (Gantrisin)

Action on liver enzymes
sulthiame (Conadil)

Metabolic inhibition and/or impairment

chloramphenicol (Chloromycetin)
chlordiazepoxide (Limbitrol)
chlorpromazine (Thorazine)
diazepam (Valium)
disulfiram (Antabuse)
ethosuximide (Zarontin)
halothane (Fluothane)

isoniazid (Laniazid)
nitrazepam (Mogadon)
phenobarbital (Phendex)
phenylbutazone (Butazolidin)
prochlorperazine (Compazine)
proxyphene (Darvon)

The following drugs may cause a decrease in test results:

Reduction in half-life of Dilantin
chlorophenothane (DDT)
ethanol (grain alcohol)

Miscellaneous
folate (Folvite); stimulates metabolism of folate-deficient patients

Related Lab Studies: Monitor response to Dilantin and observe for signs and symptoms of toxicity.

BUN
creatinine, creatinine clearance
*EKG
ALT (SGPT)
alkaline phosphatase
AST (SGOT)
bilirubin
electrolytes

IMPLICATIONS FOR NURSING CARE
PRETEST: Factors related to the test
Nursing Diagnosis: Potential for injury related to changes in chemical balance

Guide to assessment	Guide to planning and intervention	Guide to evaluation
Assess patient factors that may influence test results: 1. Comprehensive drug history See Drug Influences	1. Report to lab and physician drugs the patient is receiving that may influence lab results.	1. Drugs patient is currently receiving that may influence lab results are identified and

*Not discussed in this book.

Guide to assessment	Guide to planning and intervention	Guide to evaluation

Note time, amount, and route of last dose of Dilantin
2. Preexisting conditions (See Increases/Decreases)
3. Knowledge deficit
	Record date, time, amount, and route of last dose of Dilantin on lab slip.
	2. Record preexisting conditions on lab slip.
	3. Explain test to patient.
	  a. Define Dilantin levels (See Description).
	  b. Explain procedure (See Procedure).
		the proper people are notified.
		
		2. Patient's preexisting conditions are noted on lab slip.
		3. Patient demonstrates knowledge of test by defining and stating procedure.

Patient Preparation Checklist

1. √ Date, time, amount, and route of last dose of Dilantin noted on lab slip.
2. √ Influencing drugs noted and reported (See Drug Influences).
3. √ Preexisting conditions noted on lab slip (See Increases).
4. √ Patient knowledge; explain test and procedure (See Description and Procedure).

IMPLICATIONS FOR NURSING CARE
POSTTEST: Factors related to the results of the test
Nursing Diagnosis: Alterations in chemical balance related to phenytoin level

Guide to assessment	Guide to planning and intervention	Guide to evaluation

Assess patient factors that may be influencing test results:
1. Dilantin toxicity
  Nystagmus on a lateral gaze
  Nystagmus
  Drowsiness
  Lethargy
  Ataxia
  Slurred speech
  Nausea
  Rash
  Gingival hyperplasia
	1. Implement plan of care to correct and prevent Dilantin toxicity by:
	  a. Being alert to signs/symptoms of Dilantin toxicity.
	  b. Discontinuing or reducing amount of Dilantin as ordered by physician (if Dilantin is used for seizure control, another anticonvul-
		1. The patient does not demonstrate signs and symptoms of Dilantin toxicity.
		
		  The patient identifies signs and symptoms of Dilantin toxicity to be reported to physician.

Guide to assessment	Guide to planning and intervention	Guide to evaluation
Peripheral neuropathies Lupus erythematosus-like syndrome Morbilliform rash	sant needs to be started). c. Teaching patient signs/ symptoms of Dilantin toxicity to be reported to physician. d. Teaching name, amount, and time to take Dilantin. e. Instructing the patient not to take over-the-counter drugs without consulting physician.	

Test: Estriol, free estriol (serum)

Abbreviation: E_3, serum or urine

Reference Values: Serum—levels depend upon week of gestation. Range during pregnancy is 6–34 ng/ml, showing a gradual rise. Serial tests are required for comparison.

Urine—levels depend upon week of gestation. Range during last 6 weeks of pregnancy is 10–24 mg/day. Serial tests are required for comparison.

Specimen: Serum (or plasma)
24-hour urine collection

Description: Estriol is a metabolite of estrogen. During pregnancy the fetal adrenals produce steroid precursors, DHEA and 16-OHDHEA, that are synthesized into estriol in the placenta. It is conjugated in the maternal liver and excreted in maternal urine. Estriol levels show a progressive rise during pregnancy. Measurements of estriol levels are of particular value during the third trimester as an index to fetal well-being and placental functioning.

Serum and urine estriol can be measured. Urinary estriol is affected by certain drugs, maternal diseases, and incomplete urine collection. Serum estriol radioimmunoassay is less affected by maternal influences than urinary estriol measurements and does not require a timed urine collection.

Procedure: (red top tube)

Serum

1. No food or fluid restrictions.
2. Approximately 5 ml of blood is drawn from the patient.
3. Serial evaluations are required.
4. Observe puncture site for bleeding or evidence of hematoma.

Urine
(24-hour collection)

1. No food or fluid restrictions.
2. Interfering drugs should be withheld, as possible, several days prior to and during urine collection.
3. Collection bottle may contain preservative.
4. Urine *must* be refrigerated during entire collection.
5. Collection.
   a. Discard first voided specimen.
   b. Begin timing.
   c. For next 24 hours place all voidings into specimen container immediately after voiding.
   d. Have patient void just prior to completion of 24 hours and put sample in collection bottle.
6. Record exact start and finish times on lab slip.
7. Send to lab immediately or keep refrigerated until sent.
8. Serial evaluations are required for accurate evaluation.

Conditions Related to Increases	Rationale

Serum and Urine

1. Healthy fetus
   1. High estriol levels with a rising curve are associated with a normal pregnancy and healthy fetus.

Urine

1. Hemolytic disease of the newborn
   1. Excessive levels are sometimes observed. There is no correlation between levels and disease.
2. Multiple pregnancies
   2. In multiple pregnancies excessive increases are sometimes observed.

Conditions Related to Decreases	Rationale

Serum and Urine

1. Anencephaly
   Exogenous corticoids
   1. The estriol decrease is caused by decreased synthesis of ACTH by the fetal pituitary. The estriol level shows a persistently low curve.
2. Adrenal hypoplasia
   Retarded fetal growth
   2. The decrease is due to decreased synthesis of steroid precursors.
3. Fetal jeopardy
   3. Significant decreases from baseline in 2 consecutive days indicates placental insufficiency and impending fetal distress. A serum estriol level with a sharp drop within 1–2 hours or below 4 ng/ml may indicate fetal death.
4. Placental insufficiency
   Placental infarction
   Hydatidiform mole
   4. Decreased placental synthesis of estriol causes the low estriol levels.
5. Placental sulfatase deficiency
   5. The estriol precursor 16-OHDHEA is not hydrolyzed from 16-OHDHEA sulfate before it can be converted to estriol.
6. Malabsorption
   6. Prevents reabsorption of estriol.
7. False low results
   7. May be from drugs, incomplete urine collection, decreased maternal glomerular filtration rate, or maternal liver disease.

Drug Influences: The following drugs may influence test results. The drugs are listed alphabetically by generic name and divided into columns according to the effect of the drug. Examples of trade names are in parentheses.

The following drugs may cause an increase in test results:

Urine

Increased hydroxylation
   barbiturates

Miscellaneous
   corticotropin
   spironolactone (Aldactone)

The following drugs may cause a decrease in test results:

Plasma

Intestinal flora alteration
   ampicillin (Omnipen)
   penicillin

Following abortion
   prostaglandin F2 alpha

Urine

Decreased synthesis by Fetoplacental unit
   ampicillin (Omnipen)
   cascara sagrada
   senna

Affect on integrity of intestinal microflora
   methenamine mandelate (Mandelamine)
   neomycin
   phthalylsulfathiazole (Sulfathalidine)
   tetracyclines

Hormonal effect
   oral contraceptives

Metabolic effect
   thyroxine (Synthroid)

Blocked tubular excretion
   probenecid (Benemid)

Miscellaneous
   hydrochlorothiazide
   meprobamate
   phenazopyridine hydrochloride
   phenothiazines

Related Lab Studies: To monitor fetoplacental status:

   *amniotic fluid studies
   *fetal scalp pH
   progesterone, serum
   *total urine estrogen
   hemoglobin
   hematocrit

---

*Not discussed in this text.

urinalysis
*oxytocin challenge test (OCT)

IMPLICATIONS FOR NURSING CARE
PRETEST: Factors related to the test
Nursing Diagnosis: Potential for injury related to changes in biochemical balance

Guide to assessment	Guide to planning and intervention	Guide to evaluation
Assess patient factors that may influence test results: 1. Comprehensive drug history (See Drug Influences)	1. Identify and withhold as possible drugs that may influence test results. Note interfering drugs on lab slip.	1. Patient's lab values are accurate.
2. Preexisting conditions: High-risk pregnancy Diabetes Hypertension Toxemia	2. Record preexisting conditions on lab slip.	2. Patient's preexisting conditions do not influence test results.
3. Pregnancy	3. Encourage prenatal care.	3. Patient keeps clinic appointments and demonstrates understanding of health care by choice of diet, exercise, and general compliance to health needs.
4. Knowledge deficit, Patient	4. Explain test to patient: a. Define estriol (See Description). b. Explain procedure (See Procedure).	4. The patient demonstrates knowledge by defining estriol and explaining procedure.
5. Knowledge deficit, Staff Nonrefrigerated urine Incomplete collection	5. Follow procedure for timed urine collection exactly.	5. Patient's test values are not incorrect due to staff error.

Patient Preparation Checklist

1. √ Influencing drugs and note on lab slip (See Drug Influences).
2. √ Preexisting conditions; note condition or if high risk pregnancy on lab slip.
3. √ Patient knowledge; explain test (See Description/Procedure).
4. √ Staff knowledge about urine collection.

---

*Not discussed in this book.

CONSIDERATIONS FOR NURSING CARE RELATED TO ABNORMAL TEST RESULTS
POSTTEST: Factors related to the results of the test
Nursing Diagnosis: Alterations in biochemical balance

Guide to assessment	Guide to planning and intervention	Guide to evaluation

Assess patient factors that may be influencing test results.
Nursing history and/or physical exam suggestive of:
1. Chronic placental insufficiency
    Hypertension
    Diabetes mellitus
    Postmaturity
  Fetal distress
    Bradycardia
    Tachycardia
    Late decelerations
    Decreased or excessive
     fetal movement
	1. Minimize effects of fetal anoxia by:
	  a. Being alert to changes in fetal scalp, pH, and fetal heart tones.
	  b. Reporting changes to physician immediately.
	  c. Implementing medical plan to improve insufficiency.
		1. Infant is healthy at birth.

Test:	Ethanol, blood alcohol
Abbreviation:	$C_2 H_5 OH$
Reference Value:	Negative
	Different states have different laws governing legal blood alcohol limit for operating a motor vehicle. Usual level is 0.10%.
Specimen:	Whole blood
Description:	Ethanol, grain alcohol, or alcohol is a popular mood-changing drug. After ingestion, alcohol is absorbed either through the stomach (about 20%) or in the jejunum. Metabolism takes place mostly in the liver with the oxidizing of ethanol to acetaldehyde and then to CO_2 and water. About 10% of ethanol is excreted unchanged in urine, sweat, and breath.
	Blood alcohol levels are done to determine the cause of coma or for medicolegal reasons.
Procedure:	(red top tube)

1. Obtain signed permit.
2. Person drawing blood should understand legal ramifications and know institutional policy.
3. Puncture site is cleaned with nonalcohol antiseptic; a benzalkonium chloride or povidone-iodine solution is used.
4. About 7 ml of blood in vacuum tube is collected.
5. Observe puncture site for bleeding or evidence of hematoma.
6. Specimen must go to the laboratory immediately or be refrigerated.

Conditions Related to Increases

Rationale

1. Ethanol ingestion

1. The relationship of ethanol blood levels to alcohol ingestion and rate of intoxication depends on food in the stomach, accompanying drugs, chronic alcohol abuse, etc. A level of 0.05–0.10% wt./vol. is considered intoxicated by the National Safety Council's Committee on Alcohol and Drugs.

2. Drugs
   See Drug Influences

2. Drugs metabolized by the microsomal oxidizing system in combination with ethanol have prolonged effects and at times produce dangerously toxic levels.

3. Alcohol skin preparation

3. Alcohol from skin preparation can increase blood ethanol test values significantly.

Drug Influences: The following drugs may influence test results. The drugs are listed alphabetically by generic name and divided into columns according to the effect of the drug. Examples of trade names are in parentheses.

The following drugs may increase test results:

Interactions
    barbiturates
    chloral hydrate
    chlordiazepoxide hydrochloride (Librium)
    diazepam (Valium)
    guanethidine (Ismelin)

    isoniazid (INH)
    meprobamate (Equanil, Miltown)
    phenytoin (Dilatin)

Related Lab Studies

    *methyl alcohol
    *toxicology studies
    *urine alcohol
    *Breathalyzer
    barbiturate, serum
    ammonia, plasma

IMPLICATIONS FOR NURSING CARE
PRETEST: Factors related to the test
Nursing Diagnosis: Potential for injury related to chemical poisoning

Guide to assessment	Guide to planning and intervention	Guide to evaluation
Assess patient factors that may influence test results:		
1. Need for patient permission	1. Obtain signed permit.	1. The patient signs permit for blood ethanol test.
2. Comprehensive drug history (See Drug Influences)	2. Note drug influences on lab slip.	2. Patient's drug history is noted on lab slip.
3. Knowledge deficit	3. Explain test to patient/family:	3. The patient is able to define test and explain procedure.
	a. Define test (See Description).	
	b. Explain procedure.	

Patient Preparation Checklist

1. √ Permit signed.
2. √ Pertinent drug history noted on lab slip (See Drug Influences).
3. √ Patient knowledge; explain test (See Description/Procedure).

---

*Not discussed in this book.

Test:	Fecal Fat
Abbreviation:	None
Reference Value:	Below 7 g/24 hours
Specimen:	72-hour stool collection
Description:	Digestion of fats is mainly under the influence of the pancreatic enzyme, lipase. Bile salts, lecithin, and cholesterol emulsify the fats and encourage absorption. The principal site of absorption of fats is the small intestine. The study that is most reliable for determining fat digestion and absorption is the 72-hour collection for fecal fat. This study can document malabsorption or steatorrhea.
Procedure:	1. The patient should eat a 100 g fat diet for 3 days prior to and during the 3-day collection period. The patient should not drink alcohol during preparation or collection time.
	2. The patient collects all stool for 72 hours. Collection containers should be free of waxy surfaces.
	3. Samples are labeled with name, date, and time, and placed in the refrigerator until sent to the lab.

Conditions Related to Increases

Rationale

1. Malabsorption syndrome, examples of causes:

1. The inability of the intestinal mucosa to absorb nutrients with nutrient loss in the stool is considered malabsorption syndrome. Steatorrhea is excretion of more than 5 g of fat in 24 hours. A variety of conditions may cause this problem. The cause of malabsorption is either from pancreatic or biliary disease from intestinal malfunction.

   a. Gluten-sensitive enteropathy
      Tropical sprue
      Nonbacterial gastroenteritis
      Disaccharidase deficiency
      Abetalipoproteinemia

   a. Malabsorption is a result of disorders of the absorptive surface cells of the small bowel.

   b. Untreated pernicious anemia
      Folate deficiency
      Radiation to abdomen

   b. In these conditions the mucosal epithelium growth and repair is diminished.

c. Whipple's disease
   Food allergy
     diarrhea
   Intestinal lymphoma
   Regional enteritis
d. Gastric surgery
   Small bowel
     surgery
e. Hypothyroidism
   Diverticulitis
   Fistulas
   Chronic intestinal
     obstruction
f. Parasitic infestations

c. Damage to the connective tissue
   membrane beneath the mucous
   membrane discourages absorption
   of essential nutrients.

d. Reduced bile salts and with ileal resection.

e. Decreased intestinal motility may
   result in bacterial overgrowth. The
   overgrowth decreases bile salt and
   vitamin B_{12} availability.

f. The cause of steatorrrea with Giardia lamblia is unknown.

Drug Influences: The following drug groups may cause an increase in fecal fat:

Drug-induced malabsorption
   antibiotics; especially high dose or long term
   cathartics; chronic abuse

Related Lab Studies: Chronic malabsorption

   serum protein electrophoresis
   calcium, serum
   cholesterol
   electrolytes
   magnesium
   prothrombin time
   glucose tolerance test
   stool for trypsin
   5-HIAA

IMPLICATIONS FOR NURSING CARE
PRETEST: Factors related to the test
Nursing Diagnosis: Potential for injury related to changes in biochemical balance

Guide to assessment	Guide to planning and intervention	Guide to evaluation
Assess patient factors that may influence test results: 1. 100 g diet 3 days before test and during collection period.	1. Instruct patient about proper diet for test. Note inability of patient to consume diet on lab slip.	1. Patient consumes prescribed diet.

Guide to assessment	Guide to planning and intervention	Guide to evaluation

2. Drug history
    Antibiotics
    Cathartics
	2. Identify interfering drug groups. Note on lab slip.	2. Patient's interfering drugs are identified and noted on lab slip.

3. Preexisting conditions (See Increases)	3. Identify and note pertinent preexisting conditions on lab slip.	3. Patient's pertinent preexisting conditions are noted on lab slip.

4. Knowledge deficit	4. Explain test to patient:
	   a. Define test.
	   b. Explain procedure.
		4. The patient defines test and procedure.

5. Knowledge deficit Lost specimen	5. Communicate to staff and family members about stool collection.	5. Patient's specimens are not discarded.

Patient Preparation Checklist

1. √ Preparation diet followed; note on lab slip.
2. √ Note interfering drugs on lab slip.
3. √ Preexisting conditions (See Increases).
4. √ Patient knowledge; explain test to patient.
5. √ Staff informed to *save stools*.

CONSIDERATIONS FOR NURSING CARE RELATED TO ABNORMAL TEST RESULTS

POSTTEST: Factors related to the results of the test

Nursing Diagnosis: Alterations in nutrition related to malnutrition

Guide to assessment	Guide to planning and intervention	Guide to evaluation
Assess patient factors that may be influencing test results. Nursing history and/or physical exam that is suggestive of:		

1. Malabsorption
  Signs and symptoms
    Stools: large, frothy soft, light colored, sticky, oily appearance
    Weight loss
    Anemia
    Dependent edema
    ↓ Total protein
	1. Recognize signs and symptoms of fat malabsorption.
	  a. Describe stools carefully.
	  b. Consult with physician.
		1. The patient's malabsorption of fat is recognized.

Test:	Fibrinogen
Abbreviation:	None
Reference Values:	Newborn: 160–300 mg/dl Children and adults: 200–400 mg/dl Values vary with laboratory
Specimen:	Plasma

Description: Fibrinogen is synthesized in the liver and is at the end stage of clot formation. Thrombin splits fibrinogen to form fibrin that then normally becomes a stable clot. A test performed that determines the amount of fibrinogen available for fibrin formation is the plasma fibrinogen test. Thrombin is added to a plasma sample to form a clot. The amount of fibrinogen protein in the clot is determined. A result of under 100 mg/dl is evidence of severe fibrinogen abnormality. The test is done to evaluate clotting disorders and in the differential diagnosis of DIC and liver disease.

Procedure: (blue top tube)
1. No food or fluid restrictions.
2. Fill a vacuum blood tube completely full; gently tip the tube back and forth to mix the anticoagulant.
3. Observe puncture site carefully for bleeding or evidence of hematoma.
4. Send to laboratory immediately for analysis.

Conditions Related to Increases

1. Pregnancy
   Oral contraceptives

2. Postoperatively
   Inflammatory diseases
   Malignancies

Rationale

1. Increases, as do all plasma proteins, progressively through pregnancy. Oral contraceptives have pseudopregnancy effect.

2. Fibrinogen is considered an acute phase reactant. Acute phase reactants are proteins whose concentrations increase or decrease with inflammatory stimulus (11).

Conditions Related to Decreases

1. Factor I deficiency
   (fibrinogen)

2. Disseminated intravascular
   coagulation (DIC)
   Associated with
   Obstetrical conditions
   Neoplastic diseases

Rationale

1. This condition is marked by absence of fibrinogen or a reduction in the protein. Dysfibrinogenemia is a condition in which the protein is an abnormal variant of fibrinogen.

2. This complex condition reduces fibrinogen dramatically. This is due to alteration of fibrinolytic proteins. Plasmin is released in reaction to the presence of fibrin in microcirculation.

Hemolytic responses
Extensive tissue damage
Fat emboli
Acute infections

(Plasmin is a proteolytic enzyme.) The plasmin acts on the fibrinogen and fibrin to release fibrinogen/fibrin degradation products. The degradation products retain some anticoagulant activity and high levels of the products in the blood increase fibrinolysis.

3. Liver disease
   Congestive heart failure

3. Fibrinogen is synthesized in the liver.

Drug Influences: The following drugs may influence test results. The drugs are listed alphabetically by generic name and divided into columns according to the effect of the drug. Examples of trade names are in parentheses.

The following drugs may cause an increase in test results:

Metabolic effect
aspirin
estrogens (Premarin)
oral contraceptives
oxandrolone (Anavar)
oxymetholone (Anadrol-50)

The following drugs may cause a decrease in test results.

Metabolic effect
anabolic steroids
testosterone (Android-T)

Hepatotoxic effect
phosphorus (Thiacide tablets)

Complex formation
dextran (Macrodex)

Miscellaneous
asparaginase (Elspar)
kanamycin (Kantrex)
streptokinase (Streptase); in infarct patients
sucrose; sustained high sucrose diet
trifluoroethyl vinyl ether (Fluroxene)

Related Lab Studies: Hemostatic profile:
bleeding time
platelet count
activated partial thromboplastin time (APTT)
thrombin time
Hct
prothrombin time

IMPLICATIONS FOR NURSING CARE
PRETEST: Factors related to the test
Nursing Diagnosis: Potential for injury related to predisposition for bleeding and/or thrombus formation

Guide to assessment	Guide to planning and intervention	Guide to evaluation
Assess patient factors that may influence test results.		
1. Comprehensive drug history (See Drug Influences) Anticoagulant therapy	1. Identify influencing drugs and note on lab slip: a. Identify and note the following on lab slip: (1) Name of anticoagulant. (2) Route. (3) Dosage. (4) Time of last dosage.	1. Patient's test value is not influenced by unidentified interfering drug.
2. Preexisting conditions Known coagulation disorder See Increases/Decreases	2. Identify preexisting conditions and note on lab slip.	2. Patient's conditions pertinent to lab test are noted on lab slip.
3. Hemolysis	3. Prevent hemolysis: a. Not saturating the skin with antiseptic. b. Not probing venipuncture site or leaving the tourniquet on too long. c. Not forcefully withdrawing specimen. d. Not withdrawing specimen too slowly. e. Not agitating or handling specimen roughly.	3. Patient's values are not influenced by hemolysis.
4 Knowledge deficit Patient	4. Explain test to patient. a. Define test; anticoagulant monitoring or coagulation screening. b. Explain procedure.	4. The patient demonstrates knowledge by defining test and stating procedure.
5. Knowledge deficit Staff	5. Be informed about coagulation studies and anticoagulant medication schedule. Patients on full heparin therapy are tested at least once a day.	5. The patient's coagulation time is not abnormal due to staff error.

Patient Preparation Checklist

1. √ Interfering medications.
2. √ Anticoagulant, dose, time noted on lab slip.
3. √ Pertinent preexisting conditions noted on lab slip.
4. √ Patient knowledge; explain test to patient.

CONSIDERATIONS FOR NURSING CARE RELATED TO ABNORMAL TEST RESULTS

POSTTEST: Factors related to the results of the test
Nursing Diagnosis: Alterations in blood profile

Guide to assessment	Guide to planning and intervention	Guide to evaluation
Assess patient factors that may be influencing test results. Nursing history and/or physical exam that is suggestive of:		
1. Factor I deficiency	1. Replace deficient fibrinogen by: a. Assisting in starting plasma or concentrated preparations. b. Initiating nursing measures for successful completion of replacement therapy. c. Being alert to signs of bleeding.	1. The patient achieves a fibrinogen level of at least 80–100 mg/dl.
2. Liver disease	2. Replace deficient vitamin K to encourage synthesis of fibrinogen and other clotting factors by: a. Offering nutritious diet. b. Encouraging rest. c. Discouraging alcohol intake if appropriate.	2. The patient maintains sufficient fibrinogen level to prevent bleeding.

Guide to assessment	Guide to planning and intervention	Guide to evaluation

3. DIC
  Lab studies
    ↑ PT
    ↑ APTT
    ↓ Fibrinogen
    ↓ Platelet count
  Fibrin split products
  a. Obstetrical conditions
    Neoplastic disease
    Hemolytic responses
    Extensive tissue damage
    Fat emboli
    Acute infections
	3. Discourage consumption of coagulation factors by:
	
	a. Being alert to conditions that may stimulate DIC.
	b. Being alert to signs of bleeding.
	c. Initiating medical plan of care to treat underlying cause.
	d. Administering heparin as prescribed.
		3. Patient's lab values return to normal and patient's condition improves.

Test:	Fluorescent Treponemal Antibody Absorption Test
Abbreviation:	FTA-ABS
Reference Value:	Negative
Specimen:	Serum, CSF
Description:	Syphilis is a sexually transmitted disease caused by the spirochete *Treponema pallidum*. It is a disease that is easily treated, but sometimes diagnosis requires more than the commonly used flocculation tests.

After infection from *T. pallidum*, antibodies are formed. Identification of these specific syphilitic antibodies can be made by doing the fluorescent treponemal antibody absorption test. The test is complex and in the past has been used mostly in patients difficult to diagnose.

FTA-ABS is used to diagnose very early or very late syphilis. It is not useful following therapy because the treponemal antibodies are usually not removed by antibiotic therapy.

Procedure:	(red top tube)
	1. No food or fluid restriction.
	2. About 10 ml of blood is drawn from the patient.
	3. Observe puncture site for bleeding or evidence of hematoma.

Conditions Related to Positive Findings	Rationale
1. Syphilis	1. The identification of the treponemal antibody confirms its presence. The presence of treponemal antibody does not identify the stage of disease. The test may be done to confirm reinfection.
2. Pinta Yaws Bejel	2. These are all *Treponema* spirochetic diseases and may cause a reactive FTA-ABS result.

IMPLICATIONS FOR NURSING CARE
PRETEST: Factors related to the test
Nursing Diagnosis: Potential for injury related to changes in microbiological environment

Guide to assessment	Guide to planning and intervention	Guide to evaluation

Assess patient factors that may influence test results:
1. Knowledge deficit
    Patient
	1. Explain test to patient:
	    a. Define test (See Description).
	    b. Explain procedure (See Procedure).
		1. The patient demonstrates knowledge by defining test and stating procedure.

Guide to assessment	Guide to planning and intervention	Guide to evaluation
2. Hemolysis	2. Prevent hemolysis by: a. Not probing venipuncture site. b. Not forcefully withdrawing specimen. c. Not agitating specimen. d. Not saturating skin with antiseptic. e. Not withdrawing specimen too slowly.	2. Patient's test results are not influenced by hemolysis.
3. Knowledge deficit Public about sexually transmitted diseases (STD)	3. Promote public awareness about STD by: a. Being knowledgeable about the diseases. b. Educating patients with STD about the diseases, diagnosis, and treatment. c. Being knowledgeable about treatment facility options available (private and free clinics). d. Informing patient that while condoms afford some protection against disease, there is still risk involved. e. Informing patient that reporting the disease and case finding are important steps in preventing spread of disease. f. Advising patient that treatment of known contacts of someone with diagnosed STD is a method of prevention of spread of disease. g. Informing patients that infants of mothers with untreated syphilis are born with congenital syphilis. h. Encouraging public education about STD.	3. Statistics on STD improve.

Patient Preparation Checklist

1. √ Patient knowledge; see 1 and 3 above.
2. √ Prevent hemolysis of specimen (See 2 above).

CONSIDERATIONS FOR NURSING CARE RELATED TO ABNORMAL TEST RESULTS
POSTTEST: Factors related to the results of the test
Nursing Diagnosis: Alterations in microbiological environment

Guide to assessment	Guide to planning and intervention	Guide to evaluation

Assess patient factors that may be influencing test results:
Nursing history and/or physical exam suggestive of:
1. Syphilis
	1. Establish diagnosis and treatment of disease:
	  a. Referring patient for FTA-ABS test.
	  b. Administering antibiotic as prescribed.
	  c. Following patient response to therapy with follow-up VDRL.
	  d. See 3 Pretest.
		1. Patient's positive VDRL test results revert to negative.

Test:	Folic Acid
Abbreviation:	None
Reference Values:	2–14 ng/ml
Specimen:	Serum
Description:	Folic acid, or folacin, is a vitamin found in many food sources. Foods high in folic acid include mushrooms, dark green leafy vegetables, kidney, and liver. Folic acid is also found in yeast, dairy products, and fruits, especially oranges. Folic acid is water-soluble and heat-labile. Overcooking or prolonged boiling destroys the vitamin. Folic acid functions in the formation of nucleic acids, helps in the degradation of amino acids, in the synthesis of some nonessential amino acids, and functions as a coenzyme for numerous cellular reactions. A deficiency of folic acid causes a macrocytic normochromic anemia.
Procedure:	(red top tube) 1. Food and fluids are restricted 8 hours. 2. For folic acid test, up to 2 ml of blood is drawn from the patient. 3. Observe puncture site for bleeding or evidence of hematoma.

Conditions Related to Decreases

1. Malabsorption

2. Alcoholism

3. Pregnancy
   Infancy (rare in U.S.)
4. Malnutrition; any cause, e.g.,
   Elderly "tea and toast" syndrome
   Anorexia nervosa
   Overly cooked food
   Starvation
   Folic acid-poor diet

Rationale

1. Because folic acid absorption takes place primarily in the jejunum, malabsorption decreases metabolism and absorption of the nutrient.

2. Not only is there decreased folic acid intake due to accompanying malnutrition, but also alcohol interferes with the reduction of folic acid by intestinal enzymes to its active form. See 4.

3. Increased growth requirements require increased folic acid replacement.

4. Decreased intake of dietary folic acid leads to folic acid deficiency. Overcooking food or prolonged storage destroys the vitamin.

Drug Influences: The following drugs may influence test results. The drugs are listed alphabetically by generic name and divided into columns according to the effect of the drug. Examples of trade names are in parentheses.

The following drugs may cause an increase in test results:

Impaired absorption of B_{12}
   metformin

The following drugs may cause a decrease in test results:

Impaired absorption with possible megaloblastic anemia

anticonvulsants (many)	methotrexate (Mexate)
arsenicals	nitrofurans (Macrodantin)
barbiturates	oral contraceptives
cycloserine (Seromycin)	primidone (Mysoline)
diphenylhydantoin (Dilantin)	pyrimethamine (Daraprim)
ethanol (grain alcohol)	triamterene (Dyrenium)

Related Lab Studies: Monitor response to therapy or progress of disease and adjust nursing care accordingly. See individual tests for information.

vitamin B_{12}, serum	↓ reticulocytes
Schilling test	↑ LDH
RBC	↑ bilirubin
RBC indices	↓ WBC (slight)
↑ MCV	↓ platelets (slight)
MCH	electrolytes
MCHC	bone marrow

IMPLICATIONS FOR NURSING CARE
PRETEST: Factors related to the test
Nursing Diagnosis: Alterations in nutrition related to less than body requirements

Guide to assessment	Guide to planning and intervention	Guide to evaluation
Assess patient factors that may influence test results.		
1. NPO	1. Place patient NPO for 8 hours.	1. The patient is NPO.
2. Comprehensive drug history (See Drug Influences)	2. Identify and note on lab slip drugs that interfere with folic acid absorption.	2. Patient's medications do not interfere with test results.
3. Preexisting conditions (See Decreases)	3. Identify and note on lab slip patient's conditions that may influence test results.	3. Patient's conditions pertinent to test are identified and noted on lab slip.
4. Knowledge deficit	4. Explain test to patient: a. Define folic acid (See Description). b. Explain procedure (See Procedure).	4. The patient demonstrates knowledge by defining test and explaining procedure.

Patient Preparation Checklist

1. √ Patient NPO for 8 hours.
2. √ Interfering drugs and note on lab slip.
3. √ Preexisting conditions noted on lab slip (See Decreases).
4. √ Patient knowledge; explain test to patient.

CONSIDERATIONS FOR NURSING CARE RELATED TO ABNORMAL TEST RESULTS
POSTTEST: Factors related to the results of the test
Nursing Diagnosis: Alterations in nutrition related to nutrient deficiency

Guide to assessment	Guide to planning and intervention	Guide to evaluation
Assess patient factors that may be influencing test results. Nursing history and/or physical exam that is suggestive of: 1. Probable folic acid deficiency	1. Correct folic acid deficiency by:	1. The patient's megaloblastic anemia is corrected by folic acid replacement.

a. Patients at risk
  Pregnancy
  Infancy (rarely in U.S.)
  Aged: living alone
  Alcoholism
  Malabsorption/malnutrition problems
  Folic acid antagonist therapy
  Patients on prolonged Dilantin therapy
  Oral contraceptive use
	a. Being aware of patients at high risk for development of folic acid deficiency.	

b. Signs and symptoms
  Sore inflamed tongue, "beefy" red
  Diarrhea
  Fatigue
  Pallor
  Dyspnea
  Edema of legs
Daily folic acid requirements:
  Infants 50 μg
  Gradually increase to Preadolescence 400 μg
	b. Detecting signs of folic acid deficiency. Consult with physician.
	c. Encouraging maximum dietary folic acid utilization.
	  (1) Identify for patient foods high in folic acid: fruits, leafy vegetables, grains, milk, liver, yeast, eggs, meats (See Description).
	  (2) Instruct patient not to overcook foods.	

Guide to assessment	Guide to planning and intervention	Guide to evaluation
Adults 600 µg	(3) Refer to dietician for consultation. (4) Explain to alcoholic patient interaction of alcohol on folic acid. (5) Remind parents that goat's milk is very low in folic acid and infants fed goat's milk should have commercial or dietary supplement. d. Give folic acid preparation as prescribed.	
e. Methotrexate therapy Folic acid antagonist	e. Keep calcium leucovorin on hand for emergency treatment of toxicity.	

See RBC count and MCV for more information concerning macrocytic normochromic anemia.

Test:	Gamma-Glutamyl Transpeptidase
Abbreviation:	GGTP or GGT
Reference Values:	*Males*
	12–38 milliunits/ml
	4–23 IU/liter
	Females
	9–31 milliunits/ml
	3.5–13 IU/liter (5)
Specimen:	Serum

Description: Gamma-glutamyl transpeptidase is an enzyme responsible for transport of amino acids and peptides across cell membranes. The highest concentrations are found in the kidney, pancreas, and liver. It is also found in the spleen, lungs, brain, intestine, heart, and prostate and salivary glands (5, 21). The test is a sensitive indicator of liver disease, with the most marked elevations occurring in cases of biliary obstruction and hepatocarcinoma. GGTP levels rise early in most hepatic diseases with elevations persisting as long as cellular derangements last (26). GGTP is also the most sensitive indicator of alcoholism (21). GGTP levels may be useful for those working in alcoholic rehabilitation programs to assess recent alcohol ingestion. Values do not return to normal until 2–3 weeks after regular alcohol intake ceases.

Procedure: (red top tube)
1. There are no food or fluid restrictions for this test.
2. 5–10 ml of blood is drawn from the patient.
3. Observe for bleeding at venipuncture site or for evidence of hematoma.

Conditions Related to Increases	**Rationale**
1. Cirrhosis of liver Hepatitis Carcinoma of liver Intrahepatic cholestasis	1. GGTP is derived from cells that line the smallest radicles of the biliary tract. Disturbance of these cells causes increased release of this enzyme with the greatest increases seen in obstructive liver disease.
2. Biliary duct obstruction Gallstones Obstructive tumors	2. See 1.
3. Pancreatitis	3. Some GGTP is found in the pancreas and released during cellular damage.

4. Carcinoma of head of pancreas

4. GGTP is released from the pancreas when there is tissue damage. Carcinoma may cause compression and obstruction of the common bile duct, which causes further release of GGTP from the enzyme-rich cells in the biliary tract.

5. Kidney diseases
   Nephrosis
   Renal neoplasia
   Rejection of renal transplant
   Hemodialysis

5. Elevations occur because fair amounts of GGTP exist in the brush borders of renal tubular cells.

6. Myocardial infarct and angina

6. The enzyme is present in the heart and is released when cellular damage occurs. Elevations can also reflect the effects of cardiac insufficiency on the liver. GGTP remains normal for the first 3–4 days after the MI, then rises, reaching a peak in about 10 days (5).

7. Congestive heart failure

7. GGTP is present in the heart and is released when cellular damage occurs. CHF may cause obstruction of normal hepatic blood flow leading to congestion of small bile duct radicles that contain large amounts of GGTP.

8. Cancer of prostate

8. Small amounts of GGTP are present in the prostate.

9. Alcohol ingestion

9. Alcohol is thought to cause necrosis of liver cells that then release increased amounts of GGTP when damaged. Alcohol is also thought to induce microsomial enzyme release. GGTP is a microsomial enzyme (44).

10. Epilepsy and brain tumors

10. Increase is seen in some patients with epilepsy and brain tumors. This is because small amounts of GGTP are present in brain cells.

Conditions Related to Decreases

1. Pregnancy, third trimester

Rationale

1. GGTP levels run 50% lower in pregnant women than in nonpregnant women. This is probably due to the sluggishness of the gastrointestinal system, especially during the last trimester.

Drug Influences: The following drugs may influence test results. The drugs are listed alphabetically by generic name and divided into columns according to the effect of the drug. Examples of trade names are in parentheses.

The following drugs may cause an increase in test results:

Enzyme induction
  barbiturates
  phenytoin (Dilantin)

Liver damage (other liver function tests normal)
  ethanol (grain alcohol)

Liver tumors
  metrizoate

Poisoning
  acetaminophen (Tylenol)

Miscellaneous
  streptokinase (Streptase)

No drugs have been reported to cause decreased test results (47).

Related Lab Studies: Monitor response to treatment or progression of disease and adjust nursing care accordingly. See individual tests for information.

Liver function studies, indicating liver disease
  ↑ serum bilirubin
  ↑ urine bilirubin
  ↓ albumin
  ↓ total protein
  ↑ prothrombin time (PT)
  ↑ or ↓ cholesterol
  ↑ AST (SGOT)
  ↑ ALT (SGPT)
  ↑ alkaline phosphatase
   *bile acids radio immunoassay
  ↑ serum ammonium
  ↓ *BSP excretion

---

*Not discussed in this book.

IMPLICATIONS FOR NURSING CARE
PRETEST: Factors related to the test
Nursing Diagnosis: Potential for injury related to changes in biochemical balance

Guide to assessment	Guide to planning and intervention	Guide to evaluation
Assess patient factors that may influence test results: 1. Comprehensive drug history (See Drug Influences) Ingestion of alcohol in past 2–3 weeks	1. Report to lab and physician drugs the patient is receiving that may influence lab results. Identify on lab slip and report to the physician amount of alcohol intake by the patient over the past 3 weeks.	1. Drugs and/or alcohol patient is currently receiving or has received that may influence lab results are identified and the appropriate people are notified.
2. Preexisting conditions (See Increases/Decreases) 3. Knowledge deficit	2. Record preexisting conditions on lab slip. 3. Explain test to patient: a. Define test (see Description). b. Explain procedure (see Procedure).	2. Patient's preexisting conditions are noted on lab slip. 3. Patient demonstrates knowledge of test by defining test and stating procedure.

Patient Preparation Checklist

1. √ Influencing drugs or alcohol ingestion noted and reported (See Drug Influences).
2. √ Preexisting conditions noted on lab slip.
3. √ Test explained to patient (See Description/Procedure).

CONSIDERATIONS FOR NURSING CARE RELATED TO ABNORMAL TEST RESULTS
POSTTEST: Factors related to the results of the test
Nursing Diagnosis: Alterations in biochemical balance

Guide to assessment	Guide to planning and intervention	Guide to evaluation
1. Nursing history and/or physical exam suggestive of liver dysfunction or bile duct obstruction: Liver enlargement Jaundice Clay-colored stool Dark urine Water retention/ascites Level of consciousness Irritability Seizure activity Bleeding tendencies	1. Prevent further liver damage by monitoring status and adjusting care to: a. Protect patient from excessive liver palpation by students and staff. b. Measure and adjust nutritional intake according to water retention and ascites. c. Increase protein and carbohydrate intake if status allows.	1. The patient is protected against further liver damage: a. Liver palpation is minimized. b. Water retention and ascites are controlled by the measurement and adjustment of patient intake; intake and output balanced; abdominal girth stable.
2. Nursing history and/or physical exam suggestive of pancreatic disease: Increase in peritoneal fluid Vomiting	2. Reduce pancreatic irritation by: a. Giving prescribed anticholinergic drugs and maintaining NPO, gastric suction, fluid intake treatment plan.	2. The patient demonstrates reduced pancreatic stimulation by: a. Reduced abdominal distention.
b. Pain, abdominal and back, boring, bandlike and constant in nature. Also: Flushing of face Diaphoresis Thready pulse	b. Giving pain medication and/or smooth muscle relaxants as needed (not morphine or its derivatives) and ordered; help patient assume position of comfort.	b. The patient verbalizes decreased pain sensation after medication.
3. Nursing history and/or physical exam indicative of alcohol ingestion (See 1, Liver Dysfunction)	3. Prevent further liver damage by: Teaching person importance of abstaining from alcohol and encouraging participation in alcohol rehabilitation program as necessary.	3. The patient states understanding of importance of abstaining from alcohol and expresses willingness to do so.

Test:	Glucose Tests
	   Blood Glucose
	   Random Glucose
	   Fasting Blood Sugar
	   2-Hour Postprandial Blood Sugar
	   Glucose Tolerance Test

Abbreviation:	FBS (fasting blood sugar) 2°PP or 2°PPBS (2-hour postprandial blood sugar or 2°P.C. [post-cibum]) *GTT (Glucose Tolerance Test)
Reference Values:	†Serum (11, 34) Premature infant 30–80 mg/dl Full term infant 40–90 mg/dl Child–adult 60–115 mg/dl
Specimen:	Serum
Description:	Glucose is the major monosaccharide in the body. Fructose and galactose monosaccharides are represented in much smaller proportions. These monosaccharides are the source of body fuel. They come from the breakdown of carbohydrates in the diet. Carbohydrates are consumed and then broken down by gastrointestinal enzymes from polysaccharides to monosaccharides and absorbed. Glucose is taken up by hepatic cells and stored as glycogen. Glucose is utilized by peripheral tissues as well.

The liver helps to regulate blood glucose by taking up glucose, storing glucose as glycogen, and then converting glycogen, with the help of enzymes, back to glucose. The liver is capable of converting other saccharides to glucose. It is also involved in the process of glyconeogenesis or the synthesis of glucose from protein or fat breakdown.

Several hormones are involved in blood glucose concentration. Insulin is a pancreatic hormone and lowers blood glucose by making possible the transfer of glucose across the cell membrane. Glucagon and somatostatin are also pancreatic hormones that help to regulate glucose metabolism. Other hormones in glucose metabolism are thyroid, glucocorticoids, epinephrine, and growth hormone. These hormones generally increase blood glucose.

Most glucose is metabolized to carbon dioxide and water. The glucose that is not metabolized is filtered through the glomeruli and most of that is reabsorbed in the renal tubules. If the blood sugar is above 160 mg–180 mg, the renal threshold is reached and glucose is excreted in the urine.

Several blood studies are done to determine the blood glucose level. *Fasting blood sugar* is a test done as a diabetic screening

---

*Reference values for GTT should be from local lab. Values depend on age of patient, lab method and patient preparation.

†Values on whole blood may be lower. Check local laboratory for reference values.

test or as a measure to observe control of the diabetic patient. Normal values do not rule out diabetes because research indicates that the diagnosis of about 30–40% of patients with diabetes can be missed using this method. A test more sensitive to carbohydrate metabolism imbalances is the *2-hour postprandial blood sugar test*. The patient is challenged by a high carbohydrate load. If blood glucose is not normal in 2 hours after ingesting a carbohydrate load, the test is repeated. This is a test used to detect diabetes, not hypoglycemia. The *oral glucose tolerance test* is a 3- to 5-hour test. It is used to evaluate insulin response to a carbohydrate load and can be used in the diagnosis of diabetes and hypoglycemia. The normal curve is a blood glucose peak at .5–1 hour after a glucose load with a gradual decline to fasting levels by the third hour. In finding reference values for GTT it is most important to use local laboratory values as method and age influence numerical test values.

Procedure: (gray-top tube)

Fasting Blood Sugar

1. No food or fluids other than water for 12–14 hours prior to the test.
2. Withhold insulin or antidiabetic agent until after blood is drawn.
3. Up to 5 ml of blood is drawn from the patient. Capillary blood may be utilized; values will be 2–3 mg/dl higher.
4. Observe site for bleeding or evidence of hematoma.

2-Hour Postprandial Blood Sugar

1. The patient consumes a high carbohydrate diet 2–3 days prior to test.
2. No food or fluids other than water for 12–14 hours prior to the test.
3. The patient receives either a 100 g carbohydrate diet or 100 g glucose load by mouth.
4. Exactly 2 hours after meal or glucose load is ingested, up to 5 ml of blood is drawn from the patient. Capillary blood samples after the carbohydrate load are considerably higher than venous concentration (34).
5. Observe site for bleeding or evidence of hematoma.

Glucose Tolerance Test

1. The patient consumes a high carbohydrate diet (minimum 150g/day) 2–3 days prior to testing.
2. This test should be performed on ambulatory patients.
3. Hold, if possible, drugs such as salicylates, diuretics, and anticonvulsants 3 days prior to testing. Oral contraceptives should be discontinued for one complete cycle prior to testing (11). Insulin or hypoglycemic agents should be withheld until after test. If they must be given it must be noted on lab slip.

4. Up to 5 ml of blood is withdrawn from the patient. Capillary blood may be used; after carbohydrate loading, values are considerably higher than for venous blood (34).

5. The patient is given a loading dose of glucose. Dosage is calculated by body surface area for adults and per kilograms in children.

6. Blood specimens are obtained after .5 hour and then every hour for 3–5 hours (5 specimens for 3 hour; 7 specimens for 5 hour GTT).

7. The patient may be asked to give urine samples at each blood drawing.

8. The patient should report any symptoms of headache, nervousness, lightheadedness, restlessness, sweating, and hunger.

9. The patient should refrain from smoking or exercise during the test. The patient should be encouraged to drink water.

10. Observe for bleeding or hematoma at puncture site.

Conditions Related to Increases

1. Diabetes mellitus
   Insulin dependent (Type I)
   Noninsulin dependent (Type II)
   Other types (secondary to other conditions or syndromes)

2. Stress
   Infections
   Convulsions
   Acute injury
   Emotional stress
   Hypothermia
   Severe pain
   Myocardial infarction
   Dehydration
   Shock

3. HHNK
   (Hyperglycemic hyperosmolar non-ketonic coma)
   Diabetes mellitus
   Acute stress

Rationale

1. In order to be a source of energy for the body, glucose must be within the cell. Insulin is the hormone responsible for facilitating the transport of glucose into cells. In diabetes there is insufficient insulin or there is insulin resistance to metabolize glucose properly. The result is high blood glucose. Insulin insufficiency in juvenile diabetics (Type I) is severe with wide fluctuations in blood sugar.

2. Blood glucose levels increase during periods of stress because of the body's stress adaptive mechanism. Glycogenolysis is stimulated and insulin release is blocked by the increased circulating adrenaline. This results in increased blood glucose.

3. A condition with pronounced hyperglycemia and with minimal to no ketosis present. This condition may occur in any patient with continued increased blood glucose, dehydra-

Pancreatectomy
Glucocorticoid therapy
Burns
Hemodialysis
Hyperalimentation (poorly monitored)

tion, and electrolyte imbalance. The increased blood glucose or inability to metabolize glucose completely causes hyperglycemia leading to osmotic diuresis that causes severe dehydration and plasma hyperosmolality. Because of the hypovolemia there is diminished renal blood flow and this decreases glucose excretion, further compounding the hyperosmolality.

4. Glucocorticoid excess
   Cushing's disease
   Adrenogenital syndrome
   Cortisone therapy

4. Any condition that causes an increase in glucocorticoid levels will cause an increase in blood glucose. Glucocorticoids influence the breaking down of protein to amino acids and their synthesis into glucose. Glucocorticoids may also decrease cellular utilization of glucose. See Drug Influences.

5. Hyperthyroidism
   Thyrotoxicosis

5. These conditions increase the rate of reabsorption of glucose by the intestine and kidney so blood glucose increases. In thyrotoxicosis there may also be an increase of blood glucose due to stress response. It is also possible that the thyroid hormone will increase the metabolic rate sufficiently that readily available glucose is used up, in which case there may be decreased blood glucose.

6. Acromegaly

6. Growth hormone is secreted by the anterior lobe of the pituitary gland. It is also known as somatotropic hormone. It is thought that growth hormone decreases cellular utilization of glucose and also causes the cells to be resistant to insulin. This will cause an increase in blood glucose.

7. Pituitary gland disorders
   Brain lesions

7. Trauma to the hypothalamus or the pituitary gland may result in disruption of the pituitary-adrenocortical mechanism. ACTH is released by the anterior pituitary gland. ACTH, in turn, controls the release of glucocorticoids. Glucocorticoids influence gluconeogenesis. They may also de-

crease cellular utilization of glucose and these factors will cause an increase in blood glucose. Thyroid-stimulating hormone (TSH) and growth hormone are also released by the pituitary gland.

Conditions Related to Decreases

1. Glycogen storage disease
   Glucose-6-phosphate dehydrogenase deficiency

2. Advanced liver disease
   Alcoholic cirrhosis

3. Anterior pituitary hypofunction

4. Adrenal cortical hypofunction

5. Pancreatic tumors
   (Insulinomas)

6. Excessive insulin

7. Leucine sensitivity
   Maple syrup disease

Rationale

1. In this condition certain enzymes needed for glycogenolysis are deficient. Glucose can be stored but not returned to the blood and blood glucose decreases.

2. In advanced liver disease glycogen stores are diminished and the diseased liver has a reduced capacity for glyconeogenesis.

3. The anterior pituitary gland is responsible for releasing growth hormone, ACTH and thyroid-releasing hormone (TSH). All of these hormones have an effect on carbohydrate metabolism. Decreased amounts of these hormones result in decreased renal and intestinal reabsorption of glucose, decreased gluconeogenesis, and increased insulin activity.

4. Decreased glucocorticoids decrease intestinal absorption of glucose and gluconeogenesis.

5. These tumors produce large amounts of insulin-like activity resulting in low blood glucose.

6. Hypoglycemia may result from poorly regulated insulin dosage, missed meals, and strenuous activity.

7. Due to high concentrations of leucine, which interferes with gluconeogenesis.

8. Galactosemia

8. Hypoglycemia is a characteristic of this rare inborn error of metabolism. This disease must be diagnosed at birth or the hypoglycemia can result in mental retardation. Newborn infants are screened for this disease in most states along with PKU testing.

9. Newborn hypoglycemia

9. Probably due to the rapid absorption of carbohydrates resulting in insulin release. The insulin continues to be released even after the source of peripheral glucose is gone.

10. Newborn hypoglycemia from diabetic mother

10. The newborn's pancreas may continue to secrete insulin after birth in response to maternal hyperglycemia.

11. Reye's syndrome

11. In children under 5 years of age, hypoglycemia is common with this condition. This is probably due to cellular changes within the liver and depleted glycogen stores.

12. Reactive hypoglycemia

12. This is the hypoglycemia that occurs after meals. It is classified as follows:
    a. Functional—associated with emotional stress and epinephrine release.
    b. Prediabetic—these patients may develop diabetes mellitus. Insulin release is delayed after meals but exaggerated upon release.
    c. Alimentary—occurs after gastrointestinal surgery. Rapid absorption of glucose stimulates insulin overproduction, rapid peripheral glucose depletion, and hypoglycemia.

13. Old specimen
    Unrefrigerated specimen

13. Glycolysis occurs and makes glucose values inappropriate within .5 hour if serum is used. The specimen should be taken to the lab immediately.

Drug Influences: A great many drugs interfere with glucose test values. Listed below are some of the drugs that may influence test results. The drugs are listed alphabetically by generic name and divided into columns according to the effect of the drug. Example of trade names are in parentheses.

The following drugs may cause an increase in test results:

Serum

Diabetogenic effect
chlorothiazide (Diuril)
chlorthalidone (Hygroton)
ethacrynic acid (Edecrin)
furosemide (Lasix)
glucocorticoids (Celestone)
hydrochlorothiazide (Esidrix)
hydroflumethiazide (Diucardin)

methyclothiazide (Enduron)
metolazone (Diulo)
polythiazide (Renese)
prednisone
triamcinolone (Aristocort)
trichlormethiazide (Diurese)

Hyperglycemia by glycogenolysis
dopamine
glucagon (glucagon for injection)

isoniazid (Laniazid)
levodopa (Sinemet)

Metabolic, hormonal, and/or endocrine effect
chlorprothixene (Taractan)
cyclic AMP
dextroamphetamine (Delcobese)
epinephrine (Adrenalin Chloride)
estrogens
ether
fludrocortisone (Florinef)
fluoxymesterone (Halotestin)
glucose
haloperidol (Haldol)
isoproterenol (Isuprel)
maltose

medroxyprogesterone (Depo-Provera)
meperidine (Demerol)
meprednisone (Betapar)
nicotine
nortriptyline (Aventyl)
oxyphenbutazone (Oxalid)
phenothiazines
phenylbutazone (Butazolidin)
phenytoin (Dilantin)
piperacetazine (Quide)
thyroid preparations

Decreased tolerance to glucose
aluminum nicotinate (nicotinic acid)
phenelzine (Nardil)
phenolphthalein (Phenolax)

Miscellaneous
amino acids; IV infusion only
aminosalicylic acid; prolonged therapy
anesthetic agents

chlorpromazine (Thorazine)
reserpine (Diupres)

Glucose Tolerance Test

Curve altered in diabetic direction.

Diabetogenic-like effect
chlorothiazide (Diuril)
chlorthalidone (Hygroton)
furosemide (Lasix)

hydrochlorothiazide (Esidrix)
hydroflumethiazide (Diucardin)
triamterene (Dyrenium)

Reduced insulin release
    caffeine; non diabetic
    corticotropin (Acthar)

diphenylhydantoin (Dilantin)
glucagon

Decreased carbohydrate tolerance
    dexamethasone (Decadron-LA)
    methandrostenolone (Dianabol)
    methylprednisolone (Medrol)

paramethasone (Haldrone)
niacin (nicotines), in diabetics

Gluconeogenesis
    cortisone (Cortistan)

norethynodrel (Enovid-E)

Metabolic, hormonal, and/or endocrine effect
    estrogens (Premarin)
    ethinyl estradiol (Brevicon)
    fludrocortisone (Florinef)

oral contraceptives
prednisolone (Deltasone)
triamcinolone (Aristocort)

Miscellaneous
    chlorpromazine (Thorazine)
    ethanol (grain alcohol)
    nicotinyl alcohol (Roniacol)

perphenazine (Triavil)
phenolphthalein (Sarolax)
phenothiazines (Compazine)

Urine

Diabetogenic-like effect
    chlorothiazide (Diuril)
    chlorthalidone (Hygroton)
    furosemide (Lasix)

hydrochlorothiazide (Esidrix)
trichlormethiazide (Diurese)

Fanconi-like syndrome
    mercury compounds
    tetracycline (Achromycin)

Inhibition of insulin secretion
    diphenylhydantoin (Dilantin)

Nephrotoxic effect
    lead
    turpentine

Glycosuria with induced hyperglycemia
    aminosalicylic acid
    corticosteroids (Celestone)
    dextrothyroxine (Choloxin)
    ether

growth hormone
isoniazid (Laniazid)
niacin (Nicotinex)

The following drugs may cause a decrease in test results:

Hepatotoxic effect
    allopurinol (Lopurin)
    antimony compounds
    arsenicals
    benzene
    carbon tetrachloride

chloroform
erythromycin (Ilosone)
lincomycin (Lincocin)
pargyline (Eutonyl)
phentolamine (Regitine)

Increased insulin secretion by sufonylurea derivative
acetohexamide (Dymelor)   tolazamide (Tolinase)
chlorpropamide (Diabinese)

Anabolic effect
anabolic steroids   nandrolone (Anabolin)
androgens   oxandrolone (Anavar)
methandrostenolone (Dianabol)   oxymetholone (Adroyd)

Therapeutic effect of drug
guanethidine (Ismelin)   tolbutamide (Orinase)
insulin

Metabolic effect
fluoxymesterone (Halotestin)   potassium chloride (Slow-K)

Prolongation and/or potentiation of insulin effect
hydrazine derivatives   propranolol (Inderal)
mebanazine

Hypoglycemic effect in diabetics and/or nondiabetics
aminosalicylic acid   oxytetracycline (Terramycin)
aspirin (diabetics and toxic doses)   PIDH (PIDH)
cannabis (marijuana)   sulfonylureas (Orinase)
ethanol (grain alcohol)   tromethamine (THAM)

Glucose Tolerance Test

The following drugs may cause a flattening of curve:

Metabolic effect
fluoxymesterone (Halotestin)

Anabolic effect
methandrostenolone (Dianabol)   nandrolone (Durabolin)

Miscellaneous
diphenylhydantoin (Dilantin)   pargyline (Eutonyl)
fenfluramine (Pondimin)

Urine

None reported except for methodological interference.

Related Lab Studies: Monitor current patient status and response to therapy. See individual tests for specific information.

	Diabetic ketoacidosis		HHNK
	↑	glucose, serum	↑
	↑	glucose, urine	↑
	↑	ketones, serum	normal
	↑	ketones, urine	normal
	↓	arterial pH	normal or ↑
	↑	osmolality	↑
normal or	↓	sodium, serum	↓
normal or	↓	potassium	normal
normal or	↑	BUN	↑
	↓	bicarbonate	↓

IMPLICATIONS FOR NURSING CARE
PRETEST: Factors related to the test
Nursing Diagnosis: Potential for injury related to changes in biochemical balance

Guide to assessment	Guide to planning and intervention	Guide to evaluation
Assess patient factors that may influence test results:		
1. Food and fluids	1. Order proper diet:	1. The patient's test results are not influenced by incorrect dietary preparation.
a. FBS	a. No food or fluids, except water, 12–14 hours prior to test.	
b. 2°PPBS GTT	b. Preparation diet. (1) High carbohydrate diet (100–300 g/day) 2–3 days prior to test. (2) No food or fluids, except water, 12–14 hours prior to test.	
c. Infants/children	c. Fasting time in children is 6–8 hours. d. See Procedure.	
2. Comprehensive drug history, especially Anticonvulsants Ascorbic acid, high doses Diuretics Insulin Oral contraceptives Salicylates See Drug Influences	2. Prepare patient properly by withholding or noting influencing drugs on lab slip. See Procedure and Drug Influences.	2. Drugs that may interfere with the patient's test results are withheld or noted on lab slip.
3. Preexisting conditions (See Increases/Decreases)	3. Recognize and note pertinent preexisting conditions on lab slip.	3. Patient's preexisting conditions that may influence test results are noted on lab slip.
4. Nursing staff factors influencing test results a. Patient not properly prepared b. Wrong test ordered	4. Be sure of test ordered and prepare patient correctly.	4. Patient's values are not influenced by improper preparation.
5. Knowledge deficit	5. Explain test to patient: a. Define test (See Description). b. Explain procedure (See Procedure).	5. The patient demonstrates knowledge by defining test and explaining procedure.

Patient Preparation Checklist

1. √ Patient is NPO 12–14 hours prior to test (See Procedure).
2. √ Influencing drugs are withheld or noted on lab slip if they must be given (See Procedure/Drug Influences).
3. √ Preexisting conditions and note pertinent information on lab slip (See Increases/Decreases).
4. √ Correct test ordered; correct preparations made.
5. √ Patient knowledge; explain and define test (See Description/Procedure).

CONSIDERATIONS FOR NURSING CARE RELATED TO ABNORMAL TEST RESULTS
POSTTEST: Factors related to the results of the test
Nursing Diagnosis: Alterations in biochemical balance

Guide to assessment	Guide to planning and intervention	Guide to evaluation
Assess patient factors that may be influencing test results. Nursing history and/or physical exam suggestive of:		
1. Hyperglycemia: all patients at risk (See Increases)	1. Correct or prevent increasing hyperglycemia by:	1. The patient demonstrates normal blood and urine glucose results:
Signs/symptoms		
Increased thirst		
Increased fluid intake		
Increased appetite		
Loss of weight		
Polyuria		
Fatigue		
Malaise		
Nausea/vomiting		
Restlessness		
*Fruity breath		
Dry mucous membranes		
Mental dullness		
Coma		
	a. Recognizing early signs and symptoms of hyperglycemia; consult with physician.	a. The patient experiences no further symptoms of hyperglycemia.
b. Patient at risk (See Increases)	b. Test urine or blood for glucose twice a day during good health and 3–4 times a day when under stress. Use correct testing materials. Consult with physician regarding positive findings.	b. Patient's glucose values are within normal limits.

---

*In ketoacidosis

Guide to assessment	Guide to planning and intervention	Guide to evaluation
c. Patient at risk (See Increases)	c. Test for ketone bodies as in b.	c. As above.
d. Patient under stress Diabetic Glucocorticoid therapy	d. Keep precise intake–output and daily weight records. Watch for fluid loss. Consult physician if discrepancy.	d. The patient maintains normal fluid balance.
e. Diabetic HHNK Patient under stress	e. Recognize increased insulin need. Consult with physician. Give insulin or oral diabetic agent as prescribed.	e. The patient's insulin needs are met.
f. History of glucose metabolism imbalance (See Increases)	f. Establish level of patient knowledge and make available appropriate information.	f. The patient is able to discuss condition knowledgeably, including diet, medication, exercise, complications, and how to avoid them.
g. Patient at risk (See Increases)	g. Be knowledgeable about patient's ability to metabolize carbohydrates.	g. The patient does not experience complications because of misinformed staff.
h. Medical treatment plan	h. Implement medical plan of care. Consult with physician for needed changes.	h. The patient's medical plan is carried out and physician consulted for needed changes.
i. Knowledge deficit	i. Teach patient to: (1) Test blood or urine 2 times daily in good health and 3–4 times a day in times of stress. (2) Recognize signs/symptoms of hyperglycemia. (3) Involve patient in diabetic education program.	
2. Hypoglycemia; all patients at risk (See Decreases) a. Signs and symptoms Hunger Sweating Irritability Weakness Headache Palpitations Blurred vision, diplopia Confusion	2. Control or prevent further hypoglycemia by: a. Recognizing patients at risk and early signs/symptoms of hypoglycemia and consult with physician immediately.	2. The patient demonstrates normal blood glucose results: a. The patient does not experience further symptoms of hypoglycemia.

Guide to assessment	Guide to planning and intervention	Guide to evaluation

Lethargy
Motor incoordination
Seizures
Coma
Blood sugar ↓ 50 mg
Infant:
Jittery
Eye-rolling
Hyperirritability
Cyanosis
  ↓ Blood sugar
    Low birth weight
  ↓ 20 mg
    Normal newborn
  ↓ 30 mg		

	b. Testing blood for glucose level as prescribed, or symptoms are manifested, with dipstix method. Follow directions exactly on dipstix container. Consult with physician *immediately* if level too low.	b. Patient's glucose values are within normal limits.
c. Small glycogen stores (Newborn or deficient glycogen mobilization) Adequate glycogen stores	c. Giving IV glucose (small glycogen stores) or glycogen IM as prescribed for hypoglycemic episodes.	c. The patient receives readily available glucose and glucagon as needed for hypoglycemic emergencies.
d. Hypoglycemia Need for special diet	d. Providing diet of complex carbohydrates and protein as appropriate. For inborn errors of carbohydrate metabolism give correct diet. Consult with dietician.	d. The patient receives the correct diet high in complex carbohydrates and protein.
e. Need for frequent meals	e. Providing frequent small meals; making sure the patient receives supplement if meal not eaten.	e. The patient receives adequate carbohydrates.
f. Lengthy NPO	f. Consulting with physician if patient is NPO for prolonged periods (be aware of patient's needs by age as well as diagnosis).	
g. Need for insulin or oral hypoglycemic agents	g. Managing hypoglycemic agent peaks by: (1) Providing food at peak times.	g. The patient does not experience hypoglycemia.

Guide to assessment	Guide to planning and intervention	Guide to evaluation
	(2) Teaching patient to have glucose readily available. (3) Providing protein HS snack.	
h. Knowledge deficit Patient Family	h. Teach patient/family about: (1) Signs and symptoms of hypoglycemia. (2) Keeping readily available glucose handy. (3) Use of glycogen during hypoglycemic emergencies.	h. The patient and/or family is able to state signs and symptoms of hypoglycemia and the use of readily available glucose or glycogen.

Test:	Glucose-6-Phosphate Dehydrogenase Deficiency Test
Abbreviation:	GPD, G-6PD
Reference Values:	Values are dependent upon lab methodology. Check with local lab for appropriate value.
Specimen:	Whole blood
Description:	Glucose is metabolized via two pathways. About 90 percent is metabolized by the glycolytic pathway. The rest is metabolized by the hexosemonophosphate (HMP) shunt pathway. Glucose-6-phosphate dehydrogenase is the enzyme responsible for the first reaction in the HMP shunt pathway. This particular pathway is important because the reactions lead to red blood cell protection against oxidative injury from infections, drugs, or chemicals. A deficiency in the enzyme, and an insult to the red blood cell from infection or certain drugs, result in red blood cell injury, the formation of Heinz bodies, and shortened red blood cell survival. G-6PD deficiencies are hereditary and sex-linked with the condition carried on the X female chromosome. The disease affects mostly males, but not exclusively. The purpose of testing for G-6PD is to aid in the differential diagnosis of hemolytic anemia or to diagnose G-6PD deficiency.
Procedure:	(lavender top tube) 1. No food or fluid restrictions. 2. 0.1–5 ml of blood is drawn from the patient. 3. Observe puncture site for bleeding or evidence of hematoma.

Conditions Related to Increases

1. G-6 phosphate dehydrogenase deficiency

Rationale

1. When the red blood cell is assaulted by infection, certain chemicals, or drugs, hemolytic anemia develops. This happens quickly, within 24–72 hours. If the offending agent is continued, the hemolytic anemia becomes compensated. If the offending agent is continued for a long period of time, hyperhemolysis takes place. The amount of hemolysis present depends on the type and amount of stress present. There is no specific treatment for the hemolysis. The three most important types of G-6PD deficiency in the United States are G-6PDA$^-$, found in American Blacks; G-6PD Mediterranean, found in Caucasians; and G-6PD Canton, found in Asians.

Conditions Related to Decreases

1. Hemolytic crises

Rationale

1. Depending upon the method used, hemolytic crises may give false negatives.

Drug Influences: The following drugs may influence test results. The drugs are listed alphabetically by generic name and divided into columns according to the effect of the drug. Examples of trade names are in parentheses.

The following drugs and chemicals may precipitate hemolysis:

Antimalarials
   primaquine

Antipyretics/analgesics
   acetophenetidin (Phenacetin); in G-6PDA⁻
   aminosalicylic acid
   antipyrine
   *aspirin; in G-6PDA⁻ very large doses

Nitrofurans
   nitrofurantoin (Furadantin)
   furazolidone (Furoxone)

Others
   aniline blue
   ascorbic acid; massive doses
   chloramphenicol; in Mediterranean G-6PD
   fava beans; also known as broad beans

   methylene blue; in G-6PDA⁻
   naphthalene
   probenecid
   sulfoxone
   vitamin K; water-soluble analogues

Sulfonamides
   sulfanilamide
   sulfisoxazole (Gantrisin); G-6PDA⁻
   salicylazosulfapyridine (Azulfidine)

   sulfacetamide (Sulamyd)
   trisulfapyrimidine (Sultrin)

Related Lab Studies

   Hgb
   Hct
   RBC count
   †RBC morphology; *bite* cells present
   RBC indices
   reticulocyte count
   serum bilirubin
   urinalysis

---

*Many over-the-counter drugs contain aspirin. Read labels carefully.

†Bite cells are cells that look as though they have had bites taken from them. This is probably due to splenic removal of Heinz bodies.

IMPLICATIONS FOR NURSING CARE
PRETEST: Factors related to the test
Nursing Diagnosis: Potential for injury related to changes in biochemical balance

Guide to assessment	Guide to planning and intervention	Guide to evaluation
Assess patient factors that may influence test results:		
1. Comprehensive drug history (See Drug Influences)	1. Explore drug history. Consult with physician if patient history is positive for oxidative drug usage.	1. Patient's lab values are not influenced by oxidative drugs.
2. Hemolytic anemia Jaundice	2. Inform lab if patient is experiencing hemolytic episode.	2. Patient's hemolytic anemia does not interfere with lab procedure.
3. Knowledge deficit	3. Explain test to patient/parent: a. Define test (See Description). b. Explain procedure (See Procedure).	3. The patient demonstrates knowledge by defining test and stating procedure.
4. G-6PD screening test	4. Encourage screening tests during health for: a. Black populations. b. Mediterranean or Jewish heritage populations. c. Persons donating blood.	4. Patients are screened for deficiency prior to hemolytic episode.
5. Hemolysis	5. Prevent hemolysis by: a. Not probing venipuncture site or leaving tourniquet on too long. b. Not forcefully withdrawing specimen. c. Not withdrawing specimen too slowly. d. Not agitating or handling specimen roughly. e. Not saturating skin with antiseptic.	5. Patient's test results are not influenced by hemolysis.

Patient Preparation Checklist

1. √ Comprehensive drug history for oxidative drugs (See Drug Influences).
2. √ Hemolytic episode noted on lab slip.
3. √ Patient knowledge; define test, explain procedure (See Description/Procedure).

CONSIDERATIONS FOR NURSING CARE RELATED TO ABNORMAL TEST RESULTS
POSTTEST: Factors related to the results of the test
Nursing Diagnosis: Alterations in blood profile

Guide to assessment	Guide to planning and intervention	Guide to evaluation

Assess patient factors that may be influencing test values:
1. Hemolytic anemia
	1. Prevent further hemolytic episodes by:
	  a. Teaching patient to avoid oxidative drugs, chemicals, and foods by:
	    (1) Providing patient with complete list of drugs and chemicals that can cause hemolytic episode.
	    (2) Reading labels carefully on over-the-counter drugs.
	  b. Teaching patient to inform all health care givers of enzyme deficiency.
	  c. Encouraging G-6PD screening programs as part of public health program.
		1. Patients remain free of hemolytic episodes.

Test: Hematocrit

Abbreviation: Hct

Reference Values: *Hematocrit (Hct)*
                               Newborn 57–68%
                               1 week 46–62%
                               1 month 31–41%
                               3–5 months 30–36%
                               1 year 29–41%
                               2–10 years 36–41%
                               Adult
                               Male 40–54%
                               Female 37–47%
                               Values vary with laboratory.

Description: Hematocrit (Hct) is the percentage of red blood cells in the total blood volume. Changes in RBC size will make a difference in test values. In other words, if cell size is small, the Hct will be lower as the packed cells take up less room. Hct measurements are ordered to compute RBC indices as well as packed cell volume.

Turn to RBC count for discussion of:

    Procedure
    Increases
    Decreases
    Drug Influences
    Related Lab Studies
    Pretest Implications
    Posttest Considerations

Test: Hemoglobin

Abbreviation: Hgb

Reference Value: *Hemoglobin (Hgb)*
    Newborn   17–21 g/d
    1 week   15–20 g
    1 month   11–14 g
    3–5 months   10–12 g
    1 year   11–13 g
    2–10 years   11–13 g
    Adult
    Male   14–18 g
    Female   12–16 g
    Values vary with laboratory.

Specimen: Whole blood.

Description: Hemoglobin is made up of four globin chains and four molecules of heme, which contain iron atoms. Iron is essential in maintaining hemoglobin synthesis. Hemoglobin, through the red blood cell, transports O_2 and removes CO_2 throughout the body. By the process of diffusion, hemoglobin acts as an acid-base buffer. Hemoglobin is measured to determine the total amount of hemoglobin in the blood and to compute red blood cell indices.

Turn to RBC count for discussion of:
    Procedure
    Increases
    Decreases
    Drug Influences
    Related Lab Studies
    Pretest Implications
    Posttest Considerations

Test: Hepatitis B Surface Antigen

Abbreviation: HB_sAg

Reference Value: Negative

Specimen: Serum

Description: There are three types of viral hepatitis. Hepatitis A, often referred to as infectious hepatitis, is seen most frequently in young children. Non-A, non-B hepatitis is associated with hepatitis following blood transfusions. Hepatitis B, also known as serum hepatitis, is spread generally by innoculation with contaminated blood or blood products. It is a virus composed of a core protein with an identifiable surface antigen. This test is done as part of a hepatitis screen to identify the hepatitis type, as a screen for all blood donors to prevent transmission of the disease from a carrier, and as a screen for high-risk health workers. A positive HB_sAg means that the patient has hepatitis B or is a carrier.

Procedure: (red top tube)
1. No food or fluid restrictions.
2. Up to 7 ml of blood is drawn from the patient.
3. Observe puncture area for bleeding or evidence of hematoma.

Conditions Related to Increases

1. Hepatitis B

2. Chronic positive test

Rationale

1. Hepatitis B may be transmitted through as little as 0.00004 ml of blood (17). Those at highest risk for the disease are people who are closely associated with blood and blood products. This includes patients as well as hospital personnel. Hepatitis B is also transmitted by the fecal oral route, parenteral drug abuse, and sexual contact.

2. A positive HB_sAg after 3 months from onset of disease is indicative of chronic hepatitis or the carrier state. The person is still infectious.

Drug Influences: Drugs do not interfere with this test.

Related Lab Studies: Diagnosis of hepatitis:

  *anti-HAV (anti-hepatitis A virus)
  *anti-HBc (anti-hepatitis B antibody)
  *anti-HBs (anti-hepatitis B surface)
   AST (SGOT)
   ALT (SGPT)
   bilirubin, serum, and urine

---

*Not discussed in this book.

urobilinogen
CBC
alkaline phosphatase

IMPLICATIONS FOR NURSING CARE
PRETEST: Factors related to the test
Nursing Diagnosis: Knowledge deficit

Guide to assessment	Guide to planning and intervention	Guide to evaluation
Assess patient factors that may influence test results: 1. Knowledge deficit	1. Explain test to patient: a. Define HB$_s$Ag. b. Explain procedure.	1. The patient demonstrates knowledge by defining HB$_s$Ag and stating procedure.

CONSIDERATIONS FOR NURSING CARE RELATED TO ABNORMAL TEST RESULTS
POSTTEST: Factors related to the results of the test
Nursing Diagnosis: Alterations in microbiological environment

Guide to assessment	Guide to planning and intervention	Guide to evaluation
Assess patient factors that may be influencing test results. Nursing history and/or physical exam that is suggestive of: 1. Positive test	1. Provide supportive care to encourage return to health: a. Encourage nutritious meals. b. Encourage adequate rest. c. Explain to patient that recovery is slow; stress need for rest, well-balanced meals, and medical follow-up.	1. The patient recovers as evidenced by negative test.
2. Positive test Possible spread of infection Community Hospital personnel	2. Prevent spread of disease by: a. Explaining mode of transmission to patient. b. Administering hepatitis B immune globulin to those exposed. c. Administering hepatitis B vaccine as appropriate.	2. The disease is confined to a single patient.

Guide to assessment	Guide to planning and intervention	Guide to evaluation
	d. Informing those at risk about mode of transmission: (1) Suggest the use of gloves when handling blood-contaminated articles. (2) Report and treat immediately any skin injuries to hospital personnel in contact with patient. e. Reporting disease to Public Health Department for epidemiological follow-up.	

Test: 17-Hydroxycorticosteroids

Abbreviation: 17-OHCS

Reference Values: Baseline levels
Children to 16 years 3.1 ± 1.0 mg/M^2/24 hours
Adults
Male   4.5–12 mg/24 hours
Female   2.5–10 mg/24 hours

Specimen: 24-hour urine collection

Description: 17-hydroxycorticosteroids (17-OHCS) are steroid compounds excreted in the urine and representative of cortisol secretion. Cortisol is secreted by the adrenal cortex in response to the influences of ACTH, stress, and a diurnal rhythm.

Measurements of 17-OHCS require a complete 24-hour urine collection because of significant diurnal variation. Along with serum cortisol, 17-OHCS are tested to assess adrenocortical function or pituitary-adrenal activity. Baseline evaluations are made as well as 17-OHCS measurements after dexamethasone suppression. The low dose dexamethasone suppression test (DST) is done primarily to confirm Cushing's syndrome, while high dose DST helps to identify patients with adrenal tumors.

Procedure:

Baseline 17-OHCS

1. No food or fluid restrictions.
2. Excessive exercise should be avoided 24 hours prior to and during collection.
3. Attempt to avoid stressful situations during testing period.
4. Obtain collection container with boric acid preservative. If not, urine collection *must* be kept refrigerated.
5. Collection:
   a. Discard first voided specimen.
   b. Begin timing.
   c. For next 24 hours place all voidings into specimen container immediately after voiding.
   d. Have patient void just prior to completion of 24 hours and put sample in collection bottle.
6. Record exact start and finish times on lab slip.
7. Send to lab immediately.

Low Dose Dexamethasone Suppression Test

1. Follow procedure as above.
2. Give 0.5 mg of dexamethasone every 6 hours for 2 days.
3. Each day urine is collected and measured for 17-OHCS. Urine is measured for creatinine to determine renal function; urinary-free cortisol is also measured.

High Dose Dexamethasone Suppression Test

1. Follow the same procedure as for low dose DST, but give 2 mg of dexamethasone every 6 hours for 2 days.

Conditions Related to Increases

Rationale

1. Cushing's disease

1. In this disease there is a hypothalamic disorder that allows an increased rate of corticotropin-releasing factor (CRF) to be released that stimulates ACTH release and subsequently increases plasma cortisol levels. The increased cortisol secretion is demonstrated in increased levels of 17-OHCS.

2. Cushing's syndrome

2. Cushing's syndrome is caused by an adrenal tumor. Because of the tumor, cortisol secretion is mostly ACTH-independent. There is no dexamethasone suppression.

3. Stress
   Hospitalization
   Surgery
   Fever
   Hypoglycemia
   Examinations
   Difficult blood drawing episode (especially pediatrics)
   Anesthesia
   Activity, etc.

3. The transient, moderate increases in cortisol secretion are part of the adaptive response mechanism to stress. The increased cortisol secretion is detected in the urine measurement.

4. Diurnal rhythm

4. There is a circadian pattern to ACTH release and, so, to cortisol release. Plasma cortisol levels are highest early morning (between 6 A.M. and 8 A.M.) and at the lowest level between 9 P.M. and 4 A.M. Urinary 17-OHCS correlates with the plasma cortisol.

5. Medical exclusion list for DST*
   Major physical illness
   Trauma, fever, nausea, dehydration
   Temporal lobe disease
   Pregnancy
   High dose estrogen therapy
   Cushing's disease
   Unstable diabetes
   Malnutrition

5. All these conditions interfere with the hypothalamic-pituitary-adrenal axis in some way and so are apt to cause false positive results.

---

*Taken from James C. Ritchie and Bernard J. Carroll, "A New Test to Identify Depression," *Lab World*, September 1981.

Anorexia nervosa
Heavy alcohol use
Alcohol withdrawal
Electroconvulsive therapy
Other endocrine diseases are questionable

6. Hyperthyroidism

6. Increased metabolism increases excretion of dexamethasone, and a failure to suppress cortisol secretion is possible.

7. Congenital adrenal hyperplasia 11-hydroxylase deficiency

7. There is a deficiency of one of the five enzymes needed for synthesis of cortisol, which leads to an increase in 11-deoxycortisol levels leading to increased 17-OHCS levels.

Conditions Related to Decreases

1. Adrenocortical insufficiency
   Addison's disease

Rationale

1. This is a disease of primary adrenal cortical insufficiency. The adrenal gland does not respond to ACTH stimulation and cortisol is not released and 17-OHCS levels are normal or decreased.

2. Anterior pituitary hypofunction
   Hypophysectomy
   Postpartum pituitary necrosis
   Space-occupying tumors
   Starvation
   Severe anemia

2. The decreased cortisol levels in these conditions are due to the failure of the pituitary gland to produce adequate amounts of ACTH either because of gland removal, destruction, obliteration due to tumor, or an inadequately nourished gland.

3. Congenital adrenal hyperplasia
   21-Hydroxylase deficiency

3. Due to the enzyme deficiency there is diminished synthesis of cortisol.

Drug Influences: The following drugs may influence test results. The drugs are listed alphabetically by generic name and divided into columns according to the effect of the drug. Examples of trade names are in parentheses.

The following drugs may cause an increase in test results:

Normal effect of drug
  corticotropin (Acthar)
  diethylstilbestrol (Stilphostrol)
  metyrapone (Metopirone)

Hormonal effect
  gonadotropin (Pergonal)

Effect on release from adrenals
  histamine (histamine phosphate)

Miscellaneous
  betamethasone (Celestone)
  chlorthalidone (Hygroton)

cortisone (Cortistan)

The following drugs may cause a decrease in test results:

Inhibition of steroid biosynthesis
   aminoglutethimide (Aminoglutethimide)
   medroxyprogesterone (Depo-Provera)
   metyrapone (Metopirone)
   SKF-12185

Inhibition of release of steroid hormones and/or metabolites
   ethinyl estradiol (Brevicon)   pentazocine (Talwin)
   norethynodrel (Enovid-E)   phenothiazines (Compazine)
   oral contraceptives

ACTH suppression
   chlorpromazine (Thorazine)   morphine
   dexamethasone (Decadron)   perphenazine (Triavil)
   levodopa (Bendopa)   promazine (Sparine)
   meperidine (Demerol)   propoxyphene (Darvon)

Cortisol metabolism diverted to 6-B-OH cortisol
   diphenylhydantoin (Dilantin)   phenobarbital
   estrogens (Premarin)   phenylbutazone (Butazolidin)

Miscellaneous
   carbon disulfide, dependent on   rauwolfia (Harmonyl), depressed central
     exposure time   synthesis
   MAO inhibitors (Eutonyl, depressed   reserpine (Diupres), depressed central
     central synthesis)   synthesis
   mitotane (Lysodren)
   progesterone (Progesterone in oil)

Related Lab Studies

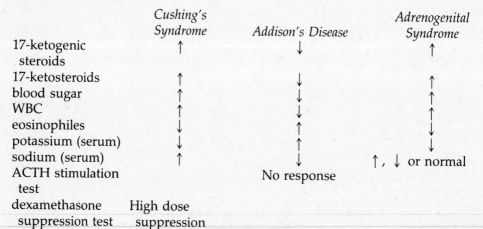

	Cushing's Syndrome	Addison's Disease	Adrenogenital Syndrome
17-ketogenic steroids	↑	↓	↑
17-ketosteroids	↑	↓	↑
blood sugar	↑	↓	↑
WBC	↑	↓	↑
eosinophiles	↓	↑	↓
potassium (serum)	↓	↑	↓
sodium (serum)	↑	↓	↑, ↓ or normal
ACTH stimulation test		No response	
dexamethasone suppression test	High dose suppression		

IMPLICATIONS FOR NURSING CARE
PRETEST: Factors related to test
Nursing Diagnosis: Potential for injury related to changes in biochemical balance

Guide to assessment	Guide to planning and intervention	Guide to evaluation
Assess patient factors that may influence test results:		
1. Comprehensive drug history (See Drug Influences)	1. Withhold interfering drugs for 2 weeks, as appropriate, prior to test. Consult with physician. Note any interfering drugs on lab slip.	1. Patient's test values are not influenced by unnecessary medication.
2. Physical activity	2. Tell patient to restrict physical activity for 24 hours prior to testing and during testing period.	2. Patient's test values are not increased because of physical activity.
3. Preexisting conditions (See Increases, especially 6. See Decreases also.)	3. Consult with physician about interfering conditions.	3. Patient's test values are not influenced by interfering conditions.
4. Knowledge deficit: Patient	4. Explain test to patient: a. Define cortisol (See Description). b. Explain procedure (See Procedure).	4. The patient is able to define test and explain procedure.
5. Knowledge deficit: Staff a. Wrong test b. Incorrect procedure	5. Prevent test error by: a. Being informed of which test is to be performed. b. Following institutional guidelines carefully.	5. Patient's results are not influenced by staff error.

CONSIDERATIONS FOR NURSING CARE RELATED TO ABNORMAL TEST RESULTS
POSTTEST: Factors related to the results of the test
Nursing Diagnosis: Alterations in biochemical balance

Guide to assessment	Guide to planning and intervention	Guide to evaluation
Assess patient factors that may be influencing test results:		
1. Cushing's disease	1. Promote cortisol suppression by:	1. The patient achieves normal cortisol levels through successful management of cause of disease.
a. Anterior pituitary tumor	a. Supporting patient through all of radiation	

Guide to assessment	Guide to planning and intervention	Guide to evaluation
b. Need for hypophysectomy	treatments. b. Initiating nursing measures to prepare patient for surgery.	
c. Replacement hormonal therapy posthypophysectomy or irradiation	c. Administering pituitary-dependent hormones as prescribed.	
d. Hormonal replacement Patient education	d. Teaching patient need to continue hormone replacement.	
e. Hypothalamic disorder Plasma cortisol 24° Urine collections 17-OHCS 17-KS DST	e. Administering high dose dexamethasone as prescribed and assisting with cortisol level monitoring as necessary.	
2. Cushing's syndrome Adrenal tumor	2. Encourage control of cortisol secretion by: a. Initiating nursing measures to prepare patient for adrenalectomy and specifically: (1) Protect patient from infection; recognize only mild symptoms may be representative of serious infection.	2. The patient's cortisol secretion returns to normal as evidenced by lab studies: (1) The patient is protected from infection due to glucocorticoid suppression of immune system and inflammatory reactions.
	(2) Attempt to keep stress to a minimum. (3) Understand emotional lability and inform patient of positive physical changes after adrenalectomy. (4) Adminster pre-op cortisol preparation as prescribed. b. Administering cortisol replacement postoperatively. c. Teaching patient about cortisol replacement.	
3. Addison's disease	3. Maintain adequate cortisol levels: a. Administer cortisol. Recognize signs of excessive long-term cortisol therapy (Cushinoid signs).	3. The patient's cortisol level is normal.

Guide to assessment	Guide to planning and intervention	Guide to evaluation
	b. Attempt to maintain stress-free environment: (1) Consistency of care givers. (2) Protect from infection. (3) Consult with physician about any signs of infection, high stress situations, etc. c. Plan with patient self-medication with glucocorticoids. Include: (1) Route. (2) Dosage. (3) Action of drug. (4) Signs of overdosage and underdosage. (5) When to call physician for dosage readjustment, e.g., illness, emotional stress, minor surgery, etc. (6) Patient should wear medical alert bracelet.	

4. Acute adrenal insufficiency
   Severe hypotension
   Hyperkalemia
   Vascular collapse
	4. Initiate nursing measures to correct acute adrenal insufficiency:
	 a. Administer fluids:
	 (1) Strict I&O, hourly.
	 (2) Hourly infusion check.
	 (3) Plasma as ordered.
	 b. Administer glucocorticoid as prescribed:
	 (1) Monitor IV infusion.
	 (2) Gradually reduce dosage as prescribed.
	 c. Take vital signs to monitor hypotension.
	 d. Protect the patient from additional stress (See 3b above).
		4. The patient's severe glucocorticoid deficiency is corrected as evidenced by cortisol levels and clinical evaluation.

e. Glucocorticoid excess/ overhydration
   Generalized edema
   Hypertension
   Paralysis, flaccid
   Hypokalemia
   Psychoses
   Loss of consciousness
	e. Detect signs of overdosage with glucocorticoids and IV fluids.	e. The patient demonstrates no signs of overhydration/ glucocorticoid excess.

Guide to assessment	Guide to planning and intervention	Guide to evaluation

5. Congenital adrenal hyperplasia
  Signs/symptoms
  In 21-hydroxylase deficiency
    Dehydration
    Shock
    Pernicious vomiting
    ↓ sodium, serum
    ↑ K^+, serum
    Virilization of female genitalia
	5. Replace insufficient cortisol:
	  a. Instruct family in use of medication and technique of administration needed.
	  b. Teach family about disease and what can be done for treatment.
	  c. Refer for follow-up to community health nurse.
		5. The patient's cortisol levels are normal as evidenced by lab values.

Test:	5-Hydroxyindoleacetic Acid
Abbreviation:	5-HIAA
Reference Values:	2–10 mg/24 hours 60–100 mEq/24 hours
Specimen:	Urine
Description:	5-Hydroxyindoleacetic acid is the primary metabolite of serotonin. Serotonin is a hormone that acts in the GI tract to regulate smooth muscle contraction and peristalsis. Serotonin is produced in the argentaffin cells of the intestine and other abdominal structures. It is present in high concentrations in platelets and in smaller amounts in brain cells. The 5-HIAA test is done to diagnose carcinoid tumors composed of chromaffin tissue arising from intestinal argentaffin cells and producing large amounts of serotonin. The test is repeated if the value is negative but a carcinoid tumor is strongly suspected. This is because carcinoid tumors will vary in capacity to store and secrete serotonin.
Procedure:	1. Omit foods rich in serotonin from the diet for 4 days prior to the test (avocado, banana, eggplant, pineapple, red plums, tomatoes, and walnuts). 2. Many drugs interfere with test values. Check Drug Influences. 3. For 24-hour urine collection, the collection container should be acidified with HCl or acetic acid. 4. Urine collection should be kept refrigerated during entire collection. 5. Send the specimen to laboratory immediately.

Conditions Related to Increases	**Rationale**
1. Carcinoid syndrome	1. A syndrome that occurs as a result of malignant tumors of the intestinal enterchromaffin cells which produce excessive amounts of serotonin (21, 41).
2. Nontropical sprue	2. The theory explaining this is that there is damage to the intestinal mucosa with probable compensating intestinal cell proliferation resulting in increased serotonin production (52).

Conditions Related to Decreases	**Rationale**
1. Malnutrition	1. There is a decreased intake of tryptophan, the amino acid precursor of serotonin.

Drug Influences: The following drugs may influence test results. The drugs are listed alphabetically by generic name and divided into columns according to the effect of the drug. Examples of trade names are in parentheses.

The following drugs/food may cause an increase in test results:

High content of serotonin
Avocado
Eggplant
Pineapple
Plum
Walnut

Tissue destruction in patients with carcinoid syndrome
fluorouracil (Adrucil)
melphalan (Alkeran)

Effect of serotonin release
caffeine
nicotine
rauwolfia (Harmonyl)
reserpine (Diupres)

Miscellaneous
phenmetrazine (Preludin)

The following drugs may cause a decrease in test results:

Serotonin biosynthesis inhibition
chlorophenylalanine (Chlorophenylalanine)
ethanol (grain alcohol)

Decreased cell permeability to 5-HT
imipramine (Tofranil)

Inhibition of conversion of 5-HT to 5-HIAA
isocarboxazid (Marplan)
MAO inhibitors (Eutonyl)

Decarboxylase inhibition
isoniazid (Laniazid)
methyldopa (Aldoclor)

Miscellaneous
hydrazine derivatives
streptozotocin (Streptozotocin)

Related Lab Studies: In the diagnosis of carcinoid tumors:

↑ VMA
* ↑ serotonin, blood

---

*Not discussed in this book.

IMPLICATIONS FOR NURSING CARE
PRETEST: Factors related to the test
Nursing Diagnosis: Potential for injury related to changes in biochemical balance

Guide to assessment	Guide to planning and intervention	Guide to evaluation
Assess patient factors influencing test results: 1. Food and fluids	1. Have patient omit foods rich in serotonin from the diet for 4 days prior to the test, e.g., avocado, banana, eggplant, pineapple, red plums, tomatoes, and walnuts.	1. The patient's diet does not affect the results of the lab test.
2. Comprehensive drug history (See Drug Influences)	2. Report drugs the patient is currently receiving that may influence lab results to the patient's physician and to the lab. (It may be necessary to withhold drugs prior to exam.)	2. Drugs the patient is currently receiving that may influence test results are identified and proper personnel or department notified.

3. Preexisting conditions (See Increases/Decreases)
4. Knowledge deficit
	3. Record preexisting conditions on lab slip.
	4. Explain test to patient:
	  a. Define 5-HIAA (See Description).
	  b. Explain procedure (See Procedure).
		3. Patient's preexisting conditions are noted on lab slip.
		4. Patient demonstrates knowledge of test by defining test and explaining procedure.

Patient Preparation Checklist

1. √ Serotonin-rich foods omitted from diet for 4 days prior to test.
2. √ Influencing drugs noted and reported (See Drug Influences).
3. √ Preexisting conditions noted on lab slip (See Increases/Decreases).
4. √ Patient knowledge; explain test and procedure (See Description and Procedure).

CONSIDERATIONS FOR NURSING CARE RELATED TO ABNORMAL TEST RESULTS
POSTTEST: Factors related to the results of the test
Nursing Diagnosis: Alterations in biochemical balance

Guide to assessment	Guide to planning and intervention	Guide to evaluation
Assess patient factors influencing test results:		

Guide to assessment	Guide to planning and intervention	Guide to evaluation
1. Nursing history and/or physical exam suggestive of carcinoid tumor	1. Administer adjuvant chemotherapeutic drugs, alpha-adrenergic drugs and p-chlorphenylalanine as ordered.	1. The patient's 5-HIAA level is within normal limits.

2. Nursing history and/or physical exam suggestive of nontropical sprue
  Weight loss
  Steatorrhea
  Diarrhea
  Abdominal distention
  Secondary vitamin deficiencies
  Muscle atrophy
	2. Promote adequate nutrition by:
	  a. Providing a gluten-free diet.
		2. The patient will demonstrate decreased intestinal irritation by decreased diarrhea, steatorrhea, and abdominal distention.

	b. Teaching patient the importance of omitting gluten from the diet and the specific foods that should be omitted (e.g., wheat, rye, barley and oats).	b. The patient will demonstrate knowledge of diet by planning gluten-free meals and will express willingness to adhere to diet.

3. Nursing history and/or physical exam suggestive of malnutrition:
  Low body weight in comparison to height
  Weakness
  Peripheral neuritis
  Restlessness
  Tachycardia
  Muscle atrophy
	3. Improve nutritional status by:
	  a. Administering enteral feedings or hyperalimentation as ordered.
	  b. Providing a diet with a balance of protein, carbohydrates, fat, and other nutrients.
	  c. Allowing the patient to select desired foods as much as possible.
	  d. Providing small, frequent feedings and protein supplements.
	  e. Serving meals attractively in a pleasant environment.
	  f. Teaching the patient the importance of adequate nutritional intake, as well as teaching basic principles of nutrition as necessary.
	  g. Encouraging intake of foods high in tryptophan, e.g., avocado, banana, eggplant, pineapple, red plums, tomatoes, and walnuts.
		3. Patient demonstrates improved nutritional status and therefore tryptophan intake as shown by weight gain and increased muscle mass.
		
		  Patient demonstrates nutritional knowledge by planning well-balanced meals.

Test: Iron
Total iron-building capacity and percent saturation

Abbreviation: Fe, TIBC, percent saturation

Reference Values:

	Iron	TIBC	% Saturation
Newborn	20–157	59–175	65
6 weeks–3 years	20–115	59–175	10–55
3–10 years	53–119	250–400	20–55
Adult	87–279	250–400	20–55

Serum iron ÷ TIBC × 100 = % saturation.

Specimen: Serum

Description: Iron is a trace mineral in the body necessary for the formation of hemoglobin. About 70% of iron exists in hemoglobin or myoglobin, about 1% functions in the formation of various cellular enzymes, and the rest is stored in the nonheme ferritin protein in the spleen, liver, and bone marrow. The newborn infant has an iron store from the mother, but this store is used up in the first few months of life. Iron replacement comes from the diet. Serum iron shows a diurnal rhythm with highest serum iron concentrations in the early morning. People with abnormal sleep-wake patterns may have a different peak.

Transferrin is the iron transport protein. This protein is not assimilated by target tissues. Transferrin carries the iron liberated by recently degraded hemoglobin back to the bone marrow to the developing erythroid cells. It also carries iron absorbed from the intestines. Transferrin is indirectly measured by the amount of iron that it can bind. That is, the amount of iron that *could* be carried if transferrin were completely saturated with iron. This is called the total iron-binding capacity (TIBC). Present transferrin saturation may be determined by dividing the serum iron by TIBC and multiplying by 100. The result is the percent saturation.

These tests are done to aid in the differential diagnosis of anemia, in approximating iron stores, and in the diagnosis of iron excess. The tests should be performed together for comparison of results.

Procedure: (red top tube)
1. No food or fluid restrictions.
2. The blood is usually drawn early morning.
3. 1–5 ml of blood is drawn from the patient.
4. Observe the puncture site for bleeding or evidence of hematoma.

Conditions Related to Increases

1. Sideroblastic anemias
   Thalassemia

Rationale

1. ↑ Serum iron
   ↓ TIBC

Lead poisoning
Certain drugs
  Isoniazid
  Cycloserine
  Alcohol, ethyl
  Chloramphenicol
Pyridoxine deficiency
Idiopathic
2. Liver disease

3. Iron poisoning

4. Hemolytic anemia

5. Hemochromatosis

↑ % Saturation
These conditions are characterized by erythroid hyperplasia of the marrow with a block to heme synthesis due to an enzymatic defect that results in an accumulation of nonheme iron. These anemias may be acquired or congenital.

2. ↑ Serum iron
  ↑ TIBC
  ↑ or ↓ % Saturation
The increase in serum iron is probably a result of altered mucosal regulation of iron absorption (97).

3. ↑ Serum iron
  ↓ TIBC
  ↑ % Saturation
From the accidental ingestion of oral iron preparations. The acute stage is very serious and there may be long-term hepatic, gastric, intestinal, or neurological effects.

4. ↑ Serum iron
  normal/↓ TIBC
  ↑ % Saturation
Increased iron absorption from excessive erythrocyte destruction and ineffective erythropoiesis results in increased serum iron.

5. ↑ Serum iron
  normal/↓ TIBC
  ↑ % Saturation
This is the excessive absorption of iron. The etiology is unknown.

Conditions Related to Decreases

1. Chronic infections

2. Lack of dietary iron
  Malabsorption
  Infancy
  Pregnancy

Rationale

1. ↓ Serum iron
  ↓ TIBC
  ↓ % Saturation
In chronic infections the reticuloendothelial system (phagocytic cells) is slow to release iron for reutilization by the developing normoblasts.

2. ↓ Serum iron
  ↑ TIBC
  ↓ % Saturation
The insufficient dietary intake is usually caused by increased iron require-

3. Malignancy
   Menstruation
   Bleeding

ments necessary for growth.

3. ↓ Serum iron
   ↓ TIBC
   ↓ % Saturation
   Blood loss, whether chronic or acute, results in iron loss.

4. Nephrosis

4. The loss in nephrosis is related to the loss in the urine of the protein responsible for iron binding (97).

Drug Influences: The following drugs may influence test results. The drugs are listed alphabetically by generic name and divided into columns according to the effect of the drug. Examples of trade names are in parentheses.

The following drugs may cause an increase in test results:

Serum

GI absorption
  ethanol (grain alcohol)

Increased iron stores
  iron dextan (Imferon)   iron salts (Bilron)

Effect of drug toxicity
  chloramphenicol (Chloromycetin)
  cycloserine (Seromycin)

Miscellaneous
  blood transfusions   oral contraceptives
  estrogens (Premarin)   phenacetin (in many aspirin
  methicillin (Staphcillin)   preparations)

Urine

Miscellaneous
  iron dextran (Imferon)   penicillamine (Cuprimine)

The following drugs may cause a decrease in test results:

Serum

Therapeutic intent
  deferoxamine (Desferal)

Impaired absorption
  cholestyramine (Questran)
  metformin

Decreased binding and/or intermediate synthesis
  corticotropin (Acthar)
  cortisone (Cortistan)
  oxymetholone (Anadrol-50)

Miscellaneous
  allopurinol (Lopurin)
  aspirin
  epinephrine (Adrenalin Chloride)

Urine

None reported.

Related Lab Studies: Monitor response to therapy or progress of disease and adjust nursing care accordingly. See individual tests for information.

Hgb
Hct
*ferritin, serum
iron, serum (serial)
TIBC with % saturation
RBC count and morphology
MCV
MCH
MCHC
reticulocyte count
urinalysis
stool for occult blood

IMPLICATIONS FOR NURSING CARE
PRETEST: Factors related to the test
Nursing Diagnosis: Potential for injury related to changes in biochemical balance

Guide to assessment	Guide to planning and intervention	Guide to evaluation
Assess patient factors that may influence test results: 1. Comprehensive drug history (See Drug Influences) Current iron therapy	1. Identify drugs that may influence test results. Note them on lab slip: a. Consult with physician. b. Hold iron therapy preparation 24 hours prior to testing.	1. Patient's drugs do not interfere with test results.
2. Preexisting conditions (See Increases/Decreases) Pregnancy Infancy	2. Identify pertinent preexisting conditions and note them on lab slip.	2. Patient's preexisting conditions are noted on lab slip.
3. Knowledge deficit	3. Explain test to patient: a. Define iron (See Description). b. Explain procedure (See Procedure).	3. The patient demonstrates knowledge by defining the test and stating procedure.

*Not discussed in this book.

Patient Preparation Checklist

1. √ Influencing drugs noted on lab slip. Iron preparation held 24 hours.
2. √ Pertinent preexisting conditions noted on lab slip.
3. √ Patient knowledge; explain test to patient.

CONSIDERATIONS FOR NURSING CARE RELATED TO ABNORMAL TEST RESULTS
POSTTEST: Factors related to the results of the test
Nursing Diagnosis: Alterations in biochemical balance

Guide to assessment	Guide to planning and intervention	Guide to evaluation
Assess patient factors that may be influencing test results.		
Nursing history and/or physical exam that is suggestive of:		
1. Iron deficiency anemia	1. Be alert to signs and symptoms of iron deficiency anemia:	1. Patient's signs and symptoms are recognized. Lab values return to normal.
Mild anemia		
Usually asymptomatic		
Moderate anemia		
Pallor		
Fatigue		
Dyspnea		
Palpitations		
Diaphoresis upon exertion		
↓ % Saturation		
Normal MCHC		
a. At-risk population	a. Identify high-risk populations for iron deficiency.	
Pregnancy		
Infancy		
Women of childbearing years		
Blood loss		
Malignancy		
Nephrosis		
Chronic infections		
b. Replacement therapy	b. Promote replacement of dietary iron by:	
Dietary iron	(1) Teaching the patient about foods high in iron content:	
Iron preparations	(a) Meats: liver, heart, red meat.	

Guide to assessment	Guide to planning and intervention	Guide to evaluation

	(b) Vegetables: kidney beans, peas.
	(c) Fruits: raisins, prunes, oranges.
	(d) Encourage vitamin C food sources with meals to encourage iron absorption.
	(2) Arranging consultation with dietician.
	(3) Giving oral iron preparation:
	  (a) Teach the patient about the drug:
	    (1) Give drug between meals for best absorption.
	    (2) Explain to patient iron therapy is continued for months.
	    (3) Taper dosage to discontinue.
	    (4) Prepare patient for usual side effects (dark stools, stained teeth from liquid preparation, etc.).
	(4) Following directions for the administration of parental iron carefully.	

c. Continued iron deficiency	c. Locate, if possible, cause of continued blood loss: (1) Perform occult blood tests on stool and vomitus. (2) Check urine for occult blood.	

d. Pica
  Dirt
  Salt
  Ice
	d. Be aware of pica peculiar to patients with iron deficiency anemia.	

e. Lab work
  Serum iron
  TIBC
  % Saturation
  Hct
  Hgb
  MCV
  MCH
	e. Check ongoing lab work for lab values to return to normal.	

Guide to assessment	Guide to planning and intervention	Guide to evaluation

2. At-risk population
   Thalassemia
   Lead poisoning
   Drugs
     Isoniazid
     Cycloserine
     Alcohol, ethyl
     Chloramphenicol
   Pyridoxine deficiency
   Idiopathic
	2. Identify patients at risk for developing sideroblastic anemia.	2. Patients at risk are identified. Lab values return to normal.

a. Lead poisoning	a. Protect patient from blocked heme synthesis due to lead poisoning:
	  (1) Promote community awareness of lead poisoning. See Lead levels.
	  (2) Attempt removal of lead from body by:
	    (a) Administering saline cathartics as ordered.
	    (b) Administer chelating agents as ordered.	

b. Drug-induced sideroblastic anemia	b. Remove offending agent.	
c. Pyridoxine deficiency	c. Give pyridoxine as prescribed.	

3. Liver disease
   Hemolytic anemia
   Nephrosis
	3. Implement medical treatment plan for underlying disease process.	3. Patient's lab values return to normal.

4. Iron poisoning	4. Prevent iron poisoning by:
	  a. Educating patients about drugs in their homes.
	  b. Reminding parents and grandparents to keep drugs out of reach of children.
	  c. Encourage patients with small children to request childproof drug bottles.
	  d. Impress upon parents to keep syrup of Ipecac on hand.
	  e. Refer child for emergency treatment if accidental ingestion occurs.
		4. Iron poisoning does not occur.

5. Hemochromatosis	5. Assist with phlebotomy as needed.	5. Patient's serum iron level decreases.

Test:	Ketones
Abbreviation:	None
Reference Values:	Serum negative (11) Urine (random sample) negative
Specimen:	Serum, urine
Description:	Ketone bodies are metabolic end products of incomplete fat metabolism. They are formed in the liver and excreted in the urine. Acetoacetic acid, beta-hydroxybutyric acid, and acetone are called ketone bodies. Normally carbohydrates supply the body with its major source of energy. When carbohydrate utilization is impaired, the body utilizes increased amounts of fats for energy, resulting in an increased ketone production. Ketones are acid bodies and are normally buffered by one of the body's buffer systems. If there is an increased production of these acid bodies due to increased fat metabolism, the buffer system becomes depleted, and acidemia results. Measurement of ketones, both in the serum and urine, are most often used in the diagnosis and management of diabetes mellitus. Tests for ketosis or ketonuria also offer a valuable diagnostic test for differentiating coma caused by ketosis from other causes, such as hypoglycemia, CVAs, uremia, or hepatic coma (5, 53). In pregnancy, early detection of ketones is essential since ketoacidosis contributes to death in the uterus (8). Generally speaking, the degree of ketonemia and ketonuria reflects the severity of the metabolic stress (5, 26, 54).

Procedure:

Urine Testing

1. Have patient void.
2. Encourage water intake and have patient void in 30 minutes after first voiding.
3. Tightly cover and store in refrigerator any urine specimen not immediately tested.
4. Utilize a testing agent that is not discolored or darkened.
5. Select a testing agent that will not produce false positive results as a result of drugs the patient is receiving.
6. Follow the manufacturer's directions for the specific testing agent.
7. Compare the test results at the exact time specified by the manufacturer and use only the color chart supplied with the agent.

Conditions Related to Increases	**Rationale**
1. Uncontrolled diabetes mellitus	1. Inadequate insulin supply causes decreased utilization of carbohydrates leading to increased fat utilization. Insulin causes lipogenesis and without

2. Vomiting

3. Starvation, cachexia, anorexia

4. Severe diarrhea or digestive disturbances

5. Conditions that greatly increase metabolic rate
   Exposure to cold
   Febrile diseases
   Violent exercise (effect noted only in untrained athletes)
   Hyperthyroidism
   Small children who have eaten little and played hard

6. Glycogen storage disease (von-Gierke's disease)

7. Ketogenic diets

8. Hypoglycemia

insulin there is increased fat breakdown (20).

2. Vomiting may lead to alkalosis, which prevents carbohydrate utilization so the body then metabolizes fat (7). Vomiting often results in a decreased carbohydrate intake.

3. Not enough carbohydrates are taken in to meet the body's energy needs so the body metabolizes fats.

4. Due to decreased carbohydrate intake and malabsorption.

5. The body's needs surpass its available glucose supply and fat is metabolized as an alternate source.

6. The enzyme primarily responsible for the synthesis of glycogen is diminished. Because of this, there is an inadequate amount of glucose produced by the liver to regulate blood glucose under fasting conditions.

7. Ketogenic diets are low in carbohydrates, high in fat and protein, and may result in an inadequate carbohydrate intake to meet energy needs; this necessitates excessive use of fats for energy.

8. Due to a lack of glucose there is increased metabolization of fats.

Conditions Related to Decreases

Rationale

1. Unknown

Drug Influences: The following drugs may influence test results. The drugs are listed alphabetically by generic name and divided into columns according to the effect of the drug. Examples of trade names are in parentheses.

The following drugs may cause an increase in test results:

Miscellaneous
   growth hormone

The following drugs may cause a decrease in test results:

Miscellaneous
   aspirin

glucose (in starvation)

Related Lab Studies: Monitor response to treatment or progression of disease and adjust nursing care accordingly. See individual tests for information.

In known diabetic
   arterial blood gases (possible acidosis as finding, ↓ pH)
   ↑ fasting blood sugar
   ↑ glucose (blood, urine)
   glucose tolerance test (abnormal finding)
   ↑ or ↓ potassium
   ↑ 2-hour postprandial blood sugar

IMPLICATIONS FOR NURSING CARE
PRETEST: Factors related to the test
Nursing Diagnosis: Potential for injury related to changes in biochemical balance

Guide to assessment	Guide to planning and intervention	Guide to evaluation

Assess patient factors influencing test results:
1. Comprehensive drug history (See Drug Influences)
	1. Report drugs the patient is receiving which may influence lab results to the patient's physician and to the laboratory.
	    Indicate on lab slip any diagnostic exams the patient has undergone that involved use of bromphthalein or phenosulfonphthalein in last 24 hours.
		1. Drugs patient is currently receiving which may influence lab results are identified and the proper people notified.
		    Lab results are not misinterpreted because of recent tests using BSP or PSP.

2. Preexisting conditions (See Increases/Decreases)
3. Knowledge deficit
	2. Record preexisting conditions on lab slip.
	3. Explain test to patient:
	   a. Define ketones (See Description).
	   b. Explain procedure (See Procedure).
	   c. Teach patient to complete the urine test accurately if it is done at home (See Procedure).
		2. Patient's preexisting conditions are noted on lab slip.
		3. Patient demonstrates knowledge of the test by defining the test, explaining the procedure, and/or accurately testing own urine for ketone bodies.

Patient Preparation Checklist

1. √ Influencing drugs noted and reported (See Drug Influences).
2. √ Preexisting conditions noted on lab slip (See Increases/Decreases).
3. √ Patient knowledge; explain test and procedure (See Description and Procedure).

CONSIDERATIONS FOR NURSING CARE RELATED TO ABNORMAL TEST RESULTS
POSTTEST: Factors related to the results of the test
Nursing Diagnosis: Alterations in biochemical balance

Guide to assessment	Guide to planning and intervention	Guide to evaluation

Assess patient factors that may be influencing test results:
1. Nursing history and/or physical exam suggestive of uncontrolled diabetes mellitus:
  a. Ketoacidosis
    Malaise
    Excessive appetite
    Thirst
    Polyuria
    Restlessness
    Mental dullness
    Fruity or acetone breath
    Nausea and vomiting
    Dizziness
    Dry mucous membranes
    Hot flushed skin
    Deep rapid respirations
    Abdominal pain
    Weight loss
    Late:
      Decreased BP and shock
      Oliguria or anuria
      Coma or stupor
	1. Correct or prevent further ketoacidosis by:
	
	  a. Promoting control of diabetes mellitus by:
	    (1) Administering IV fluids with regular insulin as ordered.
	    (2) Teaching patient to
	      (a) Test urine or blood for glucose twice a day during good health and three to four times a day in times of stress.
	      (b) Avoid persons with infections as much as possible.
	
	      (c) Protect feet from trauma by wearing cotton socks and well-fitting shoes whenever ambulating.
	      (d) Inspect feet daily for injury and clean with soap and water.
	      (e) Avoid injury by chemical irritants by wearing protective gloves when handling them.
	      (f) Treat minor injuries by washing with soap and water and applying a dry sterile dressing.
	      (g) Avoid using heat lamps, hot water bottles, or heating pads—or use them with great caution.
		1. The patient demonstrates control of disease by:
		
		  a. Blood sugar and ketone levels return to normal.
		    (a) Increased blood sugar will be identified before it becomes severe.
		
		    (b) Patient will not develop infections from unnecessary exposure to others.
		    (c) Patient will not develop an injury that might become infected.

Guide to assessment	Guide to planning and intervention	Guide to evaluation
	(h) Report to the physician any serious infections.	(h) Infections the patient develops will be identified and treated early.
	(3) Administering antibiotics as ordered. (4) Assisting patient to identify stressors and specific ways to decrease or cope with stress. (5) Teaching importance of adhering to the prescribed dietary plan and the principles of the diabetic exchange diet (or refer to dietician for teaching about diabetic diet)	(4) Patient will identify personal stressors and ways to reduce or cope with them. (5) Patient demonstrates understanding of diabetic exchange diet by planning menus for 1 week; expresses understanding of importance of consuming prescribed diet and willingness to adhere to that diet.
b. Evidence of inappropriate insulin administration Inadequate dose of insulin Omitting doses of insulin Incorrect technique of administration	b. Promoting correct administration of insulin by:	b. The patient demonstrates correct insulin balance by:
	(1) Administering insulin according to dose and times ordered by the physician. (2) Teaching patient to self-administer insulin using dosages and frequencies prescribed by the physician. (3) Teaching patient to rotate injection sites, not to administer insulin into areas of lipodystrophy and not to use outdated insulin.	(1) Patient receives insulin dose prescribed by the physician at the designated time. Patient administers correct dose of insulin to self at times prescribed by the physician, rotating injection sites and using normal skin sites for injection.
c. Evidence of inadequate dose of oral hypoglycemics	c. Promoting adequate ingestion of oral hypoglycemics by: (1) Administering oral hypoglycemics as ordered. (2) Teaching patient the importance of taking	c. The patient demonstrates adequate dose of oral hypoglycemics by: (1) Patient receives oral hypoglycemics as ordered. (2) Patient verbalizes importance of taking medi-

Guide to assessment	Guide to planning and intervention	Guide to evaluation
	medication as ordered.	cation as prescribed and expresses a willingness to do so.

d. Evidence of increased need for insulin
  Puberty
  Pregnancy
  Steroid therapy or
   Cushing's syndrome
  Febrile disease
  Trauma
  Severe emotional stress
  Surgery
	d. Promoting identification of increased need for insulin by:
	(1) Teaching patient to seek frequent physician care during puberty and pregnancy or when taking steroids or experiencing Cushing's syndrome.
	(2) Teaching patient to monitor blood glucose or urine glucose and ketones three to four times a day whenever any of the mentioned conditions exist.
	(3) Teaching patient to report to physician any infection, febrile illness, trauma, or severe emotional stress.
	(4) Monitoring urine and blood glucose every 6 hours for the patient undergoing surgery, and reporting increases to physician.
	(5) Monitoring IV glucose solutions carefully and administering insulin as ordered when the diabetic is undergoing surgery.
		d. Need for increased insulin doses will be identified and insulin dose increased to meet that need.

2. Nursing history and/or physical exam findings suggestive of hypoglycemia:
  Hunger
  Sweating
  Palpitations
  Irritability
  Faintness
  Weakness
  Tremulousness
  Anxiety
  Tachycardia
  Headache
	2. Correct or prevent hypoglycemia by:
	a. Making sure nutritional intake is adequate.
	b. Providing diet consisting of 40–45% carbohydrate, utilizing complex carbohydrates rather than refined sugars as the carbohydrate source.
	c. Providing frequent small meals and making sure the patient receives a supple-
		a. Patient will receive frequent, small meals with adequate complex carbohydrates, protein, and fat so that blood sugar will remain >90 mg/dl.

Guide to assessment	Guide to planning and intervention	Guide to evaluation
Blurred vision, diplopia Lethargy Confusion Motor incoordination	ment, if he doesn't eat a meal.	
	d. For patients on insulin, especially long-acting insulin, providing protein HS snack. e. Administering IV's or hyperalimentation as ordered, if NPO.	d. Insulin-dependent diabetic receiving long-acting insulin ingests high protein HS snack. e. Patient who is NPO will receive adequate nutritional intake so that hypoglycemia does not occur.
	f. Teaching patient the importance of frequent intake of complex carbohydrates rather than refined sugar.	f. Patient will verbalize understanding of importance of dietary restrictions and express willingness to maintain them.
3. Nursing history and/or physical exam suggestive of: Prolonged vomiting	3. Provide nursing care that will reduce or stop vomiting.	3. The patient demonstrates no further vomiting.
4. Inadequate carbohydrate intake	4. Encourage balanced carbohydrate, protein, and fat intake.	4. The patient demonstrates negative urine ketones and gradual weight gain (as appropriate).
5. Diarrhea or decreased absorption	5. Promote correction of diarrhea or prevent further diarrhea.	5. The patient demonstrates no further diarrhea.
6. Conditions that increase body metabolism (See 5 Increases)	6. Correct conditions that increase body metabolism.	6. The patient will demonstrate correction of conditions causing increased body metabolism.
7. von Gierke's disease	7. Initiate nursing measures that will provide adequate carbohydrate intake.	7. The patient will not demonstrate marked hypoglycemia and acidosis.

Test: 17-Ketogenic Steroids

Abbreviation: 17-KGS

Reference Values: Under 1 year   <1 mg/d
1–10 years   1 mg/d/year of age
Adults   Male Female
under 70   5–23 3–15
over 70   3–12 3–12

Specimen: 24-hour urine collection

Description: The urinary ketogenic steroids include the metabolites of the glucocorticoid steroid cortisol, as well as the cortisol precursor pregnanetriol. Generally, 17-KGS and 17-hydroxycorticosteroids parallel values. In the condition of 21-hydroxylase deficiency of congenital adrenal hyperplasia, however, there is a significant difference.

See 17-OHCS for complete discussion of urinary cortisol metabolites.

Procedure: See 17-OHCS.

Conditions Related to Increases

See 17-OHCS except for the following:

1. Congenital adrenal hyperplasia from 21-hydroxylase deficiency

Rationale

1. This is in contrast to 17-OHCS. The elevation is from the high pregnanetriol level measured in 17-KGS. Pregnanetriol is a cortisol precursor. Pregnanetriol is not measured in 17-OHCS.

Refer to 17-OHCS for more information.

Test:	17-Ketosteroids
Abbreviation:	17-KS
Reference Values:	Under 1 year less than 1 mg/24 hours
	1–4 years less than 2 mg/24 hours
	5–8 years less than 3 mg/24 hours
	9–12 years approximately 3 mg/24 hours
	13–16 years near adult levels
	Adult male 8–18 mg/24 hours
	Adult female 5–15 mg/24 hours
	Over 65 years 4–8 mg/24 hours
Specimen:	24-hour urine collection
Description:	17-Ketosteroids comprise a group of steroid compounds that have a ketone group on carbon-17 in the steroid nucleus. The ketosteroids are excreted in the urine and are representative of metabolites of testosterone, adrenal androgens, and small amounts of cortisol. In females they are secreted almost entirely by the adrenal cortex. In males they are secreted mostly by the adrenals with approximately one-third being secreted by the testes. In prepubertal children of either sex, the primary 17-KS source is the adrenal cortex. Measurements of urinary 17-KS are done to aid in the diagnosis of gonadal adrenal dysfunction. It is also used to aid in the diagnosis of and therapy for adrenogenital syndrome.
Procedure:	24-hour collection

1. No food or fluid restrictions.
2. The patient should try to avoid stressful situations or vigorous physical activity during collection.
3. Collection container may contain preservative; check with local lab. Keep urine refrigerated during entire collection.
4. Collection:
   a. Discard first voided specimen.
   b. Begin timing.
   c. For next 24 hours place all voidings into specimen container immediately after voiding.
   d. Have patient void just prior to completion of 24 hours and put samples in collection bottle.
3. Record exact start and finish times on lab slip.
4. Send to lab immediately.

Conditions Related to Increases	Rationale
1. ACTH therapy	1. Stimulates the entire adrenal cortex resulting in increased 17-KS or adrenosteroid output.
2. Adrenocortical dysfunction Carcinoma	2. The adrenal cortex secretes the majority of the 17-KS. If the cortex is hy-

Cushing's disease
Adrenogenital syndrome
3. Hyperpituitarism

4. Severe stress

5. Certain ovarian and testicular neoplasms

perfunctioning, it secretes increased amounts of 17-KS.

3. Hyperfunction of the pituitary results in increased amounts of ACTH, creating hyperfunction of the adrenal cortex.

4. Stress creates increased adrenal cortical activity.

5. In males, approximately one-third of the 17-KS are produced by the testicles. Very small amounts of the 17-KS are secreted by the ovaries in females. Neoplasms may create increased secretions of normally occurring substances.

Conditions Related to Decreases

1. Addison's disease or adrenalectomy

2. Hypopituitarism

3. Hypogonadism or castration

4. Advanced liver disease

5. Anorexia nervosa

6. Nephrosis

7. Kleinfelter's syndrome

Rationale

1. Hypoactivity of the adrenal gland characterized by decreased secretion of all adrenocortical hormones.

2. Hypoactivity of the pituitary results in decreased ACTH with diminished stimulation of the adrenal cortex.

3. Diminished or absent function of the gonads results in decreased release of testicular 17-KS.

4. Adrenal androgens are bound to plasma proteins, but in advanced liver disease there is decreased production of serum proteins. Androgens are conjugated in the liver but the diminished liver function disrupts this action. Also, cholesterol is essential for 17-KS formation and is manufactured by a normal liver. In advanced liver disease, cholesterol is not being made (5).

5. In this condition, a state of malnutrition eventually results. In malnutrition, there is a reduced level of plasma proteins, which are essential to bind with the adrenal androgens.

6. Androgens are excreted in the urine. In nephrosis, excessive loss may occur due to increased capillary permeability.

7. There may be a decreased release of testicular 17-KS in this syndrome.

Drug Influences: The following drugs may influence test results. The drugs are listed alphabetically by generic name and divided into columns according to the effect of the drug. Examples of trade names are in parentheses.

The following drugs may cause an increase in test results:

Metabolic effect
   cortisone (Cortistan)

Normal intended effect
   metyrapone (Metopirone)

Miscellaneous
   ampicillin (Omnipen), 14 days postinjection in postmenopausal women

The following drugs may cause a decrease in test results:

ACTH suppression
   dexamethasone (Decadron)

Estrogen-mediated decrease of cortisol secretion
   oral contraceptives

Miscellaneous
   ampicillin (Omnipen), 7 days postinjection in pregnancy

Related Lab Studies: Monitor response to treatment or progression of disease and adjust nursing care accordingly. See individual tests for information.

	Cushing's Syndrome	Addison's Disease	Adrenogenital Syndrome
17-ketogenic steroids	↑	↓	↑
17-hydroxycorticosteroids	↑	↓	↑
blood sugar	↑	↓	↑
WBC	↑	↓	↑
eosinophiles	↓	↑	↓
potassium (serum)	↓	↑	↓
sodium (serum)	↑	↓	↑, ↓, or normal
ACTH stimulation test		No response	
Dexamethasone suppression test	High dose suppression		

IMPLICATIONS FOR NURSING CARE
PRETEST: Factors related to the test
Nursing Diagnosis: Potential for injury related to changes in biochemical balance

Guide to assessment	Guide to planning and intervention	Guide to evaluation

Assess patient factors that may influence test results:
1. Exercise and stress
	1. Tell patient and assist to:
	  a. Avoid excessive physical activity while 24-hour urine sample is being collected.
	  b. Avoid stressful situations during 24-hour sample col-
		1. The patient's lab results are not influenced by exercise or stress.

Guide to assessment	Guide to planning and intervention	Guide to evaluation
	lection time.	
2. Menstruation in female	2. Delay scheduling of 24-hour urine collection until after menses.	2. The female patient's urine specimen is not contaminated with menstrual blood.
3. Comprehensive drug history (See Drug Influences)	3. Report to the lab and physician drugs the patient is receiving that may influence lab results. (Drugs may be withheld for 48 hours prior to the procedure.)	3. Drugs that patient is receiving that may influence lab results are identified and the appropriate people are notified.
4. Preexisting conditions (See Increases/Decreases) Pregnancy, third trimester	4. Record preexisting conditions on lab slip. Also note if patient is in third trimester of pregnancy, since this may elevate 17-KS.	4. Patient's preexisting conditions are noted on lab slip.
5. Knowledge deficit	5. Explain test to the patient: a. Define 17-ketosteroids. b. Explain procedure (See Procedure).	5. Patient demonstrates knowledge of test and procedure. 24-hour urine specimen is collected accurately.

Patient Preparation Checklist

1. √ Decrease activity and stress during 24-hour collection period.
2. √ Note menses.
3. √ Influencing drugs noted and reported (See Drug Influences).
4. √ Preexisting conditions noted on lab slip (See Increases/Decreases).
5. √ Patient knowledge; explain test and procedure (See Description and Procedure).

CONSIDERATIONS FOR NURSING CARE RELATED TO ABNORMAL TEST RESULTS
POSTTEST: Factors related to the results of the test
Nursing Diagnosis: Alterations in biochemical balance

Guide to assessment	Guide to planning and intervention	Guide to evaluation
Assess patient for factors that may be influencing test results.		

Guide to assessment	Guide to planning and intervention	Guide to evaluation
Nursing history and/or physical exam suggestive of: 1. ACTH treatment	1. Report increased 17-KS to physician for possible adjustment in dose of ACTH.	1. Medication dose is adjusted as necessary to permit return to normal 17-KS levels.
2. Adrenocortical dysfunction or hyperpituitarism	2. Promote decreased secretion of adrenocorticosteroids by:	2. Patient demonstrates increased energy levels, normal blood sugar, and return to normal appearance:
a. Carcinoma or Cushing's syndrome	a. Administering chemotherapeutic drugs as ordered for patients with adrenal carcinoma: (1) Administering drugs that interfere with pituitary ACTH production (cyproheptadine or bromocriptine mesylate) or drugs that inhibit synthesis of cortisol in the adrenals (metapyrone, mitotane, or aminoglutethimide) in patients with Cushing's syndrome or hyperpituitarism who are not candidates for surgery.	
b. Adrenogenital syndrome	b. Promoting decreased ACTH production by: (1) Administering glucocorticoids as ordered. (2) Teaching the child and parents the importance of taking the medication as prescribed.	b. The patient demonstrates linear growth slowed and puberty occurring at usual age.

3. Stress	3. Reduce stress by:
	a. Providing a restful, quiet environment.
	b. Explaining all procedures prior to their initiation.
	c. Encouraging verbalization of fears and concerns.
	d. Assisting the patient to identify specific stressors and possible ways of eliminating or coping with those stressors, e.g., physical activity, relaxation techniques, etc.
		3. Patient appears outwardly calm with relaxed facial muscles and states feeling relaxed.
		  Patient identifies stressors in own life and describes ways of eliminating or coping with those stressors.
		  Patient states the importance of receiving medical treatment for physiological stressors.

Guide to assessment	Guide to planning and intervention	Guide to evaluation
	e. Teaching patient the importance of receiving treatment for any condition producing stress on the system, e.g., severe infection, surgery, etc.	
4. Ovarian tumors Testicular tumors	4. Promote decrease in size of tumor by: a. Administering ordered chemotherapeutic drugs.	4. Tumor will demonstrate decrease in size.
5. Liver dysfunction	5. Promote increased transport of 17-KS in the patient's body by: a. Increasing dietary protein intake at meals and with supplements if status allows. b. Administering salt-poor albumin as ordered.	5. Patient demonstrates increase in 17-KS.
6. Addison's disease or post-adrenalectomy	6. Promote normal hormone balance by: a. Administering glucocorticoids, mineralocorticoids and testosterone as ordered. b. Teaching patient the importance of taking medications on time, and notifying the physician when experiencing any unusual physical or emotional stress so medication dose can be increased.	6. a. The patient ingests appropriate amounts of medication to prevent serious symptoms. b. The patient states understanding of the need to report physical or emotional stress.

Test: Lactic Dehydrogenase

Abbreviation: LDH or LD

Reference Values: Birth   290–501 U/L
1 day–month   185–404 U/L
1 month–2 years   110–244 U/L
<4 years   60–170 U/L
3–17 years   85–165 U/L
Adult   30–90 U/L

LDH isoenzymes   % of total
LDH_1 (heart)   24–34
LDH_2 (heart, RBC)   35–45
LDH_3 (muscle)   15–25
LDH_4 (liver, trace muscle)   4–10
LDH_5 (liver, muscle)   1–9

Specimen: Serum

Description: Lactic dehydrogenase is an enzyme found in the cytoplasm of nearly all body tissue. Five isoenzymes have been identified. In myocardial infarction, LDH isoenzyme 1 showing greater concentration than LDH isoenzyme 2 is referred to as flipped. The flipped LDH_1 value, along with elevated CPK-MB and AST (SGOT), is a good indicator of myocardial infarction.

For a more complete discussion see CPK.

Drug Influences: The following drugs may cause an increase in test results:

Cholestatic effect
anabolic steroids   norethandrolone (Nilevar)
imipramine (Tofranil)   propxyphene (Darvon)

Hepatotoxic effect
carbenicillin (Geocillin)   methotrexate (Mexate)
clindamycin (Cleocin)   mithramycin (Mithracin)
copper   quinidine (Cardioquin)
ethanol (grain alcohol)   Xylitol
floxuridine (FUDR)

Increased intrabiliary pressure
codeine   morphine
meperidine (Demerol)

Hemolytic anemia
nitrofurantoin (Macrodantin)   sulfisoxazole (Gantrisin)
sulfamethoxazole (Azo Gantanol)

Miscellaneous
anesthetic agents
clofibrate (Atromid-S)
dicumarol (Dicumarol)
oxyphenisatin (Isocrin)

The following drugs may cause a decrease in test results:

Inhibition of in vivo production
    aldrin
    benzene
    dieldrin
    fluorides

Refer to Creatine Phosphokinase (CPK, CK) for
    Related Lab Studies
    Pretest Implications
    Posttest Considerations

Test:	Lead Level
Abbreviation:	PbB (blood lead) PbU (urine lead)
Reference Values:	*Serum* Children less than 30 mcg/dl Adults less than 40 mcg/dl *Urine* less than 80 mcg/l/24-hour urine collection
Specimen:	Whole blood, timed urine collection (length varies with lab)
Description:	Lead is a toxic substance. It is found in dust and soil mainly from automotive exhaust and lead processing smelters. It is also found in powdering paint from old buildings and a variety of other sources. It enters the body by ingestion or inhalation and accumulates in bone and soft tissues. Since the rate of lead excretion is very slow, it accumulates in the body. Accumulation of excessive quantities results in acute or chronic poisoning. Lead does not serve any purpose in the body and has a number of harmful effects. Primarily, lead has an inhibitory effect on all the enzymatic steps involved in heme synthesis (21). Many of the clinical manifestations of lead toxicity are similar to those of anemia. More severe toxicity can cause severe neurological symptoms, mental retardation, and death. Lead levels show current absorption of lead, but lead mobilization methods are necessary to give a picture of lead accumulation.

Procedure:

Serum (heparinized lead-free container)

1. No food or fluid restrictions are necessary.
2. The patient's puncture site and the phelebotomist's hands must be carefully cleansed (34).
3. A heparinized lead-free container *must* be used.
4. 0.5–10 ml of venous blood is drawn from the patient.
5. Observe puncture site for bleeding or evidence of hematoma.

Timed Urine Collection

1. The patient may be placed on a low-calcium diet 3 days prior to collection.
2. Collection container must be acidified and lead-free.
3. Collection.
   a. Discard first voided specimen.
   b. Begin timing.
   c. For remainder of collection period place all voidings into specimen container immediately after voiding.
   d. If possible, have patient void just prior to completion of collection and put sample in collection container.
4. Record exact start and finish times on lab slip.
5. Send specimen to lab.

Conditions Related to Increases

Serum and Urine

1. Persons exposed to lead and its compounds
   a. Children who chew paper, make spitballs
   b. Children who chew on toys or furniture
   c. Industrial workers

   d. Manufacturing of ceramics

   e. Manufacturing insecticides and lubricants

Rationale

1. Increased exposure facilitating increased ingestion or inhalation.
   a. Newsprint contains lead.

   b. Paint may contain lead, especially if from old buildings.
   c. Exposure to battery fumes, acetyline torch fumes, paint fumes, and lead processing, which all contain lead.
   d. Improperly lead-glazed earthenware.
   e. Many contain lead.

Drug Influences: The following drugs may cause an increase in test results:

Urine

Lead-poisoning–related effect
    dimercaprol (BAL in oil)   penicillamine (Cuprimine)
    edetic acid

The following drug may cause a decrease in test results:

Whole Blood

Miscellaneous
    edetic acid; if lead poisoning is present

Related Lab Studies

Diagosis of lead poisoning:
    ↑ ESR
    ↑ *urine delta-aminolevulinic acid
    ↑ urine coproporphyrin
    ↓ RBC (stippled RBCs)
    ↑ urobilinogen and uroporphyrin
    ↑ CSF protein with normal cell count in encephalopathy
    CBC (Hct, Hgb ↓)
    ↑ reticulocyte count
    urinalysis
  * Calcium disodium edetate (EDTA) mobilization test (increased levels of lead)

---

*Not discussed in this book.

IMPLICATIONS FOR NURSING CARE
PRETEST: Factors related to the test
Nursing Diagnosis: Potential for poisoning

Guide to assessment	Guide to planning and intervention	Guide to evaluation
Patient factors that may influence test results: 1. Food	1. Place patient on low calcium diet, as ordered, for 3 days prior to testing to mobilize lead stores from bone.	1. Inappropriate diet does not result in false negative test results.
2. Comprehensive drug history (See Drug Influences)	2. If possible, withhold all calcium-containing drugs for 3 days prior to exam. Report to physician and lab any drugs that may influence test results.	2. Drugs that may influence test results are identified and the proper people are notified. Unnecessary drugs do not interfere with lab results.

3. Knowledge deficit	3. Explain test to patient:
	  a. Define lead (See Description).
	  b. Explain procedure (See Procedure).
		3. Patient demonstrates knowledge of test by defining test and explaining procedure.

Patient Preparation Checklist

1. √ Omission of calcium from diet for 3 days prior to test.
2. √ Influencing drugs noted and reported (See Drug Influences).
3. √ Patient knowledge; explain test and procedure (See Description and Procedure).

CONSIDERATIONS FOR NURSING CARE RELATED TO ABNORMAL TEST RESULTS
POSTTEST: Factors related to the results of the test
Nursing Diagnosis: Alterations of biochemical balance related to poisoning

Guide to assessment	Guide to planning and intervention	Guide to evaluation
Nursing history and/or physical exam suggestive of lead poisoning: Signs and symptoms Facial pallor Anorexia Weight loss Abdominal colic Constipation Muscle pains Weakness Anemia Depression Convulsions Delirium Mental changes	1. Promote excretion of lead by: a. Administering saline cathartics as ordered to promote elimination from gastrointestinal tract. b. Administering chelating agent (e.g., calcium disodium edetate) as ordered. 2. Promote lowered levels of lead by: a. Assisting to determine the cause of the increased levels and teaching patient/ parent to avoid ingestion or inhalation of lead.	1. Patient demonstrates decreased blood levels of lead. 2. Source of lead ingestion and/or inhalation is determined and eliminated from the patient's environment.

Test:	Lipase
Abbreviation:	None
Reference Values:	Less than 1.5 μ/ml 32–80 μ/L
Specimen:	Serum
Description:	Lipase is a digestive enzyme secreted from the pancreas through the pancreatic duct into the duodenum. Its function in the body is to split emulsified fats and triglycerides into fatty acids and glycerol. When the pancreas is damaged or there is obstruction to pancreatic duct flow, lipase, like amylase, is absorbed into the blood. Some lipase is excreted from the body in the urine but normally in negligible amounts. Lipase levels are useful in the diagnosis of pancreatic disorders, especially acute pancreatitis. They are also useful in the late diagnosis of pancreatitis as early elevations usually parallel elevations of amylase, though lipase levels remain elevated approximately 1 week longer than amylase. Another form of lipase, called lipoprotein lipase, exists but has different sites of storage, production, and action. Its major action is to hydrolyze protein-bound triglycerides in the serum (7).
Procedure:	(red top tube) 1. Food and fluids are withheld for 12 hours or as ordered. 2. 2–5 ml of venous blood is withdrawn from the patient. 3. Observe for bleeding at puncture site or for evidence of hematoma.

Conditions Related to Increases

1. Pancreatitis

2. Obstruction of pancreatic duct flow:
   Pancreatic duct obstruction
   High intestinal obstruction
   Pancreatic carcinoma
   Acute cholecystitis
3. Cirrhosis

4. Renal disease

Rationale

1. When the pancreas is damaged or greatly inflamed, the enzyme flow is obstructed and the enzymes are absorbed into the blood.

2. Any obstruction, primary or secondary of the pancreatic duct or common bile duct system, blocks the normal pathway of lipase secretion and the lipase is absorbed into the blood.

3. There may be biliary cirrhosis due to biliary duct obstruction that will cause a secondary pancreatic duct obstruction.

4. Some lipase is excreted from the body by the kidneys. When the kidneys' excretory function is impaired, lipase backs up into bloodstream.

5. Perforated duodenal ulcer

5. An ulcer in the duodenum may perforate the pancreas, causing a secondary pancreatitis (7).

6. Patients receiving opiates or cholinergics within 24 hours of test

6. Opiates may cause spasms of the sphincter of Oddi. Spasm of this sphincter acts like an obstruction to normal digestive enzyme flow.

7. Conditions causing increased serum lipid levels
   Hyperlipoproteinemia
   Fat embolism
   Crush injury

7. Increased serum fat levels cause increased release of lipoprotein lipase, which functions to clear triglycerides from the plasma (24, 27).

Conditions Related to Decreases

1. Viral hepatitis

Rationale

1. In hepatitis the liver may be unable to form bile salts, which are necessary for activation of pancreatic lipase in the intestines.

2. Congenital absence of lipase

2. This is a congenital defect resulting in the inability of the pancreas to form lipase (21).

3. Protein malnutrition

3. Severe malnutrition may cause structural damage to the pancreas resulting in decreased production of lipase.

4. Cystic fibrosis

4. This is a disease in which the pancreas is unable to secrete normal amounts of digestive enzymes.

5. Extrahepatic biliary obstruction

5. If obstruction is above the pancreatic duct and does not block pancreatic flow into the intestine but does block flow of bile salts (necessary or normal lipase activity), there will be low levels of serum lipase.

Drug Influences: The following drugs may cause an increase in serum lipase. The drugs are listed alphabetically by generic name and divided into columns according to the effect of the drug. Examples of trade names are in parentheses.

Impaired excretion due to spasm of sphincter of Oddi

bethanechol (Urecholine)
cholinergics
codeine
meperidine (Demerol)

methacholine (mecholyl chloride)
morphine
pentazocine (Talwin)
secretin (Secretin)

Pancreatitis (chemical or physical)
ethanol (grain alcohol)
sulfisoxazole (Gantrisin)

Release of tissue lipase into plasma
heparin (150% increase 10 minutes after injection; 27)

The following drugs may cause a decrease in serum lipase:

protamine (Protamine Sulfate)
saline

Related Lab Studies: Monitor response to treatment or progression of disease and adjust nursing care accordingly. See individual tests for information.

Pancreatitis:
   amylase, urine and serum
   blood glucose
   calcium
   potassium
   AST (SGOT)
   LDH
   *trypsin, serum
   hematocrit

IMPLICATIONS FOR NURSING CARE
PRETEST: Factors related to the test
Nursing Diagnosis: Potential for injury related to changes in biochemical balance

Guide to assessment	Guide to planning and intervention	Guide to evaluation
Assess patient factors that may influence test results:		
1. Food and fluids	1. Maintain patient NPO from midnight until the test is completed as ordered.	1. The patient's food and fluid intake will not cause inaccurate lab results.
2. Comprehensive drug history (See Drug Influences and Increases/Decreases)	2. Report drugs patient is receiving that may influence lab results to the lab and the patient's physician. (Withhold codeine, meperidine, morphine, and cholinergics for 24 hours preceding the test, if possible.)	2. Drugs the patient is currently receiving that may influence lab results are identified and the proper people notified.
3. Preexisting conditions (See Increases/Decreases) Pregnancy	3. Record preexisting conditions on lab slip.	3. Patient's preexisting conditions are noted on lab slip.
4. Knowledge deficit	4. Explain test to patient: a. Define lipase (See Description). b. Describe procedure (See Procedure).	4. The patient demonstrates knowledge by defining test and stating procedure.

*Not discussed in this book.

Patient Preparation Checklist

1. √ NPO 8 hours or as ordered.
2. √ Influencing drugs noted and reported (See Drug Influences).
3. √ Preexisting conditions noted on lab slip (See Increases/Decreases).
4. √ Patient knowledge; explain test and procedure (See Description and Procedure).

CONSIDERATIONS FOR NURSING CARE RELATED TO ABNORMAL TEST RESULTS
POSTTEST: Factors related to the results of the test
Nursing Diagnosis: Alterations in biochemical balance

Guide to assessment	Guide to planning and intervention	Guide to evaluation

Assess patient factors influencing test results:
1. Nursing history and/or physical exam suggestive of: Pancreatic disease
    Increase in peritoneal fluid
    Vomiting
	1. Reduce stimulation of pancreatic secretions by:
	
	a. Giving prescribed anticholinergic drugs and maintaining NPO, gastric suction, fluid intake treatment plan.
		1. The patient demonstrates reduced pancreatic stimulation by:
		a. Reduced abdominal distention.

Pain (abdominal and back) that is boring, bandlike, and constant in nature	b. Giving pain medication as needed (not morphine or its derivatives) and help the patient assume position of comfort. c. Administering nitroglycerine, Papaverine, or other smooth muscle relaxants as ordered.	b. Verbalizing decreased pain sensation after pain medication. c. Verbalizing that episodes of pain are less frequent.
2. Spasms of sphincter of Oddi Acute, severe, deep cramping pain	2. Reduce spasms of sphincter of Oddi by: a. Withholding cholinergic or opiate drugs if possible. b. Giving nonopiate pain medications. c. Administering antispasmodic drugs as ordered. d. Encouraging low-fat diet. e. Discouraging use of alcoholic beverages.	2. The patient verbalizes pain relief after pain medications and verbalizes decreasing episodes of pain.

Guide to assessment	Guide to planning and intervention	Guide to evaluation

3. Increased serum lipid levels
   Hyperlipoproteinemia
   Fat embolism
   Crush injury
	3. Decrease serum lipid levels by:
	  a. Providing diet low in animal fat.
	  b. Administering hypolipidemic drugs as ordered.
	  c. Teaching patient the importance of low animal fat diet, as well as the specific foods that need to be restricted.
		3. The patient will demonstrate decreased serum lipid levels.
		  The patient will verbalize understanding of the importance of low animal fat in the diet and express willingness to observe dietary restrictions

4. Viral hepatitis	4. Prevent further liver damage by:
	  a. Withholding hepatotoxic drugs as ordered.
	  b. Instructing patient to abstain from alcohol intake and explaining the importance of this.
		4. The patient will not receive hepatotoxic drugs or ingest alcohol.

5. Cystic fibrosis
   Congenital absence of lipase
6. Protein malnutrition
	5. Promote normal digestion by administering pancreatic enzymes as ordered.
	6. Promote increased protein intake by:
	  a. Providing a diet high in protein.
	  b. Explaining the importance of increasing protein intake and identifying specific foods high in protein.
	  c. Utilizing nursing measures to increase dietary intake toward well-balanced nutrition.
		5. The patient will demonstrate decrease in the amount of fat in the stool.
		6. The patient will increase protein intake with evidence of improved nutritional status.

Test:	Lupus Erythematosus Cell Preparation Indirect Immunofluorescent Antibody Radioimmunoassay Method
Abbreviations:	LE prep., IIFA, RIA
Reference Value:	Negative (at least two LE cells needed for positive test)
Specimen:	Clotted blood
Description:	Antinuclear antibodies are antibodies that react against some portion of the nucleus of body cells. The LE factor is an autoimmune antinuclear antibody. The LE preparation test is done in order to identify LE cell activity. The LE preparation test is positive in about 75–85% of patients with active lupus erythematosus. It is also positive in patients with dieases other than systemic lupus erythematosus (SLE). A more specific test to determine LE cell activity is the indirect immunofluorescent antibody test. The advantage of this test is that it can detect LE activity during antiinflammatory or immunosuppressive therapy. One of the most specific diagnostic tests is the radioimmunoassay method. This method detects an antibody that is fairly specific to lupus erythematosus (5). The tests for LE cell activity are done to aid in the diagnosis and management of SLE.
Procedure:	(red top tube) 1. No food or fluid restrictions. 2. 5–7 ml of blood is drawn from the patient. 3. Observe puncture site for bleeding, evidence of hematoma, or infection.

Conditions Related to Increases

1. Lupus erythematosus
   Dermatomyositis/polymyositis
   Rheumatoid arthritis
   Hepatitis
   Hemolytic anemias
   Drugs (See Drug Influences)
   Scleroderma

Rationale

1. In the laboratory, blood cells of the patient are challenged with an antigen (a specially treated protein nucleus). If the LE factor (antibody) is present, it reacts to the antigen and damages the nucleus. The nucleus is surrounded by phagocytes and ingested. The phagocyte that ingests the damaged nucleus is known as an LE cell.

Drug Influences: The following drugs may influence test results. The drugs are listed alphabetically by generic name and divided into columns according to the effect of the drug. Examples of trade names are in parentheses.

The following drugs may cause a positive test result:

LE-like syndrome

acetazolamide (Diamox)	methimazole (Tapazole)
aminosalicylic acid	oral contraceptives

anticonvulsants
chlorprothixene (Taractan)
digitalis
gold preparation (Myochrysine)
griseofulvin (Fulvicin, Grifulvin V)

phenylbutazone (Azolid, Butazolidin)
propythiouracil
sulfonamides
tetracycline
thiazides

May precipitate or activate disease
corticosteroids
hydantoin derivatives
(Dilantin)

hydrazine derivatives (Apresoline,
Hydralazine, Serpasil)

Related Lab Studies: Monitor response to therapy or progression of disease and adjust nursing care accordingly. See individual lab tests for specific information.

In SLE:
CBC
platelet count
sedimentation rate
protein electrophoresis
urinalysis
creatinine clearance
*serum complement studies
radioimmunoassay, LE factor
serology (false positive)
indirect immunofluorescent antibody
ANA

IMPLICATIONS FOR NURSING CARE
PRETEST: Factors related to the test
Nursing Diagnosis: Potential for injury related to changes in biochemical balance

Guide to assessment	Guide to planning and intervention	Guide to evaluation

Assess patient factors that may influence test results:
1. Comprehensive drug history (See Drug Influences), especially
  Hydralazine
  Procainamide
  Isoniazid
  Oral contraceptives
2. Knowledge deficit
	1. Note interfering drugs on lab slip.
	
	2. Explain test to patient:
	  a. Define LE cells (See Description).
	  b. Explain procedure (See Description and Procedure).
		1. Patient's drugs do not interfere with test results.
		
		2. The patient demonstrates knowledge of test by defining test and stating procedure.

*Not discussed in this book.

Patient Preparation Checklist

1. √ Interfering drugs noted on lab slip (See Drug Influences).
2. √ Patient knowledge; explain test to patient (See Description/Procedure).

CONSIDERATIONS FOR NURSING CARE RELATED TO ABNORMAL TEST RESULTS
POSTTEST: Factors related to the results of the test
Nursing Diagnosis: Alterations in biochemical balance

Guide to assessment	Guide to planning and intervention	Guide to evaluation
Assess patient factors that may be influencing test results. Nursing history and/or physical exam suggestive of: 1. Positive ANA test Drug therapy that causes SLE-like syndrome (See Drug Influences) 2. Systemic lupus erythematosus	1. Recognize drugs that cause SLE-like syndrome and consult with physician. 2. Promote disease remission: a. Prevent precipitation of disease by: (1) Initiating nursing measures to prevent infection. (2) Advising patient to use sunscreen if in sun. (3) Advising patient to consult with physician before using over-the-counter drugs. (4) Exploring positive ways of responding to stress. (5) Seeking mental health help as needed. (6) Advising patient to keep well rested and eat a well-balanced diet. (7) Administering antibiotics as prescribed.	1. Patient's lab values are normal. 2. Patient achieves remission:

Guide to assessment	Guide to planning and intervention	Guide to evaluation
b. Drug therapy Corticosteroids Salicylates Nonsteroidal antiin- flammatory agents Antimalarial drugs Immunosuppressive drugs	b. Decrease inflammation by: (1) Administering drugs as prescribed. (2) Educating patient to side effects and precautions of steroids. (3) See a 1–7 above.	b. The patient's inflammatory process is diminished as evidenced by lab studies, physical exam, and subjective data.
c. Lupus Foundation of America, Inc. Arthritis Foundation	c. Encourage participation in support groups.	c. The patient is able to name support groups and state the help received from them.

Test:	Magnesium
Abbreviation:	Mg
Reference Values:	*Serum* Newborn 1.52–2.33 mEq/L Child 1.4–1.9 mEq/L (46) Adult 1.3–2.5 mEq/L *Urine*, 24-hour collection 6.0–8.5 mEq/24 hours
Specimen:	Serum Urine, 24-hour collection
Description:	Magnesium is, along with potassium, one of the most abundant intracellular ions. The majority of magnesium is found in bone, within cells and cartilage. Magnesium is absorbed by the small intestine and excreted in the urine and feces (42). Plasma levels are regulated by the endocrine and urinary systems. Like calcium, approximately half of magnesium is bound to protein. Magnesium is essential for normal neuromuscular function, as well as for normal metabolism of carbohydrates, lipids, proteins, and nucleic acid synthesis (5, 8). It is also known to be required for activation of a large number of enzymes. Magnesium is needed for clotting and is essential in maintaining normal transport of sodium and potassium across cell membranes (42). Magnesium has a major effect on calcium balance, mainly by influencing parathyroid hormone secretion and by increasing the absorption of calcium from the intestines. Serum and urine magnesium levels are done to determine causes of neurological symptoms or to help evaluate renal function and determine electrolyte balance. Magnesium depletion is clinically more significant and frequent than an excess but it is still relatively uncommon (2). Hypermagnesemia may occur at birth due to treatment of the mother with magnesium salts before delivery. Urine levels were rarely done in the past but have become more popular because magnesium deficiencies are detectable in the urine before serum changes occur (42).
Procedure:	(red top tube)

Serum

1. Alcohol consumption should be omitted for 3 days prior to the test.
2. Magnesium-containing antacids or cathartics should be omitted 3 days prior to the test.
3. 10–15 ml of blood is withdrawn from the patient.
4. Observe for bleeding at the puncture site or for evidence of hematoma.

Urine

1. 24-hour urine collection.

a. Discard first voided specimen.

b. For next 24 hours place all voidings into specimen container immediately after voiding.

c. Have patient void just prior to completion of the 24 hours and put sample in collection bottle.

2. Record exact start and finish times on lab slip.
3. Send to lab.
4. No preservative is needed in collection container.

Conditions Related to Increases	Rationale
	Serum
1. Acute or chronic renal failure	1. Much of magnesium is excreted by the kidney and when kidney function is diminished, magnesium cannot be excreted as well.
2. Addison's disease or postadrenalectomy	2. In Addison's disease, an extracellular fluid volume depletion may exist secondary to excessive sodium loss. This makes serum magnesium appear higher due to the state of dehydration (40). Renal blood flow may be compromised in Addison's disease secondary to decreased ECF volume and this may decrease renal excretion of magnesium. There is also decreased aldosterone secretion in this disease, which also results in decreased magnesium.
3. Dehydration Excessive exercise	3. A state of dehydration makes the relative level of magnesium appear higher.
4. Hypothyroidism	4. Thyroid hormone causes stimulation of bone reabsorption or bone-forming activity. In a hypothyroid state, bones do not have this normal stimulus from the thyroid and they break down faster, leading to a release of calcium, phosphorus, and magnesium (49). There may be diminished renal blood flow in hypothyroidism that leads to magnesium retention (49). Calcitonin, which is released by the thyroid gland, has been found to increase magnesium clearance from the kidney. In hypothyroidism, there are decreased levels of calcitonin, resulting in decreased magnesium excretion and higher serum magnesium levels (40).

5. Chronic ingestion of magnesium-containing antacids
   Use of MgSO$_4$
   Neonatal hypermagnesemia

6. Hyperparathyroidism

7. Untreated diabetic acidosis

5. Excessive intake of magnesium. In the newborn there may be an increase due to treatment of the mother with magnesium salts before delivery.

6. The parathyroid hormone (PTH) causes increased renal tubular reabsorption of magnesium. In states of increased levels of PTH there is increased serum magnesium (7, 40).

7. Magnesium is elevated due to the existing dehydration (which is due to osmotic diuresis occurring with marked hyperglycemia).

Conditions Related to Decreases

1. Malabsorption disorders
   Gastroenteritis and colitis
   Celiac sprue disease
   Regional enteritis
   Faulty absorption following intestinal bypass surgery
   Diarrhea
2. Hyperthyroidism

3. Vomiting or continuous bowel or gastric aspirations
4. Nephrotic syndrome and acute poststreptococcal glomerulonephritis

5. Use of diuretics (thiazides and ethacrynic acid)

6. Malnutrition
7. Alcoholism

Rationale

1. Magnesium is normally absorbed in the small intestine. In disorders where there is impaired absorption, magnesium does not get absorbed and so serum levels are low.

2. The decrease is probably related to the associated increased renal blood flow and increased glomerular filtration rate present in hyperthyroidism. Magnesium is excreted by the kidneys and this increased activity leads to low serum levels (49). Diarrhea is often a problem in thyrotoxicosis, resulting in diminished absorption of magnesium from the small intestine.
3. Magnesium is unable to be absorbed due to loss from the body.
4. In the nephrotic syndrome and glomerulonephritis, excessive albumin is lost through the kidney. Since some magnesium is bound to albumin, there is a concomitant magnesium loss.
5. These groups of diuretics prevent renal tubular reabsorption of magnesium as well as a number of other electrolytes.
6. Inadequate intake.
7. Decrease is due to the usual malnutrition associated with alcoholism.

8. Prolonged intravenous feeding with magnesium-poor solutions

8. Inadequate intake and replacement.

9. Hyperaldosteronism

9. Aldosterone increases urinary excretion of magnesium. Too much aldosterone causes excessive magnesium loss. Hyperaldosteronism also causes fluid retention, resulting in a state of relative hypomagnesemia.

10. Hypoparathyroidism

10. The parathyroid hormone increases reabsorption of magnesium by the kidneys. In hypoparathyroidism, there are low levels of parathyroid hormone, resulting in decreased magnesium reabsorption.

11. Hyperparathyroidism

11. Low magnesium levels have been found in about 14% of patients with hyperparathyroidism (21, 5, 9).

12. Diabetes mellitus

12. Magnesium may be decreased secondary to osmotic diuresis due to hyperglycemia (before a state of severe dehydration exists).

13. Chronic dialysis and chronic renal disease

13. Magnesium is not absorbed without vitamin D, and vitamin D cannot be activated unless the kidneys function. Magnesium may be dialyzed out in excessive amounts.

14. Inappropriate ADH syndrome

14. In this syndrome, there is excessive secretion of ADH, causing fluid retention and a relative or dilutional hypomagnesemia.

15. Severe osteoporosis

15. Much of the body's supply of magnesium is found in bone. If bones are severely broken down there is a decreased body level of magnesium.

16. Pancreatic diseases

16. In many pancreatic diseases, fat digestion is impaired due to a lack of enzymes. Excessive intestinal fats bind with calcium and magnesium and reduce their absorption (54).

17. Liver failure

17. In liver disorders there may be low magnesium levels because of decreased absorption. This is due to higher than normal ammonia levels that bind with the magnesium in the intestines and produce an insoluble nonabsorbable complex (7). Also, in liver disease, there may be defective hepatic synthesis of 25-hydroxycho-

lecalciferon (vitamin D precursor) that results in decreased magnesium absorption (54). Vitamin D is essential for magnesium absorption.

18. Treatment of diabetics in coma

18. Treatment with insulin may lower serum magnesium because magnesium moves with potassium back into the cells.

Conditions Related to Increases

Rationale

Urine

1. Diabetes mellitus

1. Osmotic diuresis secondary to hyperglycemia causes increased excretion of many substances, including magnesium.

2. Hyperthyroidism

2. In the hyperthyroid state there is increased renal blood flow and increased glomerular filtration rate leading to increased renal excretion of magnesium.

3. Nephrotic syndrome

3. A fair amount of magnesium is normally bound to albumin. In this syndrome excessive amounts of albumin are lost through the kidney, and the magnesium bound with albumin is also lost.

Conditions Related to Decreases

Rationale

1. Hypoparathyroidism

1. Initially, values may show an increased urine level due to low parathyroid hormone (PTH) and decreased renal reabsorption of magnesium. (PTH normally increases renal reabsorption of magnesium.) Eventually, serum magnesium depletion results and the urine magnesium levels will be low.

2. Hypothyroidism

2. Levels may be low due to decreased renal blood flow and glomerular filtration rates that result in decreased excretion of magnesium.

3. Acute poststreptococcal glomerulonephritis

3. Due to the hypoproteinemia associated with this disease there is often a fall in both serum and urine magnesium.

Drug Influences: The following drugs may cause an increase in serum and urine magnesium levels. The drugs are listed alphabetically by generic name and divided into columns according to the effect of the drug. Examples of trade names are in parentheses.

Serum Increases

Affects membrane transport system
lithium carbonate (Eskalith, Lithane, Lithobid)

Decreases renal excretion
parathyroid extract

Increased magnesium intake
magnesium products (antacids, magnesium sulfate, Milk of Magnesia)
The following drugs may cause a decrease in magnesium serum and urine levels:

Increased renal excretion
aldosterone
ammonium chloride (Triaminicol)
amphotericin B (Fungizone, Mysteclin-F)
insulin
mercurial diuretics

Increased GI excretion
neomycin (Coly-Mycin S, Cortisporin, Mycolog, Polymyxin B, Neosporin)

Related Lab Studies: Monitor response to treatment or progression of disease and adjust nursing care accordingly. See individual tests for information.

serum electrolytes
CBC
osmolality (urine and serum)
blood sugar
*Lactic acid
BUN
creatinine, serum; creatinine clearance

IMPLICATIONS FOR NURSING CARE
PRETEST: Factors related to the test
Nursing Diagnosis: Potential for injury related to changes in biochemical balance

Guide to assessment	Guide to planning and intervention	Guide to evaluation

Assess patient factors influencing test results:
1. Comprehensive drug history
  See Drug Influences
  Alcohol ingestion
  (See Increases/Decreases)
	1. Report drugs the patient is receiving that may influence lab results to the patient's physician and to laboratory:
	  a. Report to the laboratory if patient is receiving "gluconate" drug, since this drug may affect one
		1. Drugs the patient is currently receiving that may influence test results are identified, and the proper people notified.

*Not discussed in this book.

Guide to assessment	Guide to planning and intervention	Guide to evaluation
	method of laboratory analysis. b. Instruct patient to omit all magnesium-containing antacids or cathartics and all alcohol for 3 days prior to the exam.	
2. Preexisting conditions (See Increases/Decreases) Exercise, menses, pregnancy	2. Record preexisting conditions on laboratory slip. Also note on lab slip whether patient has been involved in heavy exercise over prolonged time prior to exam (leads to increase in lab result); whether female patient is menstruating (leads to increased value); or whether female patient is pregnant (produces decreased value).	2. Patient's preexisting conditions are noted on lab slip.
3. Knowledge deficit	3. Explain test to patient: a. Define magnesium (see Description). b. Describe procedure (see Procedure).	3. The patient demonstrates knowledge of test by defining test and stating procedure.

Patient Preparation Checklist

1. √ Influencing drugs noted and reported (See Drug Influences).
2. √ Preexisting conditions noted on lab slip (See Increases/Decreases).
3. √ Patient knowledge; explain test and procedure (See Description and Procedure).

CONSIDERATIONS FOR NURSING CARE RELATED TO ABNORMAL TEST RESULTS
POSTTEST: Factors related to the results of the test
Nursing Diagnosis: Alterations in biochemical balance

Guide to assessment	Guide to planning and intervention	Guide to evaluation
Assess patient factors that may influence test results. 1. Nursing history and/or physical exam suggestive of	1. Promote decreased magnesium levels by:	1. The patient's magnesium levels are lowered:

Guide to assessment	Guide to planning and intervention	Guide to evaluation
a. Hypermagnesemia Diminished reflexes Muscle weakness Flaccid paralysis Respiratory muscle paralysis (may cause respiratory distress) Drowsiness Flushing Confusion Lethargy Bradycardia Weak pulse Hypotension Heart block Cardiac arrest	a. Detecting signs and symptoms of increased magnesium and reporting them to physician immediately.	a. The patient does not demonstrate signs or symptoms of hypermagnesemia.
b. Dehydration	b. Maintaining fluid balance.	b. The patient is hydrated.
c. Renal failure	c. Questioning giving magnesium to a patient with renal failure: (1) Withholding magnesium-containing medication as ordered. (2) Administering calcium gluconate as ordered when high levels of magnesium are present.	c. The patient's magnesium level is within normal limits: (1) Unnecessary magnesium is withheld. (2) Calcium gluconate is given as ordered.
d. Chronic ingestion of magnesium-containing antacids and cathartics	d. Identifying and teaching patient about: (1) Nonmagnesium-containing antacids or cathartics. (2) Appropriate nonmedication methods of controlling constipation.	(1) The patient identifies nonmagnesium-containing antacids and cathartics. (2) The patient describes methods for decreasing constipation without medication.
e. Prenatal $MgSO_4$ administration (mother and newborn)	e. Giving calcium gluconate as ordered.	e. The patient maintains normal muscle tone, level of consciousness, and pulse and respiration.
f. Hypothyroidism	f. Administering thyroid medication as ordered.	f. The patient receives thyroid medication as ordered.
2. Nursing history and/or physical exam suggestive of	2. Promote increased levels of magnesium by:	2. The patient does not demonstrate signs or symptoms of hypomagnesemia.

Guide to assessment	Guide to planning and intervention	Guide to evaluation

a. Hypomagnesemia
Symptoms:
  Hyperirritability
  Tetany
  Leg and foot cramps
  Chvostek's sign
  Confusion
  Delusions
  Hallucinations
  Convulsions
  Arrhythmias
  Vasodilation
  Hypotension
  Possible hypertension
	a. Detecting signs and symptoms of decreased magnesium and reporting them immediately to physician.
	  Administering magnesium as ordered.
		The patient receives magnesium as ordered.

b. Malnutrition	b. Assisting in improvement of nutrition status.	b. The patient demonstrates normal nutrition by height, weight, and general appearance.
c. Primary aldosteronism	c. Administering spironolactone (Aldactone) as ordered.	c. The patient demonstrates increased sodium and water output, and signs and symptoms of hypomagnesemia do not occur.
d. Hyperglycemia Diabetic acidosis	d. Assisting in the correction or prevention of ketoacidosis and promoting correct administration of insulin or oral hypoglycemics as ordered.	d. The patient's blood sugar and ketone levels are normal.

e. Inappropriate ADH syndrome	e. Assisting in the correction of fluid balance by:
	  (1) Restricting fluids as ordered by the physician.
	  (2) Administer, in severe cases, hypertonic saline solution IV and administration of IV diuretics.
		e. Patient will demonstrate balanced fluid intake and output, increased urinary output, and decreased weight.

f. Severe osteoporosis	f. Administering calcitonin, calcium, vitamin D, estrogen, and/or anabolic steroids as ordered.	f. The patient does not demonstrate progressive bone decalcification.
g. Pancreatic disease	g. Administering pancreatic enzymes as ordered.	g. The patient demonstrates improved absorption as shown by decrease in amount of fat in stools.

Test:	Mean Corpuscular Hemoglobin
Abbreviation:	MCH
Reference Values:	Newborns　32–34 pg All others　27–31 pg
Specimen:	Whole blood
Description:	The mean corpuscular hemoglobin (MCH) is determined by dividing the hemoglobin by the red blood cell count. This is a measurement of the average weight of hemoglobin in a red blood cell. The results generally parallel mean corpuscular volume (MCV) results as cell size dictates the amount of hemoglobin the cell holds. Increases in MCH are seen in macrocytic anemias; decreases are seen in microcytic anemia. This test, along with MCV and mean corpuscular hemoglobin concentration (MCHC), makes up the red blood cell indices or index. Indice measurements aid in the identification of anemias. This test should include RBC morphology.

Turn to RBC count for discussion of:

Procedure
Increases
Decreases
Drug Influences
Related Lab Studies
Pretest Implications
Posttest Considerations

Drug Influences: The following drug may cause a slight increase in MCH after continued use:

oral contraceptives

Also refer to RBC count, Drug Influences.

Test: Mean Corpuscular Hemoglobin Concentration

Abbreviation: MCHC

Reference Values: Newborn 30–34 g/dl
1 month 33–37 g/dl
All others 32–36 g/dl

Description: This test measures the concentration of hemoglobin in 1 dl (100 ml) of packed red cells. Calculation is determined by dividing the hematocrit value into the hemoglobin value. If the result is within normal limits, the finding is *normochromic*; if the finding is decreased, it is *hypochromic*. Because the red blood cells normally hold the maximum hemoglobin concentration, MCHC values are not usually elevated. An increase in MCHC is seen only in spherocytosis. Decreased values are seen in conditions of reduced hemoglobin. This test, with MCH and MCV, makes up red blood cell indices. RBC morphology should be included. RBC indices are measured to aid in the identification of anemia.

Turn to RBC count for discussion of:
Procedure
Increases
Decreases
Related Lab Studies
Pretest Implications
Posttest Considerations

Drug Influences: The following drugs may influence test results and may cause a decrease in test results:

Hemolytic anemia
lead

Hypochromic anemia
penicillamine

Also refer to RBC count, Drug Influences.

Test:	Mean Corpuscular Volume
Abbreviation:	MCV

Reference Values: Newborn   110–128 μm^3
1 month   93–109 μm^3
thereafter   82–101 μm^3
Values vary with laboratory

Specimen: Whole blood

Description: Dividing the hematocrit by the red blood cell count gives the mean corpuscular volume (MCV). This is a way of measuring the volume of a red blood cell. An increase in MCV means the red blood cells are large, or *macrocytic*; a decrease means the red blood cells are small, or *microcytic*. Sometimes the MCV may give a falsely high result. This is because of possible variations in cell size and results in a normal MCV. It is important that an RBC morphology smear be done in connection with this test. This test, along with mean corpuscular hemoglobin (MCH) and mean corpuscular hemoglobin concentration (MCHC), makes up the red blood cell indices or index. The indices are measured to aid in the identification of anemias.

Turn to RBC count for discussion of:

Procedure
Increases
Decreases
Drug Influences
Related Lab Studies
Pretest Implications
Posttest Considerations

Drug Influences: The following drugs may influence test results. The drugs are listed alphabetically by generic name and divided into columns according to the effect of the drug. Examples of trade names are in parentheses.

The following drugs may cause an increase in test values:

Megaloblastic anemia

aminobenzoic acid (Cetacaine, Pabalate, Potaba)
aminosalicylic acid
anticonvulsants
barbiturates
colchicine
cycloserine (Seromycin)
estrogens
glutethimide (Doriden)

mefenamic acid
nitrofurantoin (Furadantin)
nitrofurazone (Furacin)
pentamidine
phenacetin
pyrimethamine (Daraprim)
triamterene (Dyrenium)
trimethoprim

Effect on folic acid metabolism

ethotoin (Peganone)
phenformin (DBI)

The following drugs may cause a decrease in test results:

Hemolytic anemia
   lead

Megaloblastic anemia/hypersensitivity
   nitrofurantoin, in conjunction with G-6-PD

Microcytic hypochromic anemia
   warfarin (Coumadin)

Test: Monospot, Monotest, Monoscreen

Abbreviation: Monotest, HAT (heterophile antibody titer)
                     IM test (infectious mononucleosis test)

Reference Value: Negative

Specimen: Serum (or plasma)

Description: In patients infected with Epstein-Barr virus of infectious mon-
                     onucleosis, heterophile antibodies appear early in the disease.
                     The heterophile antibodies are antibodies that will react to the
                     red blood cells of other animals. These specific infectious mon-
                     onucleosis (IM) antibodies are now able to be identified by fast
                     hemagglutination slide tests. These tests use specially processed
                     horse erythrocytes that act as antigens. In the presence of IM
                     heterophile antibodies the erythrocytes will agglutinate. These
                     tests are considered 90–95% accurate for identifying IM heter-
                     ophile antibodies.

Procedure: (red top tube)
                     1. No food or fluid restrictions.
                     2. 2 ml of blood is drawn from the patient.
                     3. Observe for bleeding from the puncture site or for evidence
                     of hematoma.

Conditions Related to Increases

1. Infectious mononucleosis

2. False positive

Rationale

1. The heterophile antibody is present early in the disease. The disease is most commonly seen in patients between 15 and 25 years of age. It is not very contagious and transmission is probably by oropharyngeal secretions.

2. This reaction may occur in patients with lymphoma, hepatitis, leukemia, or cancer of the pancreas. False positives are very rare.

Conditions Related to Decreases

1. Heterophile negative

Rationale

1. In about 10% of patients with IM, no IM heterophile antibody is present. This is especially true in pediatric patients. Diagnosis is substantiated in these cases by identification of Epstein-Barr virus antibodies.

Drug Influences: The following drugs may influence test results and may cause a positive test result:
Possible positive result
  aminosalicylic acid
  phenytoin (Dilantin)

Related Lab Studies

CBC
↑ WBC; differential, 50–60% of WBCs are lymphocytes and monocytes, 10% of lymphocytes are atypical
↑ ALT (SGPT)
↑ AST (SGOT)
↑ bilirubin, serum

IMPLICATIONS FOR NURSING CARE
PRETEST: Factors related to the test
Nursing Diagnosis: Potential for injury related to changes in microbiological environment

Guide to assessment	Guide to planning and intervention	Guide to evaluation
Assess patient factors that may influence test results.		
1. Comprehensive drug history (See Drug Influences)	1. Note drugs the patient is receiving that may influence test results on lab slip.	1. Patient's drugs that may influence test results are noted on lab slip.
2. Knowledge deficit	2. Explain test to patient: a. Define mono tests (See Description). b. Explain procedure (See Procedure).	2. The patient demonstrates knowledge of test by defining test and stating procedure.

Patient Preparation Checklist

1. √ Drug history (See Drug Influences).
2. √ Patient knowledge; explain test to patient (See Description/Procedure).

CONSIDERATIONS FOR NURSING CARE RELATED TO ABNORMAL TEST RESULTS
POSTTEST: Factors related to the results of the test
Nursing Diagnosis: Alterations in microbiological environment

Guide to assessment	Guide to planning and intervention	Guide to evaluation

Assess patient factors that may be influencing test results.
Nursing history and/or physical exam suggestive of:
1. Infectious mononucleosis symptoms
   15–25 years old
   General malaise
   Fever (38.5°C or ↑)
   Sore throat
   Lymphadenopathy
   Splenomegaly
	1. Protect patient from continued disease process or relapse by:
	  a. Encouraging sufficient rest.
	  b. Encouraging well-balanced meals.
		1. The patient does not experience prolonged illness or relapse of disease.

Test:	Occult Blood, Hemoccult, Hematest, Quaiac Test
Abbreviation:	None
Reference Value:	Negative
Specimen:	Feces (this test may also be done on emesis)
Description:	The test for occult blood is a method of determining hidden bleeding, most frequently of the bowel. The most common tests are generally simple and not unpleasant for the patient. The results are obtained by chemical reaction to blood in which a color change takes place. A green reaction indicates a negative test, a blue reaction indicates a positive test.
Procedure:	1. (Variable) The patient is instructed to observe the following dietary directions for 3 days prior to testing and during the stool testing period: a. Meat-free diet. b. No horseradish or turnips. c. High residue foods should be eaten: prunes, grains, peanuts, raw vegetables. 2. Collect a small stool sample. A wooden applicator is usually provided if commercial testing kit is used. 3. Smear a thin coating of stool on filter paper. 4. Allow to dry. 5. Apply specified amount of developing solution to filter paper. 6. Time results for period specified and read results. 7. Follow directions on kit exactly.

Conditions Related to Increases

1. Gastrointestinal disease:
   Carcinoma of the bowel
   Gastritis
   Ulcers
   Esophagitis
   Varices
   Diverticulitis
   Portal hypertension
   Severe diarrhea
   Pancreatitis
   Neoplasms
2. Meat
   Fish
   Poultry
   Turnips
   Horseradish

Rationale

1. Normally the body loses 2–2.5 ml of blood from the gastrointestinal tract daily. Screening tests for occult blood are designed to detect a higher percentage of blood loss than the usual daily loss. The most frequent reason for testing for occult blood is screening for colonic carcinoma.

2. These foods contain peroxidases and cause false positive test results. Because the screening tests depend on the peroxidase activity of hemoglobin for the chemical color reaction, it is necessary to remove the exogenous sources for test accuracy.

Drug Influences: The following drugs may influence test results. The drugs are listed alphabetically by generic name and divided into columns according to the effect of the drug. Examples of trade names are in parentheses.

The following drugs may cause a positive occult blood test:

Gastrointestinal symptoms/bleeding

acids
alcohol
alkalies
amphotericin B
aspirin
benzene
chloramphenicol (Chloromycetin)
chlorophenothane (DDT)
digitalis; GI hemorrhage
ergot preparations; with overdose

lipomul
methotrexate
nalidixic acid (NegGram)
novobiocin (Albamycin)
phenylephrine (Neo-Synephrine)
procarbazine (Matulane)
pyrazolones (Narone)
tetracycline

Ulceration

amphetamine
corticosteroids
ibuprofen (Motrin)
indomethacin (Indocin)

phenolphthalein
potassium
reserpine
triamcinolone (Aristocort, Kenacort)

Severe diarrhea

chlorpropamide (Diabinese)
cyclophosphamide (Cytoxan)
iodides; also interferes with methodology
lincomycin

Miscellaneous

aminopyrine; impaired platelet aggregation
aminosalicylic acid; gastritis
colchicine; toxic manifestation
dicumarol; intramural hemorrhage
fluorouracil; toxic manifestation
gold; trombocytopenia
histamine sub q; gastric mucosal bleeding
pyrvinium (Povan); stains bright red, does not interfere with test results
warfarin; intramural hemorrhage

The following drug may cause a false negative test result: vitamin C (large doses)

Related Lab Studies

*radioactive chromium-51
CBC
urinalysis

---

*Not discussed in this book.

IMPLICATIONS FOR NURSING CARE
PRETEST: Factors related to the test
Nursing Diagnosis: Potential for injury related to changes in biochemical balance

Guide to assessment	Guide to planning and intervention	Guide to evaluation
Assess patient factors that may influence test results:		
1. Dietary restrictions	1. Explain dietary restrictions to patient. (Sometimes test is done without dietary restrictions): a. No meat, fish, poultry. b. No turnips or horseradish. c. High residue foods should be eaten. d. Restrictions are for 2–3 days prior to testing and all during testing. If dietary restrictions are not followed, note pertinent diet history on lab slip.	1. Patient's test values are not influenced by exogenous sources of peroxidase enzyme.
2. Comprehensive drug history (See Drug Influences)	2. Hold influencing drugs for 2–3 days prior to testing, as possible. Note influencing drugs patient is receiving on lab slip.	2. Patient's influencing drugs are noted on lab slip.
3. Knowledge deficit	3. Explain test to patient: a. Define occult blood (See Description). b. Explain procedure (See Procedure).	3. The patient demonstrates knowledge by defining test and explaining procedure.

Patient Preparation Checklist

1. √ Dietary restrictions followed; if not, note pertinent diet history on lab slip.
2. √ Influencing drugs; note on lab slip.
3. √ Patient knowledge; explain test to patient.

CONSIDERATIONS FOR NURSING CARE RELATED TO ABNORMAL TEST RESULTS
POSTTEST: Factors related to the results of the test
Nursing Diagnosis: Knowledge deficit of public about Occult Blood Screening Programs

Guide to assessment	Guide to planning and intervention	Guide to evaluation
1. Occult blood screening program	1. Encourage detection of occult blood screening programs: a. Teach patient how to collect specimen for specific test used.	1. Patient occult blood screening is successful as demonstrated by participation, collection, and follow-up of positive screening tests.
b. Healthy patients over 40	b. Encourage patients over 40 to have routine occult blood testing.	
c. Screening programs Nursing order	c. Promote community awareness by patient and family health education.	

Test:	O_2 Saturation
Abbreviation:	O_2 sat, S_aO_2, SO_2
Reference Value:	94–100% (arterial blood)
Specimen:	Arterial blood
Description:	Oxygen is transported largely by hemoglobin and is known as oxyhemoglobin. The oxygen saturation test is the measurement of oxygen in the blood that is combined with hemoglobin. Oxygen saturation is affected by the pH of the blood and the amount and type of hemoglobin. pO_2 is the more common test to measure oxygen delivery and follows oxygen saturation quite closely. Oxygen saturation is measured generally as part of the cardiac catherization workup.

See Arterial Blood Gases for a discussion of pO_2.

Drug Influences: Oxygen saturation and oxygen content are lineally related through the oxygen capacity. Oxygen capacity depends on the amount and type of hemoglobin in the blood. The following drugs may influence test results. The drugs are listed alphabetically by generic name and divided into columns according to the effect of the drug. Examples of trade names are in parentheses.

The following drugs may increase test results:

Respiratory depression
  narcotics

propoxyphene (Darvon)

O_2 saturation increase, miscellaneous
  atropine (Probocon)
  cobalt
  corticotropin (ACTH)

histamine
oral contraceptives
vitamin B_{12}

The following drugs may cause a decrease in test values:

Hemolytic anemia with G-6PD deficiency
  acetothexamide (Dymelor)
  aminopyrine (Pyramidon)
  antipyrine (Phenazone)
  chloroquine (Aralen)
  dimercaprol (BAL in oil)
  furazolidone (Furoxone)
  melarsonyl (Trimelarsan)
  methylene blue (Prosed)
  nalidixic acid (NegGram)

naphthalene
nitrofurantoin (Macrodantin)
nitrofurazone (Furacin)
phytonadione (AquaMephyton)
primaquine (Primaquine Phosphate)
quinacrine (Atabrine)
quinidine (Cardioquin)
quinine (Quinamm)
sulfacetamide (Sultrin)

Hemolytic anemia
  aminosalicylic acid
  amphetamine (Delcobese)
  amphotericin B (Fungizone)
  aspirin
  cephalothin (Keflin)
  chlorpromazine (Thorazine)
  dapsone (Dapsone)

phenacetin (in many aspirin
  preparations)
phenazopyridine (Azotrex)
phenothiazines (Compazine)
piperazine (Antepar)
probenecid (Benemid)
procainamide (Pronestyl)

diphenhydramine (Ambenyl)
glucosulfone (Promin)
hydralazine (Apresazide)
isoniazid (Laniazid)
lead
mefenamic acid (Ponstel), autoimmune
  hemolytic anemia
mephenytoin (Mesantoin)
methyldopa (Aldoclor), autoimmune
  hemolytic anemia
niridazole (Ambilhar)
nitrobenzene
penicillin

salicylazosulfapyridine (Azulfidine)
stibophen (Fuadin)
streptomycin
sulfadiazine (Suladyne)
sulfamethizole (Azotrex)
sulfamethoxazole (Azo Gantanol)
sulfanilamide (Vagitrol)
sulfoxone (Diasone Sodium)
tetracycline (Achromycin)
thiazolsulfone (Promizole)
tripelennamine (PBZ)

Megaloblastic anemia
  aminobenzoic acid (Pabirin)
  colchicine (ColBenemid)
  cycloserine (Seromycin)
  estrogens (Premarin)
  ethanol (grain alcohol)
  methotrexate (Mexate)

neomycin
nitrofurantoin (Macrodantin)
oral contraceptives
primidone (Mysoline)
pyrimethamine (Daraprim)
triamterene (Dyrenium)

Test:	Osmolality*
Abbreviation:	None
Reference Values:	*Serum*
	270–300 mOsm/L
	Urine
	Infant 50–645 mOsm/kg
	Child-adult 50–1400 mOsm/kg
	Serum/urine ratio Above 1.0 but less than 3.0
Specimen:	Serum, urine

Description: The term osmolality is defined as the concentration of solute particles in terms of a mass of solvent (39 p. 154) or, more simply, the number of particles dissolved in serum and urine. The major solute particles contributing to the osmolality of serum are electrolytes and, to a lesser degree, glucose, urea, creatinine, and protein. Plasma osmolality is the primary regulator of ADH release. ADH acts to control water reabsorption by the kidneys and this, in turn, influences serum and urine osmolality. Serum osmolality helps to determine hydration status, as serum electrolyte values alone can be misleading. Urine osmolality is more sensitive than urine specific gravity because it measures the kidneys' ability to dilute and concentrate urine. A clear picture of the change in hydration is obtained only when both serum and urine values and intake and output are compared.

Procedure:
1. A high protein diet may be prescribed 3 days prior to the test.
2. Fluids and food will be withheld from the patient for a prescribed period of time.
3. Collection
   a. The patient voids early morning (about 6 A.M.) and the urine is discarded.
   b. The next urine is saved and refrigerated until sent to the lab.
   c. Early morning the lab will draw 0.5–5 ml blood from the patient.
4. Random osmolality samples are often ordered.

Conditions Related to Increases	**Rationale**
1. Diabetes insipidus	1. In this condition there is decreased secretion of ADH, resulting in decreased water reabsorption by the kidneys that leads to dehydration.
2. Acidosis	2. Increased amounts of circulating solutes, such as lactic acid and ketones, act to increase osmolality (26).

*Osmolality is the preferred term; also known as osmolarity.

3. Dehydration (from any cause)

3. In hemoconcentration the proportion of solutes/mass to solution is higher.

4. Hyperglycemia and/or diabetes mellitus

4. Glucose is a substance contributing to osmolality. Increased amounts increase the osmolality. Increased glucose also acts as an osmotic diuretic leading to dehydration (see 3).

5. Primary aldosteronism

5. Aldosterone acts to reabsorb sodium in the renal tubules. Increased sodium levels create increased serum osmolality.

6. Uremia

6. Retention of many electrolytes and other solutes, such as urea, creatinine, and glucose, occurs in uremia and this increases serum osmolality.

7. High protein diet

7. Excessive protein intake and the products of protein breakdown increase the ratio of solutes.

8. Electrolyte excesses

8. Excessive solutes increase serum osmolality.

9. Shock

9. Shock often creates a state of extracellular volume depletion due to fluid loss or fluid shift. Shock may also create lactic acidosis due to hypoxia (see 2).

10. Advanced liver disease with hyperbilirubinemia

10. Excessive bilirubin contributes to solute concentration.

11. Alcohol ingestion

11. Alcohol inhibits ADH secretion, resulting in decreased water reabsorption leading to dehydration (see 3).

Conditions Related to Decreases

Rationale

Serum

1. Malignant neoplasm of bronchus and lung

1. There is an ectopic production of ADH in some cases. The excessive ADH causes increased reabsorption of water to hemodilution and hypoosmolality.

2. Inappropriate ADH syndrome caused by
Pain
Trauma, including surgery
Anesthetics and narcotics
IPPB treatments

2. In this syndrome there is an increase in ADH levels leading to water retention and a hypoosmolar state.

3. Addison's disease

3. In this disease the adrenal cortex secretes decreased levels of corticosteroids. Because of the decreased amounts of these hormones secreted,

the body is unable to reabsorb normal amounts of sodium and this results in hypoosmolality.

4. Compulsive (psychogenic) polydipsia

4. Excessive water intake creates hemodilution.

5. Any condition causing fluid retention
   Congestive heart failure
   Liver failure
   Renal failure

5. Fluid overload decreases the solute-to-solution ratio and this causes hypoosmolality.

Conditions Related to Increases

Rationale

Urine

1. Addison's disease

1. This condition results in lower levels of corticosteroids, especially aldosterone, so that the body is unable to reabsorb sodium normally and excessive sodium is lost in the urine.

2. Conditions where the serum osmolality is increased due to excessive solutes
   Hyperglycemia
   Uremia
   Acidosis or shock
   Electrolyte excesses
   Dehydration

2. In these conditions there are excessive solutes present in the blood that will be lost in excessive quantities in the urine.

3. Conditions with increased ADH levels
   Postsurgery
   Posttrauma
   Use of anesthetics and narcotics

3. Increased ADH secretion causes greater water reabsorption without affecting electrolyte excretion. In effect, electrolyte excretion remains the same but with less water and this makes the urine more concentrated.

Conditions Related to Decreases

Rationale

Urine

1. Renal disease

1. The kidneys are unable to concentrate the urine normally.

2. Diabetes insipidus

2. Lowered secretion of ADH results in lowered reabsorption of water by the kidneys. Excessive water is lost through the kidneys, resulting in low urine osmolality.

3. Compulsive (psychogenic) polydipsia

3. The kidneys normally compensate for overhydration by excreting excessive water (dilute urine). (See 4 Serum Decreases.)

4. Primary aldosteronism

4. Increased secretion of aldosterone causes increased reabsorption of sodium in the kidneys. As a result, the urine has fewer solutes.

5. Multiple myeloma

5. Kidney involvement is often a complication in multiple myeloma, which results in a decreased renal concentrating ability.

Drug Influences: The following drugs may cause a change in serum or urine osmolality. The drugs are listed alphabetically by generic name and divided into columns according to the effect of the drug. Examples of trade names are in parentheses.

Serum Osmolality Increases

Solute increase
  corticosteroids
  glucose

Hemoconcentration
  ethanol
  glycerin
  mannitol

Impaired renal tubular function
  methoxyflurane (Penthrane)

Urine Osmolality Increases

Diuretic effect
  anesthetic agents
  chlorpropamide (Diabinese)
  cyclophosphamide (Cytoxan)
  metolazone (Diulo, Zaroxolyn)
  phlorizin
  vincristine (Oncovin)

Serum Osmolality Decreases

Diuretic effect
  thiazides and related diuretics

Urine Osmolality Decreases

Nephrotoxic effect
  methoxyflurane (Penthrane)

Related Lab Studies:
Monitor response to treatment and adjust nursing care accordingly.

In dehydration
  ↑ hematocrit
  ↑ serum sodium and chloride
  ↑ urine sodium and chloride
  ↑ urine specific gravity

In diabetes insipidus
  ↓ *ADH
    *dehydration test
  ↓ urine specific gravity

---

*Not discussed in this book.

IMPLICATIONS FOR NURSING CARE
PRETEST: Factors related to the test
Nursing Diagnosis: Potential fluid volume alterations

Guide to assessment	Guide to planning and intervention	Guide to evaluation
Patient factors influencing test results:		
1. Food and fluids	1. If possible and as ordered prior to urine osmolality test, place the patient on a high protein diet for 3 days; provide a dry supper the evening before the test; withhold all fluids from 6 P.M. until the test is completed the following morning.	1. The patient's food and fluid intake does not produce inaccurate lab results.

2. Comprehensive drug history
  a. See Drug Influences
  b. Alcohol ingestion in past
	2. Report to lab and physician drugs the patient is receiving that may influence lab results.
	  Report to lab and physician any alcohol ingestion by the patient in the past 24 hours and delay test if ordered.
		2. Drugs and/or alcohol patient is receiving, or has received, that may influence lab results are identified and the appropriate people are notified.

3. Preexisting conditions (See Increases/Decreases)
4. Knowledge deficit
	3. Record preexisting conditions on lab slip.
	4. Explain to patient:
	  a. Define osmolality (See Description).
	  b. Explain test procedures (See Procedure).
		3. Patient's preexisting conditions are noted on lab slip.
		4. Patient demonstrates knowledge of test by defining test and stating procedure.

Patient Preparation Checklist

1. √ Food and fluid restrictions prior to urine osmolality (See 1 above).
2. √ Influencing drugs or alcohol ingestion noted and reported (See Drug Influences).
3. √ Preexisting conditions noted on lab slip (See Increases/Decreases).
4. √ Patient knowledge; explain test and procedure (See Description and Procedure).

CONSIDERATIONS FOR NURSING CARE RELATED TO ABNORMAL TEST RESULTS
POSTTEST: Factors related to the results of the test
Nursing Diagnosis: Alterations in fluid volume

Guide to assessment	Guide to planning and intervention	Guide to evaluation

Assess patient factors that may be influencing test results.
Nursing history and/or physical exam suggestive of:
1. Diabetes insipidus
  Signs and symptoms
    Polydipsia
    Polyuria
    Inability to increase urine specific gravity and osmolality when fluids are withheld
    Anorexia
    Weight loss
	1. Maintain water balance by:
	
	a. Administering vasopressin correctly and as ordered.
	b. Teaching the patient to:
	  (1) Check urine specific gravity or
	  (2) Observe for polydipsia and polyuria.
	  (3) The importance of reporting to the physician indications for medication.
	c. Administering nonhormonal drugs as ordered (e.g., thiazide diuretics, chlorpropamide, clofibrate, carbamizine).
		1. The patient's 24-hour urinary output remains below 3500 cc:
		a. The patient receives correctly prepared and administered vasopressin.
		b. The patient identifies signs/symptoms indicative of need for medication and reports them to physician.

2. Hypoglycemia or diabetic acidosis.
  a. IV fluids
 	
  b. Knowledge deficit
	2. Correct or prevent further ketoacidosis by:
	a. Administering IV fluids with regular insulin as ordered.
	b. Teaching patient to:
	  (1) Test urine or blood for glucose twice a day during good health and three to four times a day in times of stress.
	  (2) Avoid any injury, skin breakdown, burn, or infection.
	
	  (3) Adhere to the prescribed dietary plan and the principles of the dia-
		2. The patient demonstrates normal osmolality ratio by:
		a. Blood sugar and ketone levels decreasing to normal.
		b. Increased blood sugar being identified before it becomes severe.
		
		(2) The patient does not develop infections from unnecessary exposure to others or from trauma to skin.
		(3) The patient demonstrates an understanding of diabetic exchange diet

Guide to assessment	Guide to planning and intervention	Guide to evaluation
	betic exchange diet (or refer to dietician for teaching about diabetic diet).	by planning menus for 1 week.
c. Personal stressors	c. Assisting the patient to identify stressors and specific ways to decrease or cope with stress.	c. The patient will identify personal stressors and ways to reduce or cope with them.
d. Need for insulin	d. Administering insulin correctly and following nursing measures specific to insulin administration.	d. The patient receives correctly administered insulin at designated time.
e. Need for oral hypoglycemic agent	e. Administering oral hypoglycemic agent as ordered.	e. The patient receives oral hypoglycemics as ordered.
f. Evidence of increased need for insulin: Puberty Pregnancy Steroid therapy Cushing's syndrome Febrile illness Trauma Severe emotional stress Surgery	f. Detecting increased need for insulin.	f. The patient's need for increased insulin is identified.
3. Fluid balance disorder Dehydration (from any cause) Primary aldosteronism Shock Inappropriate ADH syndrome Compulsive or psychogenic polydipsia Conditions causing fluid retention, e.g., Liver failure CHF Renal failure	3. Promote fluid/electrolyte balance by: a. Administering fluids as ordered. b. Detecting and reporting signs and symptoms of over/underhydration. c. Keeping accurate I&O records, daily weights.	3. The patient's fluid and electrolyte balance is maintained by: a. Fluids administered as ordered. b. Reporting early signs and symptoms of fluid imbalance. c. Recording I&O and weights accurately.
d. Dehydration	d. Administering antiemetics, antidiarrheals, or antipyretics as ordered and as needed to prevent dehydration.	d. The patient's cause of dehydration is corrected.
e. Primary aldosteronism	e. Promote sodium and water excretion by administering spironolactone (Aldactone) as ordered.	e. Serum and urine sodium are within normal limits.

Guide to assessment	Guide to planning and intervention	Guide to evaluation
f. Inappropriate ADH syndrome	f. Administering, in moderate to severe cases, hypertonic saline IV, IV diuretics and lithium carbonate (inhibits ADH).	f. The patient demonstrates balanced I&O with appropriate specific gravity and osmolality ratio.
h. Compulsive or psychogenic polydipsia	h. Promoting decreased fluid intake by reinforcing patient's attempts to restrict fluid intake <3000 cc/day, teaching patient to take small amounts of liquid at a time, and seeking psychotherapy if necessary.	h. The patient will demonstrate decreased fluid intake by stating willingness to attempt a self-restricted fluid intake, and a decreased urine out.
i. Fluid retention	i. Administering diuretics as ordered.	i. The patient demonstrates decreased fluid retention by decreased body weight, edema, neck vein distention, and pulmonary fluid.
g. Addison's disease	g. Promoting normal hormone balance by administering corticoids as ordered.	g. The patient will receive appropriate amounts of medication.

4. Electrolyte excess
    Sodium
    Potassium
    Chloride
	4. Reduce electrolyte excess by:
	a. Adjusting diet to electrolyte needs of patient.
	b. Encouraging adequate fluid intake.
	c. Administering IV solutions as ordered.
	d. Administering diuretics, corticosteroids, or mitramycin as ordered.
	e. Assisting with renal dialysis or plasmapheresis as ordered.
		4. The patient demonstrates normal electrolyte levels and a normal osmolality ratio.

Test:	Ova and Parasites
Abbreviation:	O and P
Reference Value:	Negative
Specimen:	Feces
Description:	Intestinal ova and parasites are most frequently diagnosed by microscopic examination of the parasite ova, cysts, larvae, or trophozoites from a fresh stool specimen. Some intestinal parasites are fairly constant in the observed forms and shed in the feces day to day, but some parasites are shed irregularly. It is for this reason that several stool specimens are collected with a day or two between collection.
Procedure:	1. No food or fluid restriction. 2. Stool sample is collected in clean container. If collected into a bedpan, the stool should be removed with tongue blades and placed in a stool cup. Cover container securely. Do not contaminate with urine. 3. Send entire stool specimen. If entire specimen cannot be sent and visible worm segments are present, send worm segment section. 4. Send stool specimen to lab immediately. If it cannot be sent, follow local procedure; refrigerate specimen or place some of it in preservative. 5. Collect subsequent stool specimen 2–3 days apart.

Conditions Related to Increases

Protozoa
  Giardia lamblia
  Entamoeba histolytica
  Dientamoeba fragilis

Nematodes
  Ascaris lumbricodes (roundworm)
  Trichuris trichiura (whipworm)
  Enterobius vermicularis (pinworm)
  Necator americanus (hookworm)
  Ancylostoma duodenale (hookworm)

Trematodes
  Clonorchis (Opisthorchis sinensis)
   (Chinese liver fluke)
  Schistosoma mansoni (blood fluke)

Cestodes
  Hymenolepis nana (dwarf tapeworm)
  Taenia saginata (beef tapeworm)
  Taenia solium (pork tapeworm)

Rationale

Intestinal parasites are transmitted by hand to mouth contamination, swallowing airborne eggs, penetration of skin by larvae in contaminated soil, ingestion of contaminated water or food, or penetration of skin or oral mucosa by larvae in fresh water.

Drug Influences: Some types of drugs interfere with examination of feces for ova and parasites. Listed below are drug types and their effect.

Crystalline residue
    antidiarrheal agents
    antacids
    barium
    bismuth

Interferes with examination
    oily laxatives

Decreased number of organisms
    antibiotics
    contrast media

Related Lab Studies:

    CBC (anemia and eosinophilia possible)
    serology (rarely)

IMPLICATIONS FOR NURSING CARE
PRETEST: Factors related to the test
Nursing Diagnosis: Potential for injury related to changes in microbiological environment

Guide to assessment	Guide to planning and intervention	Guide to evaluation
Assess patient factors that may influence test results: 1. Drug interferences	1. Prevent drugs from interfering with test results by:	1. Patient's test results are not incorrect due to drug interferences.

a. Antidiarrheal agents
   Antacids
   Barium
   Bismuth
   Oily laxatives
	a. Advising patient not to use drugs listed in left-hand column.	

b. Antibiotics	b. Note on lab slip if patient is on antibiotics.	
c. Barium	c. Collect specimen after barium is expelled, or before barium exam.	
2. Travel history	2. Note patient's travel on lab slip.	2. Patient's travel is noted on lab slip.
3. Knowledge deficit	3. Educate patient: a. Define ova and parasites (See Description). b. Explain procedure (See Procedure). c. Stress good handwashing technique.	

Patient Preparation Checklist

1. √ Interfering drug history (See Drug Influences). Note if antibiotics on lab slip.
2. √ Travel history: note on lab slip.
3. √ Patient knowledge (See Description/Procedure).

CONSIDERATIONS FOR NURSING CARE RELATED TO ABNORMAL TEST RESULTS

POSTTEST: Factors related to the results of the test
Nursing Diagnosis: Alterations in microbiological environment

Guide to assessment	Guide to planning and intervention	Guide to evaluation

Assess patient factors that may be influencing test results:
1. Positive stool for O and P
	1. Teach patient about condition and prevent reinfestation:
	  a. Administer mebendazole (Vermox) or anthelmintic as ordered.
	  b. Test all members of family on same day.
	  c. Wash perianal area daily.
	  d. Wear clean underwear daily.
	  e. Change bedding daily.
	  f. Wash hands and clean fingernails after every bowel movement.
	  g. Wash hands carefully before meals.
	  h. Keep fingernails short; avoid nail biting.
	  i. Apply vaseline to anus to hinder deposit of eggs.
	  j. Encourage child-patient to wear wide-crotch, snug-legged cotton underpants to prevent contact with perianal area.
	  k. Inform patient/parent that infestation is not a reflection on family hygiene or housekeeping practices.
		1. Patient is free of parasites.

Test:	Activated Partial Thromboplastin Time
Abbreviation:	APTT (PTT)
Reference Values:	APTT 16–40 seconds
	PTT 30–45 seconds
	Each laboratory establishes its own normal values.
Specimen:	Whole blood

Description: The intrinsic and common pathways of coagulation are evaluated by the activated partial thromboplastin time (APTT) study. This test determines the time it takes to form a fibrin clot after adding an activating agent, calcium, and phospholipid. The partial thromboplastin time (PTT) is a similar, less sensitive test. Normally, the blood contains all of the procoagulants necessary for intrinsic pathway clot formation. (See Figure 1.) This test, along with prothrombin time (PT) and thrombin time (TT), is used in the diagnosis of specific coagulation disorders. It is also used for monitoring heparin therapy.

Procedures: (blue top tube)
1. No food or fluid restrictions.
2. The vacuum tube is completely filled; the tube is gently tipped back and forth to mix the anticoagulant.
3. Observe puncture site carefully for bleeding or evidence of hematoma.

Conditions Related to Increases

Rationale

1. Deficiency in Factors
   II (prothrombin)
   V (plasma accelerator globulin)
   X (Stuart-Prower factor)

1. These are factors in the common pathway and a deficiency in any of these will result in prolonged bleeding. The deficiencies show both APTT and PT prolonged values. See Figure 1.

2. Vitamin K deficiency

2. Vitamin K is necessary for the synthesis of factors II, VII, IX, and X. Bleeding tendencies occur from any condition that diminishes the absorption, utilization, or synthesis of vitamin K. Causes of vitamin K deficiency are:
   a. Sterilization of the bowel with antibiotics. Vitamin K is gained from the diet and from gastrointestinal bacterial synthesis.
   b. Malnutrition in severely ill patients. Rationale as above in 2a.
   c. Newborn infants, because of lack of body stores and decreased synthesis.

COAGULATION, INTRINSIC AND EXTRINSIC PATHWAYS

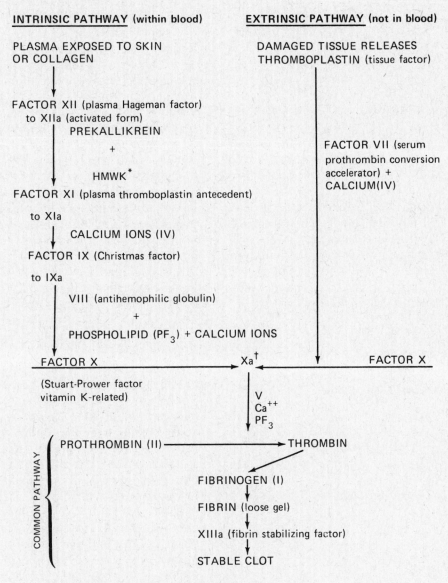

INTRINSIC PATHWAY (within blood)   EXTRINSIC PATHWAY (not in blood)

PLASMA EXPOSED TO SKIN   DAMAGED TISSUE RELEASES
OR COLLAGEN   THROMBOPLASTIN (tissue factor)

FACTOR XII (plasma Hageman factor)
   to XIIa (activated form)
          PREKALLIKREIN
                                     FACTOR VII (serum
              +   prothrombin conversion
                                     accelerator) +
          HMWK*   CALCIUM(IV)
FACTOR XI (plasma thromboplastin antecedent)

   to XIa
          CALCIUM IONS (IV)
   FACTOR IX (Christmas factor)

   to IXa
          VIII (antihemophilic globulin)
                 +
          PHOSPHOLIPID (PF$_3$) + CALCIUM IONS

FACTOR X   Xa† FACTOR X

(Stuart-Prower factor
vitamin K-related)   V
                                     Ca^{++}
                                     PF$_3$

PROTHROMBIN (II) ————————————→ THROMBIN

          FIBRINOGEN (I)

          FIBRIN (loose gel)

          XIIIa (fibrin stabilizing factor)

          STABLE CLOT

COMMON PATHWAY

*HIGH MOLECULAR WEIGHT KININOGENS.
†Xa IN ASSOCIATION WITH Ca^{++}, PF$_3$, AND FACTOR V (plasma accelerator globulin).

d. Malabsorption because of decreased vitamin K absorption. Biliary obstruction blocks bile salts and results in lack of absorption of fat-soluble vitamin K.

e. Coumarin or coumarin-like drugs cause decreased utilization of vitamin K. APTT and PT are both prolonged in this disorder.

3. Liver disease

3. The liver is an important organ in coagulation. The liver synthesizes fibrinogen, prothrombin, factors V, IX, and XI—all factors essential to normal coagulation. APTT and PT are both prolonged in liver disease.

4. Deficiency in Factors
   VIII (antihemolitic globulin factor)
   IX (Christmas factor)
   XI (plasma thromboplastin antecedent)
   XII (plasma Hageman factor)
   Prekallikrein (Fletcher factor)
   HMWK (Fitzgerald factor)

4. These factors represent the intrinsic coagulation pathway. A deficiency in any one of these factors results in a prolonged APTT. A defective factor VIII is known as hemophilia A or classic hemophilia. Abnormal factor IX is known as Christmas disease or hemophilia B. APTT is prolonged in these disorders, PT is normal. See Figure 1.

5. Lupus anticoagulant

5. Known as an inhibitor, this condition interferes with the formation of the prothrombinase complex. This complex consists of factor V, Xa, Ca, and lipid. Patients with this condition usually do not bleed unless there is a companion hemostatic defect such as thrombocytopenia. The mechanism is not clearly understood, but evidence suggests it is an in vitro reaction only. The APTT is prolonged; the PT, bleeding time, and platelet count are normal.

6. Hypofibrinogenemia
   Afibrinogenemia

6. Either low or absent levels of fibrinogen (factor I). Interestingly, patients with this condition have less difficulty with hemostasis than patients with hemophilia. APTT is prolonged, as are PT and TT.

7. DIC (disseminated intravascular coagulation)

7. This complex condition, in response to a variety of conditions, is characterized by thrombin in the circulation that results in fibrin deposits in mi-

crocirculation, irreversible platelet aggregation, increased fibrinolysis, and consumption of coagulation factors (152). APTT, PT, and TT are abnormal.

8. Heparin therapy

8. Full dose heparin therapy is often monitored by APTT. The usual range is an APTT 1.5–2.5 times the control. Mini dose heparin therapy (5000 USP units every 12 hours) need not be monitored by APTT.

Drug Influences: Many drugs interfere with normal clotting. Listed below are some general drug classifications that may influence test results.

Increase in test results
androgens
anesthetic agents
antibiotics
anticoagulants
barbiturates
cathartics
corticosteroids
diuretics

MAO inhibitors
narcotic antagonists
narcotics
oral contraceptives
radioactive compounds
radiographic agents
sulfonamides

Decrease in test results
anabolic steroids
antacids
antihistamines
barbiturates
caffeine

corticosteroids
diuretics; with anticoagulant therapy
oral contraceptives
vitamin K

Related Lab Studies: Hemostatic profile:

platelet count
bleeding time
prothrombin time (PT)
thrombin time (TT)
Hct
APTT

IMPLICATIONS FOR NURSING CARE
PRETEST: Factors related to the test
Nursing Diagnosis: Potential for injury related to changes in biochemical balance

Guide to assessment	Guide to planning and intervention	Guide to evaluation
Assess patient factors that may influence test results.		

1. Comprehensive drug history (See Drug Influences)	1. Identify influencing drugs and note on lab slip:
	  a. Identify and note the following on lab slip:
	    (1) Name of anticoagulant.
	    (2) Route.
	    (3) Dosage.
	    (4) Time of last dosage.
		1. Patient's test value is not influenced by unidentified drug that may influence test results.

2. Preexisting conditions
  Known coagulation disorder
  (See Increases/Decreases)
	2. Identify preexisting conditions and note on lab slip.	2. Patient's condition pertinent to lab test are noted on lab slip.

3. Hemolysis	3. Prevent hemolysis by:
	  a. Not saturating the skin with antiseptic.
	  b. Not probing venipuncture site or leaving the tourniquet on too long.
	  c. Not forcefully withdrawing specimen.
	  d. Not withdrawing specimen too slowly.
	  e. Not agitating or handling specimen roughly.
		3. Patient's values are not influenced by hemolysis.

4. Lack of patient knowledge	4. Explain test to patient:
	  a. Define test; anticoagulant monitoring or coagulation screening.
	  b. Explain procedure.
		4. The patient demonstrates knowledge by defining test and explaining procedure.

5. Lack of staff knowledge	5. Be informed about coagulation studies and anticoagulant medication schedule. Patients on full heparin therapy are tested at least once a day.	5. The patient's coagulation time is not abnormal due to staff error.

Patient Preparation Checklist

1. √ Interfering medications.
2. √ Anticoagulant, dose, time noted on lab slip.
3. √ Pertinent preexisting conditions noted on lab slip.
4. √ Patient knowledge; explain test to patient.

CONSIDERATIONS FOR NURSING CARE RELATED TO ABNORMAL TEST RESULTS
POSTTEST: Factors related to the results of the test
Nursing Diagnosis: Predisposition to bleeding and/or thrombus formation

Guide to assessment	Guide to planning and intervention	Guide to evaluation
Assess patient factors that may be influencing test values. Nursing history and/or physical exam suggestive of:		
1. Heparin therapy APTT 1.5–2 times control Hct Platelet count	1. Inhibit thrombin formation with the administration of heparin: a. Be aware of frequent lab test monitoring. b. Follow local guidelines concerning heparin use. c. Be alert to signs of bleeding.	1. The patient maintains anti-coagulant therapy with desired APTT.
2. Factor deficiencies Prothrombin V VIII IX X XI XII	2. Replace factor deficiencies: a. Assist with starting the administration of plasma products. b. Initiate nursing measures that will promote successful plasma administration completion.	2. The patient's bleeding stops and lab results are adequate.
3. Vitamin K deficiency See with: Antibiotic therapy, long term Severe malnutrition Newborn Malabsorption syndromes Coumarin or coumarin-like drugs Liver disease	3. Replace deficient vitamin K for synthesis of coagulation factors: a. Recognize conditions that may encourage vitamin K deficiency. b. Consult with physician. c. Administer vitamin K as prescribed.	3. The patient's PTT is normal. The patient does not experience bleeding.
4. DIC Lab Studies: ↑ PT ↑ APTT ↓ Fibrinogen ↓ Platelet count Fibrin split products a. Obstetrical conditions	4. Discourage consumption of coagulation factors. a. Be alert to conditions that may stimulate DIC.	4. Patient's lab values return to normal and the patient's condition improves.

Guide to assessment	Guide to planning and intervention	Guide to evaluation
Neoplastic disease Hemolytic responses Extensive tissue damage Fat emboli Acute infections, etc.	b. Be alert to signs of bleeding. c. Initiate medical plan to treat underlying cause of DIC. d. Administer heparin as prescribed.	

Test:	Serum Phenylalanine
Abbreviation:	PKU test, Guthrie test
Reference Value:	Below 4 mg/dl
Specimen:	Serum

Description: An inborn error of metabolism, classical phenylketonuria (PKU) is caused by the absence of the liver enzyme phenylalanine hydroxylase. Because of this absence, phenylalanine is not oxidized to tyrosine, an essential step in protein metabolism. Phenylalanine and other metabolites accumulate in the blood and urine. The phenylalanine accumulation causes irreversible damage to the central nervous system by interfering with biochemical maturation of neural tissue. Treatment is a low phenylalanine diet. Phenylalanine levels are measured in almost all states by law before the fourth day of life and again before the fourth week of life. If the disease is diagnosed, serum levels are closely monitored to ensure that the diet does not contain too much phenylalanine. Children who are diagnosed during the first few weeks of life and begun on treatment right away (first 2–3 weeks of life) will have normal intelligence.

Since 1975, six variants of hyperphenylalaninemia have been described. Not all of these variants are responsive to treatment with a low phenylalanine diet. Differential diagnosis is essential to treatment.

Procedure: Guthrie test.
1. Fill out lab slip completely.
2. Cleanse infant's heel with an antiseptic solution. Air-dry.
3. A heel puncture is done.
4. Collect blood on lab slip on special section. Saturation is essential for accuracy.
5. Air-dry blood sample.
6. Insert sample into envelope and mail to state laboratory (or designated laboratory).
7. Follow instructions on lab slip precisely.

Conditions Related to Increases	Rationale
1. Phenylketonuria	1. Early diagnosis is made by newborn blood levels. The level rises to abnormal after ingestion of protein-containing feedings (breast or prepared formula) (9).
2. Viral hepatitis	2. In hepatic encephalopathy there is amino acid balance disturbance which will show an increase in phenylalanine levels (9).

Drug Influences: Drugs do not interfere with serum phenylalanine levels.

Related Laboratory Studies: For diagnostic purposes or for following blood levels, these lab tests may be done.

Classical PKU

↑ Serum phenylalanine levels
↑ *Blood tyrosine levels
↑ *Urine phenylalanine metabolites

IMPLICATIONS FOR NURSING CARE
PRETEST: Factors related to the test
Nursing Diagnosis: Potential for injury related to changes in biochemical balance

Guide to assessment	Guide to planning and intervention	Guide to evaluation
Assess patient factors that may influence test results:	Guthrie Test	
1. Food and fluids	1. Indicate how long infant has been on milk or formula feeding (3–4 days is preferable). Indicate type of milk or formula.	1. The infant's protein intake is sufficient to make serum PKU levels accurate.
2. Age	2. Perform follow-up specimen no later than 6 weeks of age.	2. The infant's follow-up specimen is sent to state lab.
3. Knowledge deficit: Parents	3. Explain Guthrie test: a. Define phenylalanine and phenylketonuria (See Description). b. Explain procedure (See Procedure).	3. The parents demonstrate knowledge of screening test for PKU by defining the test and stating procedure.

Patient Preparation Checklist

1. √ Length and type of protein intake.
2. √ Follow-up specimen done.
3. √ Parent knowledge; explain test (See Description/Procedure).

---

*Not discussed in this book.

CONSIDERATIONS FOR NURSING CARE RELATED TO ABNORMAL TEST RESULTS
POSTTEST: Factors related to the results of the test
Nursing Diagnosis: Alterations in biochemical balance

Guide to assessment	Guide to planning and intervention	Guide to evaluation

Assess patient needs that may influence test results:
1. Diagnosis of PKU
	1. Promote management of patient with PKU through regional treatment center by:
	  a. Providing support to family and child.
	  b. Encouraging treatment center visits as ordered.
	  c. Seeking clarification if instructions are not clear.
		1. The infant's phenylalanine levels are enough to ensure needed protein synthesis.

Test:	Phosphates
Abbreviation:	P
Reference Values:	Newborn 4.0–10.5 mg/dl
	1 year 4.0–6.8 mg/dl
	5 years 3.6–6.5 mg/dl
	Adult 2.5–4.5 mg/dl
Specimen:	Serum

Description: Phosphate is a principal cellular electrolyte that is mostly combined with calcium in the bones. Phosphate is replaced by dietary intake. Phosphorus deficiency is very rare because phosphorus is found in many foods, including carbonated beverages. Phosphate is closely aligned with calcium, and together with parathormone and vitamin D, increases or decreases serum calcium. As calcium levels increase, phosphate levels decrease and the electrolyte in excess is excreted by the kidney. Phosphates also function in the building of skeletal tissue, as cellular buffers, in cellular energy production and in carbohydrate and fat metabolism.

Because of the close relationship with calcium the two electrolytes are measured together. *Conditions that cause serum calcium levels to increase will cause serum phosphate levels to decrease.*

Refer to Calcium for discussion.

Drug Influences: The following drugs may influence test results. The drugs are listed alphabetically by generic name and divided into columns according to the effect of the drug. Examples of trade names are in parentheses.

The following drugs may cause an increase in test results:

Serum

Nephrotoxic effect
tetracycline (Achromycin)
methicillin (Staphcillin)

minocycline (Minocin)

Miscellaneous
anabolic steroids; increased retention
androgens; augments balance
ergocalciferol (Vi-Penta F); increases
 reabsorption

furosemide (Lasix); temporary increase
growth hormone
hydrochlorothiazide (Aldactazide)
phosphates; increased intake

Urine

Inhibits tubular reabsorption
acetazolamide (Diamox)
acetoacetate
aspirin
cadmium

calcitonin (Calcimar)
glycine
tryptophan (Amina 21, Tryptacin)

Metabolic effect
bicarbonates
corticosteroids

hydrochlorothiazide (Aldactazide)
tetracycline

The following drugs may cause a decrease in test results:

Serum

Increased phosphorylation
epinephrine glucose
fructose insulin

Miscellaneous
acetazolamide (Diamox); defective phosphate/calcium reabsorption
aluminum salts; binds PO_4
anesthetic agents (ether, chloroform)
anticonvulsants; disturbs vitamin D metabolism
calcitonin (Calcimar); causes urinary loss
mithramycin (Mithracin); decreased bone reabsorption of calcium phenobarbital;
  increases clearance

Urine

Increased reabsorption
phlorizin

Test:	Pinworms
Abbreviation:	None
Reference Value:	Negative
Specimen:	Perianal smear

Description: Enterobius vermicularis, or pinworms, are found all over the world. Infection is by contamination of food and drink from contaminated hands and fingernails or from biting fingernails. Children are infected more often than adults.

Pinworms are small white worms that, upon infestation, live in the upper part of the large intestines. The pregnant female worm migrates to the rectum, usually at night, and deposits ova around the anal area.

The test is done by microscopic visualization of the ova to confirm infestation.

Procedure: Scotch tape slide.
1. Early morning before bath or bowel movement is best collection time.
2. Use prepackaged slide or tongue blade with scotch tape, sticky side out, and press about anus. Do not put the tongue blade or slide in anus.
3. Cover slide per kit instruction. From tongue blade put scotch tape sticky side down.
4. Send slide to laboratory.
5. Wash hands well with disinfectant soap and water. Clean fingernails.

Conditions Related to Increases	Rationale
1. Pinworms	1. Female worm is 9–12 mm long and may be visible around anus.

Drug Influences: Drugs do not interfere with test.

Related Lab Studies: Stool for O&P.

IMPLICATIONS FOR NURSING CARE
PRETEST: Factors related to the test
Nursing Diagnosis: Potential for injury related to changes in microbiological environment

Guide to assessment	Guide to planning and intervention	Guide to evaluation
Assess patient factors that may influence test results:		
1. Travel	1. Note on lab slip known contacts, such as nursery school outbreak, etc.	1. Patient's contacts are noted on lab slip.
2. Knowledge deficit	2. Educate patient/parent:	2. Patient/parent demon-

Guide to assessment	Guide to planning and intervention	Guide to evaluation
	a. Define pinworms (See Description). b. Explain procedure (See Procedure). c. Stress good handwashing technique.	strates knowledge by defining test, stating procedure and need for good handwashing.

CONSIDERATIONS FOR NURSING CARE RELATED TO ABNORMAL TEST RESULTS

POSTTEST: Factors related to the results of the test
Nursing Diagnosis: Alterations in microbiological balance: pinworm infestation

Guide to assessment	Guide to planning and intervention	Guide to evaluation
Assess patient factors that may be influencing test results: 1. Positive pinworm slide	1. Teach patient about condition and prevent reinfestation: a. Order or give appropriate anthelmintic and be aware of precautions about drug. b. Treat all members of family on same day. c. Wash perianal area daily. d. Wear clean underwear daily. e. Change bedding daily; gather up bedding without shaking, to avoid depositing eggs on floor. f. Wash hands and clean fingernails after every bowel movement. g. Wash hands carefully before meals. h. Keep fingernails short; avoid nail biting. i. Apply vaseline to anus to hinder deposit of eggs. j. Encourage child-patient to wear wide-crotch, snug-legged cotton underpants to prevent contact with perianal area.	1. Patient is free of pinworms.

Guide to assessment	Guide to planning and intervention	Guide to evaluation
	k. Support patient/parent that infestation is not a reflection on family hygiene or housekeeping practices. l. Encourage parent to vacuum or mop floor to prevent reinfestation of children who play on floor.	

Test:	Platelet (Thrombocyte) Count
Abbreviation:	None
Reference Values:	150,000–400,000/μl
Specimen:	Heparinized blood
Description:	Platelets are produced almost completely in the bone marrow as fragments of very large cells called megakaryocytes. Platelets are granular and disk-shaped and they are the smallest of the cellular bone marrow elements. Platelet function is for vascular repair and maintenance of hemostasis. This is accomplished by platelets adhering to each other and to the vessel wall and releasing ADP (an aggregating agent); by releasing the potent vasoconstrictor serotonin; by releasing platelet factor 3 (PF3) and other factors that accelerate coagulation; and by releasing the platelet contractile protein actomyosin, which causes the clot to shrink and grow firm. About 90% of platelets are in circulation and 10% remain in reserve in the spleen. An increased platelet count is known as thrombocytosis. It is caused by increased production of megakaryocytes in the bone marrow or from a release of platelets into circulation from splenic storage pool. A decreased platelet count is called thrombocytopenia. Thrombocytopenia occurs because platelet production is diminished or platelet destruction has increased.

Platelet counts are done to evaluate platelet production, assess patient effects of chemotherapy or radiation therapy, and to aid in the diagnosis of thrombocytic disease.

Procedure:	(lavender top tube)

1. There are no food or fluid restrictions.
2. Up to 7 ml of blood may be drawn from the patient.
3. Apply pressure to puncture site as needed.
4. Observe puncture site for bleeding or evidence of hematoma. Report and record prolonged bleeding.

Conditions Related to Increases	Rationale
1. Chronic myelogenous leukemia Idiopathic thrombocytosis Carcinoid syndrome Sickle-cell anemia	1. The increase in platelets in these conditions is due to the myeloproliferation of megakaryocytes. Because platelets are abnormal in these conditions there is both bleeding and thrombosis.
2. Polycythemia (primary and secondary)	2. This disease is characterized by an increase in bone marrow activity. There is an increased supply of precursor cells, including megakaryocytes, which are the cells from which the platelets are derived. Platelet counts may be higher than 1 million and

3. Collagen diseases
   Posthemorrhage
   Postsurgery
   Infections
   Iron deficiency anemia
   Malignancies
   Trauma
   Hypoxia
4. Postsplenectomy

5. Exercise, strenuous
   Stress, e.g.
   High altitudes, persistently cold environment, etc.

platelets may be abnormal. Bleeding and thrombosis may be present.

3. These conditions cause a reactive thrombocytosis. Megakaryocyte and platelet production is stimulated. After the precipitating cause is resolved, counts return to normal. In reactive thrombocytosis, platelet morphology and survival time are normal.

4. Often there is a transient thrombocytosis after splenectomy. The spleen is the major site for platelet storage and destruction. After splenectomy, platelet production continues at the same rate and this temporarily increases the platelet count. By 2 months postsplenectomy, the platelet count returns to normal.

5. A transient rise in platelets is noted immediately after strenuous exercise or stress. The increase is due to splenic release of platelets.

Conditions Related to Decreases

1. Aplastic anemia
   Malignant bone marrow diseases
   Chemotherapy
   Chlorthiazides
   Alcohol consumption
   Corticosteroids
   Estrogens
   Menstrual cycle
   Congenital megakaryocytic hypoplasia
   X-ray radiation therapy
   Infections

2. Splenic enlargement regardless of etiology
   Lymphomas
   Felty's syndrome
   Gaucher's disease
   Sarcoidosis
   Hepatic cirrhosis

3. Megaloblastic anemias
   Vitamin B$_{12}$
   Folate deficiency
   Hereditary thrombocytopenias

Rationale

1. These conditions/drugs may cause decreased thrombopoiesis, and so the platelet count is diminished. Thrombocytopenia may be profound in aplastic anemia and malignant bone marrow diseases. Platelet counts below 50,000 are associated with spontaneous bleeding; below 5,000, fatal CNS or GI hemorrhage is possible.

2. Platelets are removed from active circulation by splenic sequestration. It is possible that up to 90% of platelets can be pooled within the enlarged spleen. (The diminished peripheral circulating platelets may stress the marrow to increase production) (11).

3. These conditions affect the production of megakaryocytes. The cells are large but lobular and produce fewer platelets.

4. Idiopathic thrombocytopenia
   purpura
   Systemic lupus erythematosus
   Infectious mononucleosis
   Neonatal thrombocytopenia

4. The decrease in platelets in these conditions is caused by an immunological reaction. Autoantibodies bind to the platelets, causing defective aggregation. Macrophages in the liver and spleen are stimulated to remove the disordered platelets.

5. Drug-associated thrombocytopenia
   (See Drug Influences), especially
   Quinidine
   Quinine
   Sulfonamides
   Gold

5. Drugs may cause a drug-induced antibody production. The drug binds to a plasma protein and stimulates an antibody formation. The platelets are removed by the macrophage system.

6. Disseminated intravascular coagulation (DIC)

6. In this complication of disease, there is an acceleration of the normal clotting process that enhances platelet aggregation. This increased clotting activity consumes platelets and clotting factors to the point of depletion.

7. Prosthetic cardiovascular
   devices
   Vasculitis
   Arterial thrombosis

7. Platelet destruction takes place because of injury to platelets as they pass over abnormal arterial surfaces.

Drug Influences: Many drugs interfere with platelet production and survival. Listed below are some of the drugs that may have an effect on the platelet count. The drugs are listed alphabetically by generic name and divided into columns according to effect of the drug. Examples of trade names are in parentheses.

The following drugs may cause an increase in platelets:

Normal physiologic response
   epinephrine; see 5 Increases

Stimulates platelet production
   glucocorticoids

The following drugs may cause a decrease in platelet count:

Aplastic anemia
   acetazolamide (Diamox)
   allopurinol (Zyloprim)
   aminobenzoic acid (Pabirin, PreSun 8 Lotion)
   aminosalicylic acid
   amphotericin B
   antidiabetic agents, oral (Dymelor, Diabinese, Orinase, etc.)
   antimony compounds
   antineoplastic agents (Imuran, Cytosine Arabinoside, Methotrexate, Oncovin, etc.)
   antipyrine (Auralgan)
   asparaginase (Elspar)
   benzene
   bismuth salts

carbon tetrachloride
chloramphenicol (Chloromycetin)
chloroquine
diphenylhydantoin (Dilantin)
ethosuximide (Zarontin)
mefenamic acid (Ponstel)
mephenytoin (Mesantoin)
meprobamate (Equagesic, Equanil, Meprobamate)
methazolamide (Neptazane)
paramethadione (Paradione)
phenacemide (Phenurone)
phenothiazines (Prolixin, Quide, Sparine, Thorazine)
phenylbutazone (Butazolidin)
primidone (Mysoline)
probenecid (Benemid)
trimethadione (Tridione)
urethan

*Thrombocytopenic response *immune-induced*
   *allymid
   *amitriptyline
   *ampicillin
   *antazoline
   *apronalide
  †*aspirin; ↓ platelet aggregation
    barbiturates
   *carbamazepine
   *cardiac glycosides; rare
   *desipramine
   *diazoxide
    diethylstilbestrol
   *dipyrone
    gentamicin
    lincomycin; rare
    lipomul
    methimazole (Tapazole)
   *nitroglycerin; after prolonged use
   *novobiocin (Albamycin)
    oxyphenbutazone (Oxalid, Tandearil)
    penicillamine
    penicillin
   *phenolphthalein
    potassium iodide
   *prednisone
   *propranolol

---

†Many drugs contain aspirin even though the trade name does not make it obvious. Check patient history carefully.

*protriptyline
pyrazinamide
pyrimethamine (Daraprim)
*quinidine
*quinine
*rifampin (Rimactane)
*smallpox vaccine
*sulfonamides
thiouracil

Miscellaneous
DDT
heparin
methyldopa (Aldomet); very rare
propynyl-cyclohexanol carbamate
radioactive phosphorus
restocetin A&B
salicylates
thiazide diuretics; rare

Related Lab Studies: Monitor response to therapy and adjust nursing care accordingly. See individual tests for specific information.

In assessment of platelets:
peripheral blood smear
bleeding time
**platelet aggregation test
bone marrow
**prothrombin consumption test
CBC
direct Coombs' test
serum protein electrophoresis

IMPLICATIONS FOR NURSING CARE
PRETEST: Factors related to the test
Nursing Diagnosis: Potential for injury related to changes in biochemical balance

Guide to assessment	Guide to planning and intervention	Guide to evaluation
Assess patient factors that may influence test results:		
1. Comprehensive drug history (See Drug Influences)	1. Report drugs the patient is currently receiving that may influence lab results to the patient's physician and laboratory.	1. Drugs the patient is currently receiving that may influence test results are identified and the proper people notified.
2. Preexisting conditions (See Increases/Decreases)	2. Record preexisting conditions on lab slip.	2. The patient's preexisting conditions are noted on lab slip.

_____
**Not discussed in this book.

Guide to assessment	Guide to planning and intervention	Guide to evaluation
3. Hemolysis of specimen	3. Prevent hemolysis by: a. Not probing venipuncture site. b. Not forcefully withdrawing specimen. c. Not withdrawing specimen too slowly. d. Not agitating specimen.	3. The patient's blood sample is handled gently to avoid hemolysis.
4. Patient level of knowledge	4. Explain test to patient: a. Define platelet count (See Description). b. Explain procedure (See Procedure).	4. The patient demonstrates knowledge of a platelet count by defining the test and explaining the procedure.

Patient Preparation Checklist

1. √ Influencing drugs noted and reported (See Drug Influence).
2. √ Preexisting conditions noted on lab slip (See Increases/Decreases).
3. √ Patient knowledge; explain test and procedure (See Description/Procedure).

CONSIDERATIONS FOR NURSING CARE RELATED TO ABNORMAL TEST RESULTS

POSTTEST: Factors related to the results of the test
Nursing Diagnosis: Predisposition to bleeding and/or thrombus formation

Guide to assessment	Guide to planning and intervention	Guide to evaluation
Assess patient factors that may be influencing test results. Nursing history and/or physical exam suggestive of: 1. Thrombocytosis	1. Promote hemostasis in the patient with an increased platelet count by:	1. The patient's platelet count is within normal limits:
a. Postsplenectomy (Exercise, strenuous; stress)	a. Recognizing transient increases in platelet counts due to normal physiological processes. Report increases to physician.	a. The patient's transient increase in platelet count is recognized and reported.

Guide to assessment	Guide to planning and intervention	Guide to evaluation
b. Reactive thrombocytosis (See 3 Increases)	b. Implementing medical plan and nursing care to treat disease processes involved in reactive thrombocytosis.	b. The patient's platelet count returns to normal after treatment of the precipitating cause of increase.
c. Myeloproliferative diseases (See 1 and 2 Increases)	c. Promote lowering of the platelet count by:	c. The patient demonstrates that control of the myeloproliferative process has been established by a reduction in the platelet count.
(1) Myelosuppressive therapy	(1) Administering radioactive phosphorus as ordered.	
(2) Chemotherapy	(2) Administering chemotherapeutic agents as ordered (e.g., busulfan).	
(3) Phlebotomy	(3) Assisting with phlebotomy as needed.	
(4) Return medical checkups	(4) Encouraging follow-up care and blood studies.	(4) Follow-up visits are kept.
2. Thrombocytopenia	2. Promote hemostasis in the patient with a decreased platelet count by:	2. The patient's platelet count is within normal limits:
a. Platelet count below 100,000 Easily bruised Bleeding gums Petechiae	a. Initiating nursing care to avoid trauma: (1) Do not give IM injections unless absolutely necessary. (2) Do not use sharp objects. (3) Prevent straining at stool by giving stool softeners. (4) Provide a safe environment to prevent falls and blunt injuries. (5) Discontinue interfering drugs as ordered.	a. The patient is protected from bleeding/bruising episodes and subsequent platelet loss.
b. Platelet count below 50,000 Signs of bleeding: Mucocutaneous, soft tissue, CNS (positive neuro signs) Palpable spleen and liver	b. Initiating nursing care to avoid or detect bleeding: (1) Be alert to and report signs/symptoms. (2) Test urine and stool for occult blood. (3) Do not take rectal temperatures. (4) Apply pressure to all	b. The patient is protected from further platelet loss due to bleeding.

Guide to assessment	Guide to planning and intervention	Guide to evaluation

	puncture sites until bleeding is stopped (5–10 minutes).
	(5) Administer hormones to stop menstrual periods as ordered.
	(6) Maintain bed rest during episodes of active bleeding.
	(7) Prevent superficial capillary breaks from B/P measurements:
	  (a) Take B/P with cuff as infrequently as possible.
	  (b) Do not overinflate cuff.
	  (c) Rotate B/P sites.
	(8) Following nursing care in 2a.	

c. Need for platelet transfusion	c. Administering platelet transfusions as ordered: (1) Platelets should be room temperature when administered. (2) Use of matched platelets lessens chance of antibody formation. (3) Sensitizing platelets are reduced by using washed red cells.	c. The platelet count is increased (temporarily).
d. Acute bleeding	d. Administering adrenal corticosteroids as ordered.	d. The bleeding is stopped and the patient's platelet count is increased.

e. Thrombocytopenic purpura
  Splenomegaly
  Poor response in platelet count to medical treatment
	e. Preparing patient for splenectomy.	e. The patient's platelet count increases postsurgery.

f. Lack of knowledge	f. Teaching patient preventive measures: (1) Use electric razor. (2) Use sharp object with *extreme* caution. (3) Understand relationship of aspirin to bleed-	f. The patient states preventive measures to avoid bleeding.

Guide to assessment	Guide to planning and intervention	Guide to evaluation
	ing. Be aware of hidden aspirin in over-the-counter drugs. (4) Report any bleeding to physician.	

Test:	Porphyrins (Uroporphyrins, Coproporphyrins, Porphobilinogens)
Abbreviation:	UP, CP, PBG
Reference Values:	*Uroporphyrins (UP)* Women 1–22 μg/24 hours Men 0–42 μg/24 hours *Coproporphyrins (CP)* Women 1–57 μg/24 hours Men 0–96 μg/24 hours *Porphobilinogens (PBG)* 1.5 μg/24 hours
Specimen:	24-hour urine collection
Description:	Porphyrins are involved in the formation of hemoproteins and are important to the intermediate steps of heme synthesis. Normally, only very small amounts of porphyrins are excreted in the urine and feces. Increased excretion is suggestive of abnormal heme biosynthesis. An initial screening test using fresh voided urine may be ordered. Blood porphyrins are measured as well as the 24-hour urine collection.

Procedure:	24-hour collection.
	1. No food or fluid restrictions.
	2. Cover collection bottle to protect it from light. The collection bottle should contain a preservative.
	3. The collection should be refrigerated for the entire collection period.
	4. Collection.
	   a. Discard first voided specimen.
	   b. Begin timing.
	   c. For next 24 hours place all voidings into the specimen container immediately after voiding.
	   d. Have the patient void just prior to completion of 24 hours and put that sample in the collection bottle.
	5. Record exact start and finish times on lab slip.
	6. Send to lab immediately.

Conditions Related to Increases	Rationale

1. Congenital erythropoietic porphyria	1. ↑ UP
	   ↑ CP
	   Normal PBG
	   An autosomal recessive disorder that results in impaired conversion of porphobilinogen to uroporphyrinogen.

2. Acute intermittent porphyria	2. ↑ PBG An autosomal dominant disorder. The conversion in the liver of porphobilinogen to uroporphyrinogen is

partially blocked.

3. Variegate porphyria
   Hereditary coproporphyria

3. PBG
   CP
   UP
   All normal except during attack.
   Closely related defects with impaired heme enzyme activity.

4. Porphyria cutanea tarda

4. ↑ UP
   ↑ CP
   Normal PBG
   Diminished uroporphyrinogen enzyme activity.

5. Lead poisoning

5. ↑ CP
   Enzymes responsible for the formation of porphobilinogen are affected by lead.

Drug Influences: The following drugs may influence test results. The drugs are listed alphabetically by generic name and divided into columns according to the effect of the drug. Examples of trade names are in parentheses.

The following drugs may cause an increase in test results:

May precipitate acute porphyria
   antipyretics
   barbiturates
   carbromal (Carbrital)
   chloral hydrate
   chlordiazepoxide (Librax)
   chlorpropamide (Diabinese)
   diazepam (Valium)
   dichloralphenazone (Midrin)
   ergot preparations
   estrogens
   glutethimide (Doriden)
   hydantoin derivatives
   isopropyl dipyrone
   meprobamate (Equagesic, Equanil)
   methyldopa (Aldomet)
   metyrapone (Metopirone)
   nikethamide (Coramine)
   pentazocine (Talwin)
   progesterones
   succinimides
   sulfonamides

Synthesis of porphyrin precursor (ALA)
   aminopyrine
   ethanol
   griseofulvin
   hexachlorobenzene
   sulfomethane

The following drugs may cause a decrease in test results: oral contraceptives (in established disease).

Related Lab Studies: In the differential diagnosis of porphyria:
   *urine delta-aminolevulinic acid (ALA)
   urine porphyrins
   serum porphyrins

---

*Not discussed in this book.

IMPLICATIONS FOR NURSING CARE
PRETEST: Factors related to the test
Nursing Diagnosis: Potential for injury related to changes in biochemical balance

Guide to assessment	Guide to planning and intervention	Guide to evaluation
Assess patient factors that may influence test results: 1. Comprehensive drug history (See Drug Influences)	1. Identify drugs that may influence test results. Consult with physician. Note interfering drugs on lab slip.	1. Patient's drugs do not interfere with test results.
2. Knowledge deficit	2. Explain test to patient: a. Define porphyrins (See Description). b. Explain procedure (See Procedure).	2. Patient demonstrates knowledge by defining test and stating procedure.

Patient Preparation Checklist

1. √ Interfering drugs and note on lab slip.
2. √ Patient knowledge: explain test.

CONSIDERATIONS FOR NURSING CARE RELATED TO ABNORMAL TEST RESULTS
POSTTEST: Factors related to the results of the test
Nursing Diagnosis: Alterations in biochemical balance

Guide to assessment	Guide to planning and intervention	Guide to evaluation
Nursing history and/or physical exam that is suggestive of: 1. Lead poisoning	1. Protect patient from blocked heme synthesis due to lead poisoning: a. Promote community awareness of lead poisoning. See Lead levels. b. Attempt removal of lead from body by: (1) Administering saline cathartics as ordered. (2) Administering chelating agents as ordered.	1. Patient's lead levels are reduced.

Test:	Potassium
Abbreviation:	K
Reference Values:	*Serum* Below 10 days of age 3.5–7.0 mEq/L (46) All other ages 3.5–5.5 mEq/L *Urine* Children and adults 25–100 mEq/24 hours
Specimen:	Serum 24-hour urine collection
Description:	Potassium is the major cation of intracellular fluid. It is widely distributed throughout the body cells. The body's requirement for potassium is maintained primarily through dietary intake of 50–150 mEq of potassium per day. The cation is absorbed through the small intestine into the blood. The function of potassium in the body is to maintain the osmolality of intracellular fluids. It is necessary for nerve impulse conduction and normal excitability of muscle tissue, especially the heart muscle. Potassium plays a role in maintaining the acid-base balance of the body. As the blood pH decreases, potassium leaves the cells in exchange for extracellular hydrogen ions. Potassium is necessary for cellular growth and is involved in converting carbohydrates into energy. Potassium is excreted mostly by the kidneys but also through the intestines. Some is lost through the skin in sweat. Excretion of potassium through the kidneys is influenced by aldosterone, potassium levels, and the acid-base balance of the body. Potassium continues to be lost through the kidneys, however, even in states of low body potassium. Serum potassium levels are done to determine water and electrolyte balance and to detect changes in potassium concentrations that may cause cardiac toxicity. Although potassium is the most abundant cation in the body, it is found only in small amounts in the extracellular fluid. Urinary potassium levels are measured to determine total potassium loss in a 24-hour period and to evaluate certain endocrine disorders by comparing urinary sodium excretion to potassium excretion. Generally, urinary potassium is reflective of potassium intake.
Procedure:	(red top tube)

Serum

1. No food or fluid restrictions.
2. 0.5–10 cc of venous blood is withdrawn from the patient.
3. Observe puncture site for bleeding or evidence of hematoma.

24-Hour Urine Collection

1. No food or fluid restrictions.
2. Obtain collection container; no preservative necessary.

3. Keep urine collection refrigerated.
4. Collection.
   a. Discard first voided specimen.
   b. Begin timing.
   c. For the next 24 hours place all voidings into specimen container immediately after voiding.
   d. Have the patient void just prior to completion of 24 hours and put the sample in the collection bottle.
5. Record the exact start and finish times on lab slip.
6. Send to lab refrigerator.

Conditions Related to Increases	Rationale
	Serum
1. Hemolysis of specimen	1. Hemolysis will cause the release of intracellular potassium, resulting in false high potassium levels.
2. Tourniquet on when arm exercised (i.e., hand pumping and squeezing)	2. Venous stasis without exercise of arm does not affect potassium values. Increases are noted of up to 3 mmol/L when the arm is exercised. The increases are due to leakage of potassium into the plasma from damage to surrounding cells (11, 21).
3. Administration of massive transfusions	3. Stored plasma contains an abnormally high level of potassium due to blood cell lysis with release of potassium (82).
4. Myeloproliferative disorders Polycythemia vera Chronic granulocytic leukemia Myelofibrosis	4. The increase is related to the rapid platelet turnover resulting in release of intracellular potassium (21).
5. Extensive tissue injury Severe infections Trauma Chemotherapy Disseminated intravascular coagulation (DIC) Hemorrhage	5. Damage to a large number of body cells results in the release of intracellular potassium.
6. Acute renal disease (oliguric phase)	6. Potassium excretion is impaired. If acidosis is present there may also be a shift of potassium to extracellular fluids.
7. Acidosis Chronic obstructive lung disease	7. In acidosis the chemical-cellular buffer system moves potassium out of and hydrogen ions into the cells. This exchange is to decrease extracellular acid. This shift may cause serum potassium concentrations to

become elevated; total body potassium may be decreased.

8. Adrenal cortical hypofunction

8. The lack of aldosterone feedback results in decreased excretion of potassium.

9. Diabetes mellitus

9. Insulin promotes entry of potassium into cells. With decreased levels of insulin, potassium does not move into cells as readily. Because of this, there may be increased serum potassium.

10. Hyperparathyroidism

10. The serum potassium increase in some cases is probably due to the accompanying acidosis.

11. Heatstroke

11. Excess body heat causes cellular breakdown that results in potassium leaving cells and entering the extracellular fluid. Potassium remains in the extracellular fluid because of decreased renal excretion secondary to circulatory collapse.

12. Malignant hyperpyrexia

12. The etiology is unknown, but the reaction is believed to be part of the generalized human stress syndrome (85). See first sentence of 11 above.

13. Burns (first 48 hours)

13. Extensive cellular damage causes the release of potassium into the extracellular fluid (16).

14. Hemolysis due to sickle-cell or hemolytic anemia

14. Hemolysis of blood cells due to abnormal red cell morphology leads to increased release of potassium (83).

15. Hyperkalemic periodic paralysis

15. This condition results from an inherited autosomal dominant transmission defect. The defect causes a shift of intracellular potassium into extracellular fluid. The paralytic attacks are precipitated by strenuous exercise, cold exposure, hunger, and rapid administration of potassium.

16. IV potassium penicillin

16. Penicillin G potassium for parenteral injection contains 1.7 mEq/million U. Patients receiving high-dose penicillin therapy can have increased serum levels.

Conditions Related to Decreases	Rationale
	Serum
1. Metabolic and respiratory alkalosis	1. Extracellular potassium enters the cells in exchange for hydrogen ions and so serum potassium levels are reduced.
2. Hyperaldosteronism	2. Aldosterone acts on the cells of renal tubules to increase excretion of potassium. High levels of aldosterone cause increased amounts of potassium to be excreted through the tubules.

3. Excessive licorice ingestion:
   Licorice candy
   Licorice-containing alcoholic beverages
   Chewing tobacco
	3. Licorice contains glycyrrhizic acid, which acts on the renal tubules in a manner identical to that of aldosterone, causing increased excretion of potassium.

4. Cushing's disease	4. The excessive secretion of mineralocorticoids causes an increase in the secretion of potassium through the kidneys (36).
5. Diabetic acidosis (6–8 hours after treatment started)	5. There is an intracellular potassium deficit present due to acidosis and the increased need for potassium in cellular regrowth. As treatment is started, the improved renal flow, increased excretion of potassium, and the shift of extracellular potassium into the cells lead to a serum decrease (16).
6. Burns (4th–5th day postinjury)	6. Potassium shifts from extracellular to intracellular fluid. Renal losses of potassium increase when diuresis starts. See 3 Serum Increases.
7. Jejunoileal bypass for obesity	7. Potassium lost in feces is about three times greater than normal. Since transit time is shortened and a diarrheal state exists, intestinal potassium will escape reabsorption (87).

8. ACTH-producing tumors
   Oat cell carcinoma of the bronchus
   Pheochromocytomas
   Certain ovarian tumors
	8. Related to high blood levels of corticosterone and deoxycorticosterone, which encourages sodium retention and potassium loss (69).

9. Renal vascular hypertension Malignant hypertension	9. Excessive renin production stimulates aldosterone secretion leading to excessive urinary loss of potassium. See 2 Serum Decreases.

10. Renal tubular acidosis

10. There is an elevated rate of potassium excretion in the distal portion of the nephron caused by a rise in sodium and bicarbonate loads.

11. Laxative abuse
    Chronic diarrhea
    Sprue
    Malabsorption syndrome

11. A high rate of fecal excretion of potassium leads to a decrease in serum levels.

12. Villous adenoma of colon and rectum

12. Stool volume high in potassium may achieve levels of 1500–3500 ml/day. Source of the stool potassium may result from increased secretion of potassium-containing intestinal mucosal cells or from excessive excretion of intestinal mucosa (69).

13. Exercise with excessive perspiration

13. The potassium loss in sweat plus the urinary loss because of secondary aldosteronism cause decreased potassium levels (69). See 14.

14. Stress
    Peritonitis

14. Conditions of stress lead to increased production of aldosterone, which encourages potassium excretion.

15. Liddle's syndrome

15. An inherited defect in renal transport processes causing increased potassium loss (69).

16. Barium poisoning

16. Ingestion of soluble barium salts can cause low potassium plasma level due to a shift from the extracellular fluid to the intracellular fluid.

17. Starvation, including diets
    Diuretic therapy (especially thiazides)

17. Potassium replacement is maintained primarily through diet. 5–10 mEq of potassium may be excreted in the urine per day, even in a state of hypokalemia. Losses not replaced lead to hypokalemia.

18. Familial periodic paralysis

18. An inherited disorder of unknown etiology. With the onset of an attack, the serum potassium level falls and remains low during paralysis and then rises with recovery (69).

19. Gastric losses
    Vomiting
    Excess nasogastric drainage
    Pyloric stenosis

19. Gastric losses cause metabolic alkalosis and volume depletion, and this stimulates aldosterone production, leading to hypokalemia.

Conditions Related to Increases

1. Diabetic acidosis

2. Renal tubular acidosis

3. Starvation

4. Primary aldosteronism

5. Cushing's disease
   Cushing's syndrome

Rationale
Urine

1. Osmotic diuretic effect of hyperglycemia causes an increase in the excretion of potassium.

2. In this condition there is a decrease in potassium reabsorption in the proximal tubule and an increase in secretion of potassium from the distal portion of the nephron (69).

3. Increased breakdown of body cells releases intracellular potassium that is then excreted through the kidneys (9).

4. The adrenal gland secretes large quantities of aldosterone, which encourages sodium retention and potassium excretion.

5. The excessive secretion of mineralocorticoids causes an increase in the secretion of potassium (69).

Conditions Related to Decreases

1. Diarrhea

2. Acute renal failure

3. Adrenal cortical hypofunction

Rationale
Urine

1. High rate of fecal excretion of potassium leads to a decrease in serum levels that results in less potassium being excreted.

2. In renal failure, electrolytes and water are blocked from excretion. There is an accompanying serum increase.

3. Lack of aldosterone feedback system results in decreased excretion of potassium.

Drug Influences: The following drugs may cause a serum potassium increase. The drugs are listed alphabetically by generic name and divided into columns according to the effect of the drug. Examples of trade names are in parentheses.

Nephrotoxic effect
   aminocaproic acid (Amicar)
   amphotericin B
   boric acid (Murine)
   cephaloridine

   lipomul
   methicillin (Staphcillin)
   tetracycline

Contains potassium
   Potassium chloride (KCl)
   Potassium penicillin
   triamterene (potassium sparing)

Metabolic effect
  epinephrine
  saline
  spironolactone (Aldactone)

Miscellaneous
  cannabis
  histamine
  lithium
  mannitol
  tromethamine

Decreased renal excretion
  heparin

The following drugs may cause a decrease in serum potassium:

Diuretic effect
  acetazolamide (Diamox)
  aminosalicylic acid
  ammonium chloride
  aspirin
  carbenicillin
  chlorthalidone (Hygroton)
  clopamide
  clorexolone
  diapamide
  dichlorphenamide
  diuretics, especially thiazides,
    mercurials
  ethanol
  ethoxzolamide
  furosemide
  mefruside
  meralluride
  metolazone
  quinethazone
  sodium sulfate
  spironolactone, slight decrease
  streptozotocin
  triamterene (Dyrenium)
  urea (Debrox, Gly-oxide)

Mineralo/glucocorticoid response
  aldosterone
  carbenoxolone
  corticosteroids
  corticotropin
  cortisone
  desoxycorticosterone
  dexamethasone
  fludrocortisone
  glucocorticoids
  glycyrrhiza
  hydrocortisone
  methylprednisolone
  paramethasone
  prednisolone
  prednisone

Nephrotoxicity
amphotericin B

Fecal losses
  bisacodyl
  cathartics
  mercury compounds
  neomycin

Miscellaneous
  bumetanide
  enflurane, slight decrease
  epinephrine
  methazolamide (with prolonged use)
  phosphates
  polystyrene sulfonate
  sodium bicarbonate

Related Lab Studies: Monitor response to therapy and adjust nursing care accordingly. See individual tests for specific information.

electrolytes (Na, K, Cl, CO_2)
osmolality, serum, urine
creatinine, creatinine clearance
aldosterone
*renin
ABGs
FBS
Hct

IMPLICATIONS FOR NURSING CARE
PRETEST: Factors related to the test
Nursing Diagnosis: Potential for injury related to changes in biochemical balance

Guide to assessment	Guide to planning and intervention	Guide to evaluation
Patient factors influencing test results:		
1. Comprehensive drug history (See Drug Influences)	1. Report drugs the patient is receiving that may influence lab results to the patient's physician and laboratory.	1. Drugs patient is currently receiving that may influence test results are identified and the proper people notified.
2. Preexisting conditions	2. Record preexisting conditions on laboratory slip.	2. Patient's preexisting conditions are noted on lab slip.
3. Hemolysis	3. Prevent hemolysis by: a. Not saturating skin with antiseptic. b. Not probing venipuncture site. c. Not forcefully withdrawing specimen. d. Not withdrawing specimen too slowly. e. Not agitating or handling specimen too roughly. f. Not allowing patient to exercise arm with tourniquet on while drawing blood specimen.	3. The patient's blood sample is not hemolyzed.
4. Knowledge deficit	4. Explain test to patient: a. Define potassium (See Description). b. Describe procedure (See Procedure).	4. The patient demonstrates knowledge of test by defining test and stating procedure.

*Not discussed in this book; see Aldosterone.

Patient Preparation Checklist

1. √ Influencing drugs noted and reported (See Drug Influences).
2. √ Preexisting conditions noted on lab slip (See Increases/Decreases).
3. √ Patient knowledge; explain test and procedure (See Description and Procedure).

CONSIDERATIONS FOR NURSING CARE RELATED TO ABNORMAL TEST RESULTS
POSTTEST: Factors related to the results of the test
Nursing Diagnosis: Alterations in biochemical balance

Guide to assessment	Guide to planning and intervention	Guide to evaluation
Assess patient factors that may be influencing test results: 1. Hypokalemia Signs and Symptoms Weakness Flaccid paralysis Shallow respirations Decreased intestinal motility Abdominal distention Anorexia Paralytic ileus Arrhythmias Hypotension Irritability Confusion Paresthesia EKG changes; flattened T wave, inverted or prolonged QT interval Nursing history and/or physical exam suggestive of: 2. Low serum potassium a. Patients at risk for potassium losses. Tissue injury Wound infection b. Psychological stress: Fear Anxiety Emotional crises	1. Implement plan of care to correct hypokalemia by: a. Administering oral potassium, as ordered, with full glass of water and/or juice (depending on preparation). b. Administering IV potassium slowly, as ordered, to prevent vein irritation and potassium toxicity. c. Providing high potassium diet as needed. d. Implementing medical plan to treat underlying cause of decreased serum potassium. 2. Implement plan of care to prevent hypokalemia: a. Identify patients with increased potential for potassium loss. b. Reduce psychological stresses by providing a tranquil environment, showing sensitivity to patient's feelings, and maintaining consistent caregivers if possible.	1. The patient does not demonstrate signs of reduced serum potassium: a. The patient receives oral potassium preparation according to preparation directions. b. The patient receives IV potassium without venous irritation and at the correct speed. c. The patient receives adequate dietary potassium if appropriate. d. The patient's medical plan is implemented. 2. The patient's serum potassium remains normal: a. Patients at risk are identified. b. The patient's need for adaptation to psychological stress is reduced.

Guide to assessment	Guide to planning and intervention	Guide to evaluation
c. Diuretic therapy (especially thiazides)	c. Teach patient about their diuretics and the relationship to potassium.	c. The patient states the influence of diuretics on potassium excretion.
d. Dietary intake	d. Instruct patient which foods have high potassium content (oranges, bananas, dried fruits, whole grain breads and cereals, apples, halibut, cod, salmon).	d. The patient lists foods high in potassium content.
e. Nasogastric drainage Biliary drainage Vomiting	e. Replace, as ordered, potassium lost from gastric losses.	e. The patient does not experience hypokalemia because of gastric losses.
f. Knowledge deficit about laxatives	f. Instruct patient on proper use of laxatives.	f. The patient is able to explain appropriate use of laxatives.
g. Licorice ingestion	g. Explain relationship of licorice to potassium level (See 3 Increases).	g. The patient states how glycyrrhizic acid (licorice) increases potassium.
3. Hyperkalemia Signs and Symptoms: Bradycardia Ventricular fibrillation Intestinal colic Diarrhea Muscle twitching proceeding to weakness Flaccid muscle paralysis Oliguria Anuria ECG changes: wide to absent P wave; depressed ST segment	3. Implement plan of care to correct hyperkalemia by: a. Administering fluids if not contraindicated and as ordered. b. Withholding foods that contain large amounts of potassium. Consult with dietician. c. Administering ion exchange resins as ordered (e.g., Kayexalate). d. Administering glucose and insulin as ordered. e. Administering sodium bicarbonate as ordered. f. Discontinuing drugs that impair potassium excretion as ordered (See Drug Influences). g. Preparing patient for peritoneal or hemodialysis as ordered.	3. The patient does not demonstrate signs or symptoms of increased serum potassium: a. The patient's potassium excretion is increased by improved urinary output. b. The patient does not receive increased dietary potassium. c. The patient receives the ion exchange resin as ordered. d. The patient's corrected potassium ion exchange is demonstrated by normal serum potassium levels. e. As above. f. Drugs the patient is taking that interfere with potassium excretion are discontinued. g. The patient is prepared for dialysis.
4. Hyperkalemia At risk conditions for hyperkalemia (See Increases)	4. Implement plan of care to prevent hyperkalemia by: a. Identifying the patient at risk for increases in potassium levels.	4. The patient's serum potassium is within normal limits: a. Patients at risk are identified.

Guide to assessment	Guide to planning and intervention	Guide to evaluation
	b. Minimizing release of potassium from cells by controlling breakdown of tissue, e.g.: (1) Control infection. (2) Provide adequate intake of calories and carbohydrates.	b. The patient is protected from increased serum potassium from undue tissue breakdown.
	c. Reducing dietary intake of potassium.	c. The patient's dietary potassium intake is reduced.
	d. Checking carefully all IV infusions containing potassium.	d. The patient does not receive too much potassium from IV.
	e. Checking renal function prior to administering IV potassium.	e. The patient does not become hyperkalemic because of decreased renal function.
	f. Avoiding the use of potassium-containing salt substitutes for patients with oliguric renal problems (84).	f. Patients and their families are protected from excessive potassium intake from salt substitutes.
	g. Teaching patients to keep salt substitutes containing potassium away from children.	g. As above.
	h. Administering frozen washed cells to patients requiring many transfusions who have renal impairment.	h. Patients with renal impairment do not receive excessive potassium from stored plasma.

Test: Pregnancy Test, Beta subunit hCG

Abbreviation: None

Reference Values: Beta subunit hCG radioimmunoassay method
Serum: <3 ml U/ml nonpregnant
Pregnancy values vary with gestation
Urine: negative

Specimen: Serum, urine

Description: Human chorionic gonadotropin (hCG) is a glycoprotein hormone produced by trophoblastic tissue, usually of the placenta. The function of hCG in pregnancy is to prevent the destruction of the corpus luteum. The hormone may also be produced in certain carcinomas.

Measurements of hCG are done to diagnose early pregnancy, as tumor markers, and to evaluate hormone activity in threatened abortion.

Procedure:

Urine Pregnancy Test

1. No food or fluid restrictions.
2. Collect first morning specimen if possible. A random specimen may be used, but the first morning concentrated urine specimen is best.
3. Note date of last normal menstrual period on lab slip.
4. If unable to send to lab immediately, refrigerate specimen.

24-Hour Urine Collection for Quantitative Analysis

1. No food or fluid restrictions.
2. Collection bottle should contain boric acid. Keep urine refrigerated.
3. Collection.
   a. Discard first voided specimen.
   b. Begin timing.
   c. For the next 24 hours, place all voidings into the specimen container immediately after voiding.
   d. Have patient void just prior to completion of 24 hours and put sample in collection container.
4. Record exact start and finish times as well as date of last normal menstrual period (if appropriate) on lab slip.
5. Send to lab immediately.

Serum

1. No food or fluid restrictions.
2. Approximately 2 ml of blood is withdrawn from the patient.
3. Note date of LMP on lab slip.
4. Observe puncture site for bleeding or evidence of hematoma.

Conditions Related to Increases

1. Pregnancy

2. Trophoblastic tumors, e.g.,
   Hydatidiform mole
   Gestational trophoblastic disease

3. Testicular tumors, e.g.
   Testicular choriocarcinoma
   Teratomas
   Embryonal carcinoma

4. Nontrophoblastic tumors, e.g.
   Gastrointestinal carcinomas
   Multiple myeloma
   Leukemia
   Carcinoma of breast

Rationale

1. After implantation of the fertilized ovum (7–10 days), hCG is measurable in serum and urine. The hormone increases production until a peak level is reached at about 8–12 weeks. Levels begin to diminish during the remainder of pregnancy, and after delivery, levels decline and are undetectable in about 2 weeks. Serum levels are detectable within 24 hours of implantation.

2. Levels of hCG may be extremely high in these tumors, though sometimes levels may be the same as in a normal pregnancy. Serial levels in these diseases usually reveal irregular fluctuations rather than the fairly predictable pattern in a normal pregnancy.

3. In certain testicular tumors, hCG is found in urine and serum. This may be a result of hormone production from the choriocarcinoma.

4. The increased levels of hCG in these tumors are a result of ectopic production of the hormone. If hCG is present, it is often measured as an evaluation of therapy or indication of recurrence of disease.

Conditions Related to Decreases

1. Ectopic pregnancy

2. Threatened abortion

Rationale

1. It is possible to have false negative results in up to 50% of patients with ectopic pregnancies. Often a combination of laboratory methods is used to increase sensitivity for detection of ectopic pregnancies.

2. If the hCG level remains low or begins a descent during the first trimester of pregnancy, spontaneous abortion is almost inevitable.

Drug Influences: Drugs do not interfere with radioimmunoassay method of beta subunit hCG measurement.

Related Lab Studies: Other methods of hCG measurement:
   hemagglutination inhibition (HAI)
   latex particle agglutination inhibition (LAI)
   radioreceptor assays (RRA)

IMPLICATIONS FOR NURSING CARE
PRETEST: Factors related to the test
Nursing Diagnosis: Knowledge deficit; possible pregnancy

Guide to assessment	Guide to planning and intervention	Guide to evaluation
Assess patient factors that may influence test results: 1. Date of last menstrual period (LMP)	1. Note date of last menstrual period on lab slip as appropriate.	1. The patient's LMP is noted on lab slip.
2. Knowledge deficit	2. Explain test to patient: a. Define hCG as appropriate to diagnosis (See Description). b. Explain correct procedure (See Procedure).	2. The patient demonstrates knowledge by defining test and stating procedure.

Patient Preparation Checklist

1. √ Date of LMP noted on lab slip.
2. √ Patient knowledge; explain test (See Description/Procedure).

CONSIDERATIONS FOR NURSING CARE RELATED TO ABNORMAL TEST RESULTS
POSTTEST: Factors related to the results of the test
Nursing Diagnosis: Alterations in biochemical balance; hCG

Guide to assessment	Guide to planning and intervention	Guide to evaluation
Assess patient factors that may be influencing test results. Nursing history and/or physical exam suggestive of: 1. Pregnancy	1. Support patient with positive hCG levels indicating pregnancy by: a. Being alert to patient response to test results. b Referring patient, as necessary, to appropriate health care provider. c. Establishing early prenatal care.	1. The patient discusses test results knowledgeably.

Guide to assessment	Guide to planning and intervention	Guide to evaluation
2. Increased hCG due to tumor	2. Assist in reduction of hCG by: a. Preparing patient for surgery. b. Encouraging patient throughout radiation therapy. c. Administering chemotherapy as prescribed.	2. The patient's hCG level is normal.
3. Negative result Positive subjective signs of pregnancy	3. Repeat hCG test in 1 week.	3. The patient's hCG level is retested in 1 week.

Test:	Progesterone
Abbreviation:	None
Reference Values:	Males: <100 ng/dl
	Females: Follicular phase: <150 ng/dl
	Luteal phase: >400 ng/dl
	Pregnancy: >800 ng/dl
Specimen:	Plasma

Description: Progesterone is a hormone secreted by the corpus luteum in the nonpregnant female. During pregnancy, progesterone is secreted by the corpus luteum for about 2 months and then the trophoblastic cells (placenta) take over this function. Physiologic effects of progesterone include promoting endometrial thickening and secretory development in preparation for embryonic attachment and growth. Progesterone levels increase to peak levels at the midluteal phase, and if no implantation takes place, progesterone levels drop rapidly and about 2 days later menstruation begins. Progesterone decreases uterine contractility during pregnancy, which prevents uterine contractions from causing spontaneous abortion. The hormone also prepares breasts for lactation during pregnancy by promoting lobulealveolar growth. Other physiologic effects of progesterone are the metabolic influences on protein, fat, and carbohydrate metabolism, water and salt regulation, and increased sensitivity of the respiratory center to CO_2.

Some progesterone is excreted through the bile into the gut. The majority of progesterone is converted to pregnanediol in the liver, conjugated with glucuronide, and excreted in the urine as sodium pregnanediol glucuronide.

In males, postmenopausal women, and prepuberal girls progesterone is present in low levels in plasma. Secretion is mostly from the adrenal glands.

Progesterone measurements are used to evaluate placental function, assess ovulation, establish corpus luteum functioning, and help in the diagnosis of some congenital gonadal disorders and trophoblastic tumors.

Procedure: (green top tube)
1. No food or fluid restrictions.
2. About 5 ml of blood is drawn from the patient.
3. Observe puncture site for bleeding or evidence of hematoma.

Conditions Related to Increases	**Rationale**
1. Pregnancy	1. Progesterone levels during the first trimester range between 1,500 and 5,000 ng/dl. The levels continue to increase, and during the third trimester they range from 8,000 to 20,000 ng/dl.

2. Ovulation

2. Increased levels during midluteal stage of menstrual cycle indicate ovulation. Peak levels may be as high as 2,000 ng/dl.

3. Congenital adrenal hyperplasia

3. In this disease there is insufficient cortisol production, resulting in increased release of ACTH. The increased release of ACTH stimulates the adrenals to produce excessive amounts of other adrenal steroids, such as progesterone. In males, progesterone levels may be as high as 600–1,000 ng/dl.

4. Trophoblastic tumors

4. Certain tumor tissue can cause an increase in progesterone levels due to secretion of the hormone from the tissue origin (trophoblastic) or from ectopic hormone production.

5. Luteinizing tumors

5. The luteinized granulosa cells of the corpus luteum are the major cells of progesterone secretion except in pregnancy.

6. Ovarian cysts

6. Cysts that produce progesterone will increase plasma progesterone.

Conditions Related to Decreases

Rationale

1. Amenorrhea

1. In ovarian hypofunction or anterior pituitary hypofunction, there are low levels of progesterone. Progesterone secretion is stimulated by LH (luteinizing hormone, also called interstitial cell-stimulating hormone [ICSH]) and is required for ovulation.

2. Threatened abortion
   Intrauterine death

2. Levels of progesterone decrease to about 1,000 ng/dl. Levels may remain normal if placenta is functioning normally.

Drug Influences: The following drugs may influence test results. The drugs are listed alphabetically by generic name and may cause a decrease in test results:

Decrease in test value
   ampicillin, decreases synthesis
   estradiol
   oral contraceptives
   prostaglandin F_2 alpha

Related Lab Studies: In threatened abortion: estriol, serum or urine.

IMPLICATIONS FOR NURSING CARE
PRETEST: Factors related to the test
Nursing Diagnosis: Potential of injury related to changes in biochemical balance

Guide to assessment	Guide to planning and intervention	Guide to evaluation
Assess patient factors that may influence test results:		
1. Drug history for estrogen or progesterone therapy	1. Inform lab of recent hormone therapy. Note on lab slip.	1. Patient's values are not influenced by hormone therapy.
2. Preexisting conditions Week of gestation Date of LMP See Increases/Decreases	2. Note pertinent appropriate information on lab slip.	2. Patient's preexisting conditions are noted on lab slip.
3. Knowledge deficit	3. Explain test to patient appropriate to condition: a. Define progesterone (See Description). b. Explain procedure (See Procedure).	3. The patient demonstrates knowledge by defining progesterone and stating test procedure.

Patient Preparation Checklist

1. √ Drug history for recent estrogen/progesterone therapy; note on lab slip.
2. √ Preexisting conditions and note on lab slip.
3. √ Patient knowledge; explain procedure.

CONSIDERATIONS FOR NURSING CARE RELATED TO ABNORMAL TEST RESULTS
POSTTEST: Factors related to the results of the test
Nursing Diagnosis: Alterations in biochemical balance

Guide to assessment	Guide to planning and intervention	Guide to evaluation
Assess patient factors that may be influencing test results. Nursing history and/or physical exam suggestive of:		
1. Ovarian hypofunction	1. Promote stimulation of ovulation by administering exogenous gonadotropins as prescribed.	1. The patient ovulates.

Guide to assessment	Guide to planning and intervention	Guide to evaluation
2. Congenital adrenal hyperplasia Mineralocorticoid replacement Oral Parenteral DOCA pellets	2. Promote adequate cortisol replacement by: a. Understanding cortisol replacement. b. Administering replacement as ordered.	2. The patient's plasma progesterone is normal due to adequate cortisol replacement:
c. Adrenal crisis ↓ B/P ↑ Temperature Muscle and joint pain Malaise Hyponatremia Shock	c. Detecting signs of adrenal crisis early. Refer to physician for immediate treatment.	c. Patient does not experience adrenal crisis; or crisis is reversed.
d. Need for family education about replacement therapy	d. Instructing family about drug and administration techniques. Consult with visiting nurse for follow-up.	d. Patient's family is successful at giving medication.

Test:	Prothrombin Time
Abbreviation:	PT
Reference Values:	Patient: 9–12 seconds Control: derived from normal plasma Values vary with laboratory
Specimen:	Whole blood

Description: The extrinsic and common pathways of coagulation are evaluated by the prothrombin time, or the time needed for plasma to clot after the addition of tissue factor and calcium. (See Figure 2.) This test, along with activated partial thromboplastin time (APTT) and thrombin time (TT), is used in the diagnosis of specific coagulation disorders. It is also used to monitor oral anticoagulant therapy.

Procedure: (blue top tube)
1. No food or fluid restrictions.
2. A vacuum blood tube is completely filled; the tube is gently tipped back and forth to mix the anticoagulant.
3. Observe the puncture site carefully for bleeding or evidence of hematoma.

Conditions Related to Increases

1. Deficiency
   Factor VII (serum prothrombin conversion accelerator)

2. Vitamin K deficiency
   Seen with:
   Antibiotic therapy, long term
   Severe malnutrition
   Newborn
   Malabsorption syndromes
   Coumarin or coumarin-like drugs
3. Liver disease

4. Coumarin therapy

5. Disseminated intravascular coagulation (DIC)

Rationale

1. This is a rare inherited disease. As a factor distinctly of the extrinsic coagulation pathway, PT is prolonged but APTT is normal. See Figure 2.

2. Vitamin K is required for the synthesis of factor VII of the extrinsic pathway and factors II and X of the common pathway. A defect in any of these factors will cause bleeding. See APTT, Increases 2 for a more complete discussion.

3. The liver synthesizes factor V (plasma accelerator globulin) and fibrinogen, both of the common pathway. A deficiency of these factors leads to a prolonged PT. APTT is also prolonged.

4. Coumarin drugs interfere in the synthesis of prothrombin and factor VII and X (Stuart-Prower factor) in the liver. Usually PT time is 1.5–2.5 times normal for anticoagulation therapy.

5. This complex condition, in response to a variety of conditions, is characterized by thrombin in the circulation

EXTRINSIC COAGULATION PATHWAY

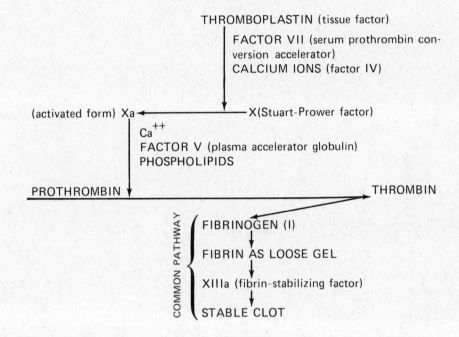

DAMAGED TISSUE RELEASES

THROMBOPLASTIN (tissue factor)

FACTOR VII (serum prothrombin con-version accelerator)

CALCIUM IONS (factor IV)

(activated form) Xa ◄─────────── X(Stuart-Prower factor)

Ca^{++}

FACTOR V (plasma accelerator globulin)

PHOSPHOLIPIDS

PROTHROMBIN ─────────────────────────────── THROMBIN

COMMON PATHWAY

FIBRINOGEN (I)

FIBRIN AS LOOSE GEL

XIIIa (fibrin-stabilizing factor)

STABLE CLOT

that results in fibrin deposits in microcirculation, irreversible platelet aggregation, increased fibrinolysis, and consumption of coagulation factors. See APTT, Increases 7 for more information.

Drug Influences: Many drugs interfere with normal clotting. Listed below are some general drug classifications that may influence test results.

Increase in test results

androgens
anesthetic agents
antibiotics
anticoagulants
aspirin
barbiturates
cathartics
corticosteroids
diuretics

MAO inhibitors
narcotic antagonists
narcotics
oral contraceptives
radioactive compounds
radiographic agents
sulfonamides

Decrease in test results

anabolic steroids
antacids
antihistamines
barbiturates
caffeine

corticosteroids
diuretics; with anticoagulant therapy
oral contraceptives
vitamin K

Related Lab Studies: Hemostatic profile:

bleeding time
platelet count
activated partial thromboplastin time (APTT)
thrombin time (TT)
Hct
PT

IMPLICATIONS FOR NURSING CARE
PRETEST: Factors related to the test
Nursing Diagnosis: Potential for injury related to changes in biochemical balance

Guide to assessment	Guide to planning and intervention	Guide to evaluation
Assess patient factors that may influence test results:		
1. Comprehensive drug history (See Drug Influences)	1. Identify influencing drugs and note on lab slip. Identify and note the following on lab slip: a. Name of anticoagulant. b. Route.	1. Patient's test value is not influenced by unidentified drug.

Guide to assessment	Guide to planning and intervention	Guide to evaluation
	c. Dosage. d. Time of last dosage.	
2. Preexisting conditions Known coagulation disorder See Increases/Decreases	2. Identify preexisting conditions and note on lab slip.	2. Patient's conditions pertinent to lab test are noted on lab slip.
3. Hemolysis	3. Prevent hemolysis by: a. Not saturating the skin with antiseptic. b. Not probing venipuncture site or leaving the tourniquet on too long. c. Not forcefully withdrawing specimen. d. Not withdrawing specimen too slowly. e. Not agitating or handling specimen roughly.	3. Patient's values are not influenced by hemolysis.
4. Knowledge deficit: Patient	4. Explain test to patient: a. Define test; anticoagulant monitoring or coagulation screening. b. Explain procedure.	4. The patient demonstrates knowledge by defining test and stating procedure.
5. Knowledge deficit: Staff	5. Be informed about coagulation studies and anticoagulant medication schedule. Patients on full heparin therapy are tested at least once a day.	5. The patient's coagulation time is not abnormal due to staff error.

Patient Preparation Checklist

1. √ Interfering medications.
2. √ Anticoagulant, dose, time noted on lab slip.
3. √ Pertinent preexisting conditions noted on lab slip.
4. √ Patient knowledge; explain test to patient.

CONSIDERATIONS FOR NURSING CARE RELATED TO ABNORMAL TEST RESULTS
POSTTEST: Factors related to the results of the test
Nursing Diagnosis: Predisposition to bleeding or thrombus formation

Guide to assessment	Guide to planning and intervention	Guide to evaluation
Assess patient factors that may be influencing test results. Nursing history and/or physical exam suggestive of: 1. Oral anticoagulant therapy PT 1.5–2.5 times the control	1. Discourage hepatic synthesis of prothrombin by the use of coumarin and coumarin-type drugs: a. Instruct patient about oral anticoagulant. b. Determine patient reliability in taking medication. c. Instruct patient about signs of bleeding, for example, overt bleeding, bruising, blood in urine, black stools, sudden back pain or GI symptoms. d. Caution patient not to take *any* drugs without consulting the physician. e. Remind patient that changes in anticoagulant status can be altered by state of health. Illness should be reported. f. Refer to general nursing care text for general nursing care surrounding patient with bleeding potential.	1. The patient maintains anticoagulant therapy with desired prothrombin time.
2. Factor deficiencies II V VII X	2. Replace factor deficiencies: a. Assist with starting the administration of plasma products. b. Initiate nursing measures that will promote successful plasma administration completion.	2. The patient's bleeding stops, and lab results are adequate.
3. Vitamin K deficiency Seen with: Antibiotic therapy, long term Severe malnutrition	3. Replace deficient vitamin K for synthesis of prothrombin and factors VII and X: a. Recognize conditions that may encourage vitamin	3. The patient's PT is normal. The patient does not experience bleeding.

Guide to assessment	Guide to planning and intervention	Guide to evaluation
Newborn Malabsorption syndromes Coumarin or coumarin-like drugs Liver disease	K deficiency. b. Consult with physician. c. Administer vitamin K as prescribed.	
4. DIC Lab studies: ↑ PT ↑ APTT ↓ Fibrinogen Platelet count Fibrin split products	4. Discourage consumption of coagulation factors by:	4. Patient's lab values return to normal and the patient's condition improves.
a. Obstetrical conditions Neoplastic diseases Hemolytic responses Extensive tissue damage Fat emboli Acute infections, etc.	a. Being alert to conditions that may stimulate DIC. b. Being alert to signs of bleeding. c. Initiating medical plan to treat underlying cause of DIC. d. Administering heparin as prescribed.	

Test:	Red Blood Cell Count with Morphology
Abbreviation:	RBC and RBC morph
Reference Values:	*Red Blood Cell Count (RBCs)*

Newborn   4.4–5.8 million/μL
2 months   3.0–3.8 million/μL
Children   4.6–4.8 million/μL

Adult
Male   4.5–6.2 million/μL
Female   4.2–5.4 million/μL
Values vary with laboratory

Specimen: Whole blood

Description: Red blood cells are produced in the bone marrow in response to stimulation by erythropoietin. Erythropoietin is a glycoprotein originating in the kidney. Red blood cell development is from the pluripotential stem cell → pronormoblast → basophilic normoblast → polychromatophilic normoblast → orthochromatic normoblast → reticulocyte (the cell is now in circulation) → erythrocyte. From one pronormoblast, 16 mature erythrocytes may develop. Red blood cells function to transport hemoglobin and other nutrients throughout the body. Hemoglobin transports O_2 and removes CO_2 and also acts as an acid/-base buffer. Normal red blood cells have a life of 120 days. As they age they decrease in size slightly, become more fragile, and suddenly fragment. Phagocytosis removes cell fragments, and hemoglobin is split into iron, heme, and biliverdin. The purpose of the red blood cell count is for RBC production evaluation and for the computation of RBC indices.

Morphology: A great deal can be learned from the study of the structure and form of red blood cells. The study is a microscopic exam of a stained blood smear and contains many diagnostic clues. Listed below is the most common information gained from red blood cell morphology.

Color Variations

Normochromic:	Normally the cells will stain reddish-orange on the outer rounded-appearing sides, with the stain dark because of high hemoglobin concentration. There is a gradual decline in color from the outer sides toward the center. The center is quite pale.
Hypochromia:	The center of the cell is larger and paler; hemoglobin content is decreased.
Hyperchromia:	More deeply stained cells. Hemoglobin content is increased.

Anisochromia:	Presence of hypochromic and normo-chromic cells on the same slide. Found after iron therapy, transfusions, and in sideroblastic anemias.

Size Variations

Microcytic:	Abnormally small red cells.
Macrocytic:	Abnormally large red cells.
Anisocytosis:	Variation in size of red cells. Seen in most anemias.

Shape Variations

Poikilocytosis:	Any abnormally shaped cell. Cells are further described by what they look like, for example, teardrop-shaped, oval, etc. See below.
Elliptocytes:	Cells have an elliptical shape. Seen in iron deficiency anemia, megaloblastic anemia, sickle-cell anemia.
Spherocytes:	Spherical shape; smaller than normal disk-shaped cell, decreased hemoglobin. Seen in spherocytosis, some acquired hemolytic anemias, direct injury to cells.
Target cells:	Have appearance of archery target, i.e., stained dark on edges and in the center; the dark edges are separated by a pale ring. Seen in obstructive jaundice, postsplenectomy, any hypochromic anemia, hemoglobin C disease.
Schistocytes:	Fragmented bizarre-shaped RBCs. Seen in hemolytic anemias.
Sickle cells:	Crescent-shaped cells as a result of deoxygenation of hemoglobin. May be seen on blood smear during hemolytic crises.

Structure Variations

Basophilic stippling:	Shows spotted or granular staining. Caused by residual cytoplasmic RNA and indicates that cells are underdeveloped. Fine stippling is seen with increased RBC production. Coarse stippling is seen with impaired hemoglobin synthesis.
Howell-Jolly bodies:	Fragments of residual DNA. These fragments are normally removed by the spleen. Seen after splenectomy or after intense RBC production.

Nucleated red cells (normoblast): The mature RBC does not contain a nucleus. Nucleated red cells are not seen in healthy individuals except in the very young infant. Usually the normoblast is in the bone marrow. The cells are seen in conditions of increased RBC destruction, such as acute blood loss, hemolytic anemia, and hemolytic disease of the newborn.

Procedure: (lavender top tube)
1. No food or fluid restrictions.
2. About 5 ml of blood is drawn from the patient. A fingerstick may be performed.
3. Observe puncture site for bleeding or evidence of hematoma.

Conditions Related to Increases

Rationale

1. Primary polycythemia (Polycythemia vera)

1. There is an excessive RBC count in this disease due to the unrestrained production of erythrocytes. The precise etiology is unknown though it is suspected to be a precursor to leukemia.

2. Secondary polycythemia, e.g.
   Cardiopulmonary disease
   High altitudes
   Cigarette smokers
   Newborn
     Small for gestational
     age
     Diabetic mother
     Hyperbilirubinemia

2. RBC counts are increased due to decreased O_2 saturation, which stimulates erythropoiesis for increased delivery of O_2 to tissues.

3. Relative polycythemia from dehydration

3. Dehydration causes an increase in RBC volume because plasma volume is diminished.

4. Renal tumors

4. A renal tumor may increase erythropoiesis either by producing erythropoietin or impinging on kidney tissue that stimulates erythropoietin.

Conditions Related to Decreases

Rationale

Anemias from Excessive Blood Loss

1. Chronic blood loss

1. Microcytic hypochromic anemia. The diminished RBC count is due to chronic loss of erythrocytes and loss of iron that may deplete iron stores.

2. Posthemorrhagic anemia

2. Normocytic, normochromic anemia. Because of excessive blood loss, RBCs are decreased.

Anemias from Reduced RBC Production

3. Aplastic anemia

3. Normocytic, normochromic anemia. The decrease in red blood cells is from depression or failure of the bone marrow.

4. Iron deficiency anemia

4. Microcytic hypochromic anemia. Causes are inadequate iron intake, impaired absorption or persistent blood loss.

5. Megaloblastic anemias
    Secondary to:
      Malabsorption syndrome
      Malnutrition
      Pernicious anemia
      Pregnancy

5. These anemias are categorized as macrocytic, normochromic anemias. In this kind of anemia, DNA synthesis is markedly reduced due to vitamin B_{12} or folic acid deficiency.

Anemias from Excessive RBC Destruction

6. Hemolytic anemias
    Cogenital:
      Spherocytosis
      Thalassemia
      Sickle-cell
      anemia
      G-6-PD
    Acquired:
      Thrombotic
      thrombocytopenia
      purpura
      Incompatible blood
      transfusion
      Disseminated
      intravascular
      clotting
    Spur cell anemia

6. Hemolytic anemias are caused by increased red blood cell destruction. This may be due to destruction of the cells directly or because the spleen is destroying RBC excessively.

Anemia from Diminished Production and Increased Destruction

7. Renal failure

7. Macrocytic, normochromic anemia. This condition causes a decrease in the production of the erythropoietin. There is also significant red blood cell destruction. Other contributing sources of anemia are from chronic blood loss and inadequate iron intake associated with renal failure.

Drug Influences: The following drugs may influence test results. The drugs are listed alphabetically by generic name and divided into columns according to the effect of the drug. Examples of trade names are in parentheses.

The following drugs may cause an increase in test results:

Increased production

androgens   corticotropin
cobalt   glucocorticoids

Hemoconcentration

epinephrine   pilocarpine

The following drugs may cause a decrease in test results:

Hemolytic anemia with G-6-PD deficiency

acetohexamide (Dymelor)   naphthalene
aminopyrine (Pyramidon)   nitrofurantoin (Macrodantin)
antipyrine (Phenazone)   nitrofurazone (Furacin)
chloroquine (Aralen)   phytonadione (Aqua-MEPHYTON)
dimercaprol (BAL in oil)   primaquine (Primaquine Phosphate)
furazolidone (Furoxone)   quinacrine (Atabrine)
melarsonyl (Trimelarsan)   quinidine (Cardioquin)
methylene blue (Prosed)   quinine (Quinamm)
nalidixic acid (NegGram)   sulfacetamide (Sultrin)

Hemolytic anemia

aminosalicylic acid   phenacetin (in many aspirin
amphetamine (Delcobese)   preparations)
amphotericin B (Fungizone)   phenazopyridine (Azotrex)
aspirin   phenothiazines (Compazine)
cephalothin (Keflin)   piperazine (Antepar)
chlorpromazine (Thorazine)   probenecid (Benemid)
dapsone (Dapsone)   procainamide (Pronestyl)
diphenhydramine (Ambenyl)   salicylazosulfapyridine (Azulfidine)
glucosulfone (Promin)   stibophen (Fuadin)
hydralazine (Apresazide)   streptomycin
isoniazid (Laniazid)   sulfadiazine (Suladyne)
lead   sulfamethizole (Azotrex)
mefenamic acid (Ponstel), autoimmune   sulfamethoxazole (Azo Gantanol)
  hemolytic anemia   sulfanilamide (Vagitrol)
mephenytoin (Mesantoin)   sulfoxone (Diasone Sodium)
methyldopa (Aldomet), autoimmune   tetracycline (Achromycin)
  hemolytic anemia   thiazolsulfone (Promizole)
niridazole (Ambilhar)   tripelennamine (PBZ)
nitrobenzene
penicillin

Megaloblastic anemia

aminobenzoic acid (Pabirin)   neomycin
colchicine (ColBenemid)   nitrofurantoin (Macrodantin)
cycloserine (Seromycin)   oral contraceptives
estrogens (Premarin)   primidone (Mysoline)
ethanol (grain alcohol)   pyrimethamine (Daraprim)
methotrexate (Mexate)   triamterene (Dyrenium)

Pancytopenia/marrow depression

arsenicals
                               meprobamate (Equagesic)

busulfan (Myleran)
chlorothiazide (Aldoclor)
diphenylhydantoin (Dilantin)
floxuridine (FUDR)
gold (Myochrysine)
hydroflumethiazide (Diucardin)
indomethacin (Indocin)

mercaptopurine (Purinethol)
phenacemide (Phenurone)
pyrazolones (Pyramidon)
sulfisoxazole (Azo Gantrisin)
tolbutamide (Orinase)
trimethadione (Tridione)
urethan (Urethane)

Related Lab Studies: Monitor response to treatment or progress of disease. Adjust nursing care accordingly. See individual tests for information.

Hct
Hgb
red blood cell indices
reticulocyte count
serum iron
total iron-binding capacity
*serum ferritin
Schilling test
serum bilirubin
urinalysis
stools for occult blood
WBC with differential
bone marrow
*osmotic fragility

IMPLICATIONS FOR NURSING CARE
PRETEST: Factors related to the test
Nursing Diagnosis: Potential for injury related to changes in biochemical balance

Guide to assessment	Guide to planning and intervention	Guide to evaluation
Assess patient factors that may influence test results: 1. Comprehensive drug history (See Drug Influences)	1. Identify drugs that may interfere with test results. Note them on lab slip. Inform physician.	1. Patient's test results are not influenced by medication.
2. Preexisting conditions Age Sex	2. Identify preexisting conditions that may influence test results and note them on lab slip.	2. Patient's preexisting conditions do not interfere with test results.
3. Hemolysis	3. Prevent hemolysis by: a. Not saturating the skin with antiseptic. b. Not probing venipuncture site. c. Not leaving tourniquet on too long.	3. Patient's values are not influenced by hemolysis of specimen.

*Not discussed in this book.

Guide to assessment	Guide to planning and intervention	Guide to evaluation
	d. Not forcefully withdrawing specimen. e. Not withdrawing the specimen too slowly. f. Not handling the specimen too roughly.	
4. Knowledge deficit	4. Explain test to patient: a. Define red blood cells and hemoglobin (See Description). b. Explain procedure (See Procedure).	4. The patient demonstrates knowledge by defining test and stating procedure.

Patient Preparation Checklist

1. √ Influencing drugs noted on lab slip (See Drug Influences).
2. √ Preexisting conditions and note on lab slip.
3. √ Hemolysis prevention (See 3 above).
4. √ Patient knowledge; explain test to patient (See Description/Procedure).

CONSIDERATIONS FOR NURSING CARE RELATED TO ABNORMAL TEST RESULTS
POSTTEST: Factors related to the results of the test
Nursing Diagnosis: Alterations in blood profile

Guide to assessment	Guide to planning and intervention	Guide to evaluation

Assess patient factors that may be influencing test results.
Nursing history and/or physical exam suggestive of:
1. Anemia
  ↓ RBC
  ↓ Hct
  ↓ Hgb
Signs and symptoms
  Mild anemia
    Asymptomatic, usually
	1. Detect signs of low red blood cell count, low hemoglobin, or hematocrit:
	a. Recognize signs and symptoms of anemia. Consult with physician.
		1. Patient's manifestations of anemia are recognized.

Guide to assessment	Guide to planning and intervention	Guide to evaluation

Moderate anemia
  Pallor
  Fatigue
  Dyspnea
  Palpitations
  Diaphoresis upon exertion
Severe anemia
  Pallor
  Exhaustion
  Severe palpitations
  Sensitivity to cold
  Anorexia
  Weakness
  Dizziness
  Headache
  Congestive failure
  Angina pectoris		

b. Patient history of:
  Poor nutrition
  Toxic drugs or chemical exposure
  Medication history in past year
  Black or tarry bowel movements
  Smoky or hazy urine
  Signs or symptoms listed in *a* above
  History of pica
  Overt blood loss
  Past medical history
	b. Recognize positive history. Consult with physician.
	c. Compare laboratory values for changes in patient's condition.	

2. Blood loss	2. Initiate nursing measures to prevent blood loss:	2. The patient does not suffer decreased RBC count due to excessive blood loss:
a. Overt bleeding At-risk patient	a. Stop bleeding by direct pressure or pressure dressing. Rarely, apply tourniquet.	a. The patient does not experience excessive RBC loss.

b. Infants
  Young children
  Bone marrow depression
  Frequent, multiple blood tests
	b. Keep track of blood loss from frequent blood drawing; record amount of blood drawn. This is especially important in children with bone marrow depression.	b. The patient's RBC count is not affected by blood loss from frequent multiple blood tests.

c. Platelet count
  ↓ 100,000
  Chemotherapy
  Aplastic anemia
	c. Protect patient from bleeding from mucous membranes:
	  (1) Use soft toothbrush.
		c. Patient's RBC loss does not occur due to bleeding.

Guide to assessment	Guide to planning and intervention	Guide to evaluation
Anticoagulation therapy	(2) Use fork carefully. (3) Avoid constipation. (4) Keep mucous membranes soft and moist, as appropriate. (5) Do not take rectal temperatures.	
d. ↓ Platelet count (below 100,000)	d. Initiate measures to avoid bleeding in patients with thrombocytopenia: (1) Do not give IM injections unless absolutely necessary. (2) Do not use sharp objects. (3) Provide a safe environment to prevent falls and blunt injuries. (4) Refer to nursing sections on Platelets and APTT.	d. Patient's RBC loss (bleeding) due to low platelet count is prevented.
e. Bleeding disorder	e. Teach patient preventive measures: (1) Use electric razor. (2) Use sharp object with extreme caution. (3) Understand relationship of aspirin to bleeding. Be aware of hidden aspirin in over-the-counter drugs. (4) Report any bleeding to physician.	e. The patient states preventive measures to avoid bleeding.
3. a. Iron deficiency anemia (Microcytic hypochromic) ↓ MCV ↓ MCH Normal MCHC ↓ Iron, serum ↑ TIBC	3. Promote RBC production: a. Iron deficiency anemia: (1) Teach patient about high-iron foods: (a) Meats: organ meats, red meat. (b) Vegetables: kidney beans, peas. (c) Fruits: raisins, prunes, oranges. (d) Miscellaneous: molasses, iron-fortified foods.	
(2) Iron preparations	(2) Administer iron preparation as prescribed: (a) Teach patient about	

Guide to assessment	Guide to planning and intervention	Guide to evaluation
	drug: (1) Give between meals for best absorption. (2) Iron therapy is continued for months. (3) Dosages may be tapered before being discontinued. (4) Prepare patient for usual side effects: dark stools, stained teeth from liquid preparation, etc.	
(b) Impaired iron absorption	(b) Follow directions for the administration of parenteral therapy carefully. (3) Locate, if possible, cause of continued iron loss (persistent blood loss).	
(4) Infants, 3–12 months Women, 15–45 years	(4) Be aware of high incidence ages.	

(5) Pica
    Ice
    Dirt
    Salt
	(5) Be aware of pica peculiar to patients with iron deficiency anemia.	

b. Megaloblastic anemia
Vitamin B_{12} deficiency
Folate deficiency
  (Macrocytic, normochromic)
  ↑ MCH
  ↑ MCV
  Normal MCHC
	b. Promote DNA synthesis.
	(1) Encourage diet high in folic acid and vitamin B_{12}.
	  (a) Meats: liver, seafood for vitamin B_{12} specifically.
	  (b) Vegetables: leafy (folic acid).
	  (c) Fruits (folic acid).
	  (d) Dairy products.
	  (e) Yeast (folic acid).	

(2) Folic acid therapy	(2) Administer folic acid as prescribed. Teach patient about drugs.	
(3) Third trimester pregnancy Alcoholics Elderly "tea and toast" syndrome	(3) Recognize those at highest risk for development of folate deficiency.	

Guide to assessment	Guide to planning and intervention	Guide to evaluation
(4) Pernicious anemia Vitamin B_{12} deficiency	(4) Administer vitamin B_{12} parenterally as prescribed: (a) Explain to patients with pernicious anemia that they must continue therapy for life. (5) Instruct patients in the need for follow-up medical visits and hematocrit measurements.	
c. Aplastic anemia (normochromic, normocytic) ↓ RBC ↓ Hct ↓ Hgb ↑ Iron, serum ↓ TIBC	c. Promote bone marrow regeneration. (1) Identify and remove toxic agent, if possible. (2) Administer RBC transfusion, as prescribed. (3) Initiate nursing measures to prepare patient for bone marrow transplant. (4) Administer steroids as prescribed. (5) Initiate nursing measures to prepare patient for splenectomy.	c. The patient experiences remission of disease process.
4. Hemolytic anemias Acquired and congenital ↓ RBC ↑ Reticulocytosis ↑ Bilirubin ↑ Red blood cell fragility ↑ Urobilinogen	4. Promote RBC integrity: a. Remove causative factors such as drugs, chemicals, infection, cold, etc. b. Maintain hydration and electrolyte balance. c. Initiate nursing measures to prevent infections. d. Maintain renal function; alkalinize urine during severe crises with sodium bicarbonate or sodium lactate. e. Give steroids as prescribed. f. Administer transfusions, cautiously, as prescribed.	4. The patient maintains RBC integrity as evidenced by clinical appearance and laboratory blood values.
5. Polycythemia ↑ RBC count ↑ Hgb ↑ Hct a. Primary polycythemia	5. Establish nonexcessive RBC levels: a. Promote reduction of RBC count by:	5. The patient's RBC count returns to normal limits:

Guide to assessment	Guide to planning and intervention	Guide to evaluation
	(1) Assisting with venesection.	
	(2) Suggesting to patient to eat low-iron diet.	
	(3) Administering myelosuppressive drugs as ordered.	
	(4) Maintaining hydration.	
b. Secondary polycythemia	b. Discourage hypoxia by: (1) Initiating nursing measures to promote oxygenation. (2) Initiating medical plan to treat underlying cause of hypoxia. (In newborns, possible partial blood exchange.)	
c. Relative polycythemia (Dehydration)	c. Replace plasma loss to reduce relative RBC count.	c. Patient's hemoconcentration is normal.

Test: Reticulocyte Count

Abbreviation: Retic count

Reference Values: % of RBCs counted
Newborn   1.8–4.6%
1 month   0.1–1.7%
Infants   0.4–2.7%
Children   0.5–1.0%

Adults
Male   0.8–2.5%
Female   0.8–4.1%

Specimen: Whole blood

Description: The reticulocyte count gives an approximate rate of red blood cell production. Reticulocytes are immature non-nucleated red blood cells. In the last phase of red blood cell development, before becoming mature red cells, reticulocytes are larger in size than mature red blood cells. They still contain ribosomal RNA as well as miscellaneous developmental cell fragments and mitochondria. Upon staining, the reticulocyte cell materials aggregate, forming reticular strands or meshwork. Reticulocytes take 24–48 hours to mature and generally make up less than 3% of red blood cells. The purpose of the test is to evaluate erythropoiesis and response to therapy.

Procedure: (lavender top tube)
1. No food or fluid restrictions.
2. Up to 7 ml of blood is drawn from the patient (may be fingerstick procedure).
3. Observe puncture site for bleeding or evidence of hematoma.

Conditions Related to Increases

1. Blood loss
   Anemia therapy, e.g.
    Iron therapy
    Vitamin B_{12} therapy
   Hemolytic disease
   Postsplenectomy

Rationale

1. An increasing reticulocyte count after blood loss or therapy for anemia indicates that the bone marrow is functioning normally. The progression from pronormoblast to reticulocyte takes 4–6 days, and it takes about a month for hemoglobin to stabilize. If reticulocytes continue to be elevated, continued blood loss should be suspected.

Conditions Related to Decreases

1. Bone marrow depression
   Hypoplastic anemia
   Aplastic anemia
   Radiation therapy

Rationale

1. Reflects reduced erythropoiesis. See 1 above.

2. Ineffective RBC production
   Pernicious anemia
   Thalassemia
   Iron deficiency anemia

2. The decrease is because of defects in red blood cell development or hemoglobin production.

Drug Influences: The following drugs may influence test results. The drugs are listed alphabetically by generic name and divided into columns according to the effect of the drug. Examples of trade names are in parentheses.

The following drugs may cause an increase in test results:

Hemolytic recovery
   antipyretics
   antipyrine
   arsenicals
   corticotropin

   nitrofurans
   phenacetin
   sulfonamides

Occurs during hemolysis
   aminopyrine
   amyl nitrate
   dimercaprol (BAL in oil)
   furazolidone (Furoxone)

   levadopa
   penicillin
   pipobroman (Vercyte)

The following drugs may cause a decrease in test results:

Decreased hemopoiesis
   azathioprine
   chloramphenicol
   dactinomycin

   methotrexate
   sulfonamides
   vinblastine

Turn to RBC count for discussion of:
   Related Lab Studies
   Pretest Implications
   Posttest Considerations

Test: Rheumatoid Arthritis Factors

Abbreviation: RAF

Reference Value: Negative

Specimen: Serum

Description: In rheumatoid arthritis as well as certain other conditions, some stimulus of unknown origin causes the production of autoantibodies. These antibodies are called rheumatoid factors and are thought to be antigammaglobulin antibodies. RAF is a specific test used in confirming the diagnosis of rheumatoid arthritis. Because many other conditions can produce a positive RAF test, a diagnosis of rheumatoid arthritis is not made solely on a positive RAF test, but in conjunction with a complete clinical workup of the patient. While a high titer (>1:60) may confirm a diagnosis of rheumatoid arthritis, about one-fourth of the patients with the disease do not have reactive titers. A negative RAF test does not rule out the disease. This test is not a useful test for following therapy because clinical symptoms and serum titers do not correlate. Patients with juvenile rheumatoid arthritis rarely have positive RAF titers.

Procedure: (red top tube)
1. No food or fluid restrictions.
2. 5–10 ml of blood is drawn from the patient.
3. Observe puncture site for bleeding, evidence of hematoma, or infection.

Conditions Related to Increases

1. Rheumatoid arthritis
   Systemic lupus erythematosus
   Viral infections
   Syphilis
   Sarcoidosis
   Endocarditis
   About 5% normal population
   Aging
2. False positives

Rationale

1. Titers in rheumatoid arthritis may be between 1:60 and 1:160. Titers are lower in other conditions.

2. May occur from poorly activated complement, high serum lipids, or cryoglobulin levels (42).

Conditions Related to False Negatives

1. Testing too soon

Rationale

1. It takes 6 months from onset of disease before RAF titers are reactive.

Drug Influences: Drugs do not influence test results.

Related Lab Studies: In diagnosis of rheumatoid arthritis:
   CBC
   sedimentation rate

serum protein electrophoresis
synovial fluid analysis

IMPLICATIONS FOR NURSING CARE
PRETEST: Factors related to the test
Nursing Diagnosis: Potential for injury related to changes in biochemical balance

Guide to assessment	Guide to planning and intervention	Guide to evaluation
Assess patient factors that may influence test results: 1. High serum lipids or cryoglobulins (seen in multiple myeloma, leukemia, and some pneumonia) Positive RAF test High fat diet 2. Knowledge deficit	1. Be alert to possible influences of fats or cryoglobulins and note on lab slip. (Test may be repeated after low-fat diet.) 2. Explain test to patient: a. Define RAF (See Description). b. Explain procedure (See Procedure).	1. Patient's test values do not need to be repeated. 2. Patient demonstrates knowledge by defining RAF and stating procedure.

Patient Preparation Checklist

1. √ High fat diet or high serum lipids. Note on lab slip.
2. √ Patient knowledge; explain test to patient.

CONSIDERATIONS FOR NURSING CARE RELATED TO ABNORMAL TEST RESULTS
POSTTEST: Factors related to the results of the test

Guide to assessment	Guide to planning and intervention	Guide to evaluation
	There are no considerations for nursing care related to increased values. Test values are not related to therapy.	

Test: Rh Factor

Abbreviation: None

Reference Values: About 85–90% of the population is Rh positive
                       About 10–15% of the population is Rh negative

Specimen: Whole blood

Description: Antibody research in the 1940s led to the discovery of the Rh factor. This factor, named for the rhesus monkey, demonstrated agglutination of human red blood cells upon the addition of rhesus monkey red blood cells. The agglutinated red blood cells were designated Rh antigen positive; those that did not agglutinate were called Rh antigen negative. Unless there is an immunizing stimulus, Rh antigens do not develop in Rh negative blood. The way Rh negative blood develops antibodies to Rh positive antigens is by blood transfusion with Rh positive blood or through the pregnancy of an Rh negative woman carrying an Rh positive fetus.

Procedure: (red top tube)
                       1. No food or fluid restrictions.
                       2. Up to 10 ml of blood is drawn from the patient.
                       3. Observe puncture site for bleeding or evidence of hematoma.

Conditions Related to Rh Positive Antibodies

Rationale

1. Rh negative person/Rh positive transfusion
   Rh negative woman/untreated Rh positive pregnancy

1. An Rh negative person receiving Rh positive blood will develop antibodies against the Rh factor.
   If a person who is sensitized to the Rh factor receives a transfusion, a hemolytic reaction occurs. Sensitization occurs either from a prior transfusion or untreated Rh positive pregnancy.

2. Hemolytic disease of the newborn

2. An Rh negative woman carrying an Rh positive baby at a first pregnancy usually results in no problems to the newborn. Subsequent infants may be affected. The Rh negative woman during her first pregnancy with an Rh positive infant develops anti-Rh antibodies. During subsequent pregnancies the transplacental passage of the anti-Rh antibodies causes fetal hemolysis of red blood cells.

Drug Influences: Drugs do not interfere with test results.

Related Lab Studies: In Rh incompatible pregnancy:

Maternal Studies	*Neonatal Studies (cord blood)*
*Rh typing	*Rh typing
*ABO typing	*ABO typing
*hemantigen test	direct Coombs'
indirect Coombs'	RBC and morphology
*amniocentesis	RBC indices
	glucose
	bilirubin, serum
	total
	direct

IMPLICATIONS FOR NURSING CARE
PRETEST: Factors related to the test
Nursing Diagnosis: Knowledge deficit related to Rh antibodies

Guide to assessment	Guide to planning and intervention	Guide to evaluation
Assess patient factors that may influence test results: 1. Knowledge deficit	1. Explain test to patient: a. Define Rh factor (See Description). b. Explain procedure (See Procedure).	1. The patient demonstrates knowledge by defining Rh factors.

Patient Preparation Checklist

1. √ Patient knowledge; explain test to patient.

CONSIDERATIONS FOR NURSING CARE RELATED TO ABNORMAL TEST RESULTS
POSTTEST: Factors related to the results of the test
Nursing Diagnosis: Potential for injury related to antigen-antibody reaction

Guide to assessment	Guide to planning and intervention	Guide to evaluation
Assess patient factors that may be influencing test results.		

---

*Not discussed in this book.

Guide to assessment	Guide to planning and intervention	Guide to evaluation
Nursing history and/or physical exam that is suggestive of:		
1. Possible transfusion reaction	1. Be certain that patient receives compatible blood:	1. The patient's blood is compatible with blood being given.
	a. Follow institutional guidelines for administering blood.	
	b. Check and recheck patient's identification and blood type.	
c. Hemolytic transfusion reaction Signs and symptoms Chills Fever Back pain Uneasiness Mild air hunger Occasionally Flushing Urticaria DIC	c. Recognize signs of hemolytic transfusion reactions. d. Stop blood drip, keep vein open with saline, consult with physician immediately should reaction occur. e. Follow institutional guidelines for emergency care following hemolytic transfusion reaction.	
2. Hemolytic disease of the newborn	2. Prevent development of anti-Rh antibodies by: a. Instructing Rh negative pregnant patients about Rh factor. b. Administer Rh immune globulin (RhIG) IM within 72 hours of patient giving birth or postabortion (therapeutic or spontaneous). c. Instruct patient that the RhIG blocks the production of antibodies against the Rh factor. (RhIG does not help if anti-Rh antibodies are already formed.)	

Test: Rubella Titer

Abbreviation: HI or HAI Test (Hemagglutination-Inhibition)

Reference Values: Titers above 1:8 indicate immunity

Specimen: Serum

Description: Generally, rubella titers are done as part of the first prenatal exam to identify women susceptible to rubella virus. A fetus exposed to rubella virus, especially during the first trimester, is in great peril of developing serious malformations.

After rubella infection, the body normally produces antibodies. To test the presence of rubella antibodies, the patient's serum is mixed with an antigen and goose erythrocytes (42). After incubation, if the cells are clumped together (hemagglutination), *no* antibodies are present and the patient is susceptible to rubella.

Rubella titers are done to diagnose congenital rubella and to identify children and females of childbearing age who are susceptible to the rubella virus.

Procedure: (red top tube)
1. No food or fluid restrictions.
2. Up to 5 ml of blood may be drawn from the patient.
3. Observe puncture site for bleeding or evidence of hematoma.

Conditions Related to Increases

Rationale

1. Congenital rubella

1. The congenitally infected infant excretes the virus for 12–14 months after birth. Due to circulating maternal antibodies, the rubella titer is not done until the infant is 6 months old. A titer of more than 1:8 in an infant older than 6 months, who has not been exposed to the virus since birth, is diagnostic of congenital rubella (42).

2. Natural immunity
   Acquired immunity

2. Seen in patients who have had the disease or who have received the rubella vaccine. Titers to some vaccines have shown significant decline over 5 years.

3. Acute rubella

3. Antibodies are present in detectable amounts about 2 weeks after exposure or within 48–72 hours after rash is first seen. These titers then increase about four times in value during the next 2 weeks. After this peak, levels begin to decline slowly but remain present in measurable amounts for life.

Drug Influences: Drugs apparently do not interfere with test results.

Related Lab Values: In diagnosis of congenital rubella:

*Rubella virus isolation

IMPLICATIONS FOR NURSING CARE
PRETEST: Factors related to the test
Nursing Diagnosis: Knowledge deficit related to communicable disease, rubella

Guide to assessment	Guide to planning and intervention	Guide to evaluation
Assess patient factors that may influence test results: 1. Knowledge deficit Public/patient	1. Promote prevention of disease: a. Be knowledgeable about disease. b. Help to educate public about disease risk to unborn children. c. Encourage immunization programs for children. d. Stress to young women that they should not get pregnant until 4 months after receiving rubella vaccine. e. Stress that history of disease is not reliable and vaccine should be given. f. Caution pregnant women without immunity about disease. g. Recognize that infants born with congenital rubella are a reservoir of disease for 2–3 years. i. Administer rubella convalescent gamma globulin IM to pregnant woman at exposure to rubella disease.	1. Patient's titers indicate immunity prior to pregnancies and health statistics show downward trend of disease.
2. Knowledge deficit	2. Explain test to patient: a. Define rubella titer (See Definition). b. Explain procedure (See Procedure). c. Listen to parents as they express fears for fetus or infants.	2. The patient demonstrates knowledge by defining test and stating procedure.

*Not discussed in this book.

Patient Preparation Checklist

1. √ Patient knowledge; explain test to patient (See Description/Procedure and 1 above).

CONSIDERATIONS FOR NURSING CARE RELATED TO ABNORMAL TEST RESULTS
POSTTEST: Factors related to the results of the test
Nursing Diagnosis: Potential injury related to changes in antigen/antibody status

Guide to assessment	Guide to planning and intervention	Guide to evaluation
Assess patient factors that may be influencing test results. Nursing history and/or physical exam suggestive of:		
1. Five years postvaccination	1. Recognize the need for periodic reevaluation of acquired immunity.	1. Patient's declines in effective acquired immunity are recognized.
2. Congenital rubella	2. Stress the need for all susceptible family members to be immunized.	2. Family members are protected against rubella infection.

Test:	Salicylate Level, Acetylsalicylic Acid (ASA)
Abbreviation:	ASA
Reference Values:	Negative

Therapeutic range (3 hours after dose)
Children up to age 10   25–30 mg/dl
Thereafter   20–25 mg/dl

Toxic
Up to age 60   >30 mg/dl
After age 60   >20 mg/dl

Specimen: Serum or plasma

Description: Salicylates are popular non-narcotic analgesics with antipyretic and antiinflammatory action. Salicylates come in oral tablet form, liquid, suppositories, or as oil of wintergreen in topical ointment or cream (skin preparations are absorbed). Acetylsalicylic acid is by far the most popular salicylate. It may be found by itself or in combination with a great many over-the-counter preparations. Though public awareness and childproof caps have made significant headway, aspirin is still the major drug involved in accidental poisoning in children.

Because salicylates may continue to be absorbed for up to 24 hours, serum levels are repeated and therapy is adjusted accordingly. Salicylates are metabolized in the liver and excreted in the urine.

Procedure: (serum—red top tube), (plasma—green top tube)
1. Permit must be signed if for medicolegal purposes.
2. At least 1 ml of blood is drawn from the patient. If microfluorometric method is used, as little as 0.1 ml may be drawn from the patient.
3. Observe puncture site for bleeding or evidence of hematoma.
4. More than one specimen several hours apart is required in monitoring salicylate poisoning.

Phenostix
1. Cleanse patient fingertip.
2. With a lancet, poke fingertip with one sharp, quick motion.
3. Place one drop of serum on test stix.
4. Read color chart.
      Tan color indicates serum level >40 mg/dl
      Brown color indicates serum level from 40–90 mg/dl
      Purple color indicates serum level >90 mg/dl
5. Follow Phenostix directions carefully.

Conditions Related to Increases	**Rationale**
1. Therapeutic overdose	1. Salicylates are used in high doses for the inflammatory action they provide. The drug is used as a mainstay of

treatment in arthritis. It is also used as an anticoagulant in patients at high risk for developing thromboembolism. Frequent salicylate levels are done on patients receiving salicylate therapy to monitor salicylate levels. Levels need to be high enough to be therapeutic but not toxic.

2. Accidental overdose

2. As a popular over-the-counter medication, ASA may be available to children for accidental ingestion. Children may also experience an overdose because of fever and dehydration with too high a dose or too frequent a dose of aspirin. See number 4. Children display a variable effect of aspirin dose to serum level. The Done Nomogram offers prognostic information about the serum salicylate level and the expected severity of reaction in young children. Adults and older children show a close correlation of serum levels to prognosis.

3. Deliberate overdose

3. In an attempt to do themselves harm, some patients may deliberately ingest large numbers of ASA. Blood levels of above 160 mg/dl are fatal.

4. Fever
   Dehydration

4. Increased aspirin levels may occur during fever even at nontoxic doses. ASA is hydrolyzed to salicylic acid and then conjugated in the liver to glucuronic acid and glycine. Aspirin is excreted in the urine as the conjugates and free salicylic acid. With decreased glycogen stores due to the body's increased metabolic needs, the process of conjugation does not take place and aspirin excretion is reduced. Toxic levels may be the result. Dehydration compounds the problem by the rapid absorption of aspirin through the stomach and small intestine.

5. Renal disease

5. Aspirin is excreted in the urine and impaired renal function interferes with aspirin excretion.

Conditions Related to Decreases	Rationale
1. Food Antacids	1. Aspirin is absorbed in the stomach and small intestine. The presence of food or antacids in the stomach will decrease absorption.

Drug Influences: The following drugs may influence test results. The drugs are listed alphabetically by generic name and divided into columns according to the effect of the drug. Examples of trade names are in parentheses.

The following drugs may cause an increase in test results. *Many drugs contain aspirin even though the trade name does not make that obvious. Check patient history carefully.*

Salicylates
   acetylsalicylic acid (aspirin, Bufferin)
   calcium carbaspirin (Calurin)
   choline salicylate (Arthropan)
   magnesium salicylate (Mobidin)
   methylsalicylate (oil of wintergreen)
   salicylamide (Salrin)
   salicylic acid
   sodium salicylate

Miscellaneous
   aminobenzoic acid (Pabirin, PreSun)
   ammonium chloride
   furosemide (Lasix)

The following drugs may cause a decrease in test results:

Miscellaneous
   antacids; decrease absorption rate
   corticosteroids

Related Lab Studies: Monitor response to treatment and adjust nursing care accordingly. See individual tests for information.

   blood glucose
   BUN
   electrolytes
   PT
   APTT
   blood gases (ABGs)
   urine pH
   urinalysis

IMPLICATIONS FOR NURSING CARE
PRETEST: Factors related to the test
Nursing Diagnosis: Potential for injury related to drug poisoning

Guide to assessment	Guide to planning and intervention	Guide to evaluation
Assess patient factors that may influence test results:		

Guide to assessment	Guide to planning and intervention	Guide to evaluation
1. Medicolegal ramifications	1. Get signed permit from family members or patient, if possible.	1. Permit is signed by patient or family member.
2. Current medication history (See Drug Influences) If possible, determine: Name of drug Dosage or number taken Time of ingestion Concurrent drug ingestion	2. Take in-depth history, as possible; note pertinent information on lab slip and in chart.	2. Patient's pertinent drug history is noted on lab slip.
3. Preexisting conditions (See Increases/Decreases) Age	3. Fill out lab slip, including pertinent preexisting conditions and the patient's age.	3. Patient's preexisting conditions and age are noted on lab slip.
4. Hemolysis	4. Prevent hemolysis by: a. Not saturating skin with antiseptic. b. Not probing venipuncture site or leaving the tourniquet on too long. c. Not forcefully withdrawing specimen. d. Not withdrawing specimen too slowly. e. Not agitating or handling specimen roughly.	4. Patient's values are not influenced by hemolysis.
5. Knowledge deficit	5. Teach family/parent: a. Define salicylate level (See Description). b. Explain procedure (See Procedure).	5. The patient does not experience salicylate toxicity.
c. Signs and symptoms of mild ASA toxicity Vomiting Hyperpnea Tinnitus Burning in esophagus and stomach Hearing loss	c. To recognize early signs/ symptoms of ASA toxicity.	
d. Febrile child	d. Suggest alternatives to aspirin: (1) Sponging. (2) Cool environment. (3) Acetaminophen.	
e. Long-term therapy	e. Stress the importance of frequent salicylate levels.	

Patient Preparation Checklist

1. √ Permit signed as needed.
2. √ Comprehensive drug history and note pertinent information on lab slip.
3. √ Patient knowledge; explain test to patient.

CONSIDERATIONS FOR NURSING CARE RELATED TO ABNORMAL TEST RESULTS
POSTTEST: Factors related to the results of the test
Nursing Diagnosis: Alterations in biochemical balance related to poisoning

Guide to assessment	Guide to planning and intervention	Guide to evaluation

Assess patient factors that may be influencing test results.
Nursing history and/or physical exam suggestive of:
1. Salicylate toxicity (See 4c Pretest for mild signs)
  Moderate to severe toxicity
    Vertigo
    Extreme lethargy
    Diaphoresis
    Hyperpyrexia
    Tetany
    Hemorrhage
    Respiratory depression
    Convulsions
    Oliguria
    Coma
	1. Recognize signs/symptoms of toxicity. Consult with physician.	1. Patient's manifestations of salicylate toxicity are recognized and physician is consulted.

2. Therapy
 	
  a. Salicylate toxicity
 	
  b. Activated charcoal
    Cathartic
  c. Mild toxicity
	2. Promote excretion of salicylates:
	  a. Administer syrup of ipecac. Lavage stomach with $NaHCO_3$.
	  b. Administer activated charcoal and cathartic as prescribed.
	  c. Administer milk and water for water diuresis as prescribed.
		2. Patient's salicylate serum levels show steady decline.

Guide to assessment	Guide to planning and intervention	Guide to evaluation
d. Urine pH ↓ 7	d. Alkalinize urine to encourage rapid excretion of free salicylate ion by administering $NaHCO_3$ IV as prescribed.	
e. Adequate urine excretion ↓ Na ↓ K	e. Replace electrolytes to ensure adequate urine flow as prescribed.	
f. Need for dialysis	f. Prepare patient for dialysis.	
3. Status monitoring	3. Initiate nursing measures to promote salicylate excretion: a. Maintain strict intake and output. b. Check urine pH and specific gravity. c. Check Phenostix salicylate levels. d. Consult with physician about changes in patient's condition.	3. The patient demonstrates lowered salicylate level by decreased salicylate blood levels and improved clinical conditions.

Test: Schilling Test

Abbreviation: None

Reference Value: 24-hour urine: greater than 8% radioactive vitamin B_{12} excreted in 24 hours

Specimen: 24-hour urine collection

Description: The Schilling test is a 24-hour urine test done to determine the amount of radioactive vitamin B_{12} excretion by the kidneys. It is expressed as a percentage of the total radioactive dose administered. The Schilling test is done in two stages. The first stage determines if there is a defect in vitamin B_{12} absorption. The second stage is done to determine if the defect is due to a lack of intrinsic factor. Intrinsic factor is a glycoprotein released by the gastric mucosa that is responsible for the absorption of vitamin B_{12} from the ileum. The disease associated with a lack of intrinsic factor is pernicious anemia. Pernicious anemia is the most common cause of a B_{12} deficiency.

If the first 24-hour urine is normal, no further testing is necessary. The patient has shown normal absorption of vitamin B_{12}. If the first 24-hour urine results reveal less than normal excretion of vitamin B_{12}, the test is repeated 3 days later with the addition of a dose of intrinsic factor. If the dose of intrinsic factor results in a normal excretion of B_{12}, the test is diagnostic for pernicious anemia. If the B_{12} excretion remains low even with the addition of intrinsic factor, malabsorption is considered the etiology of the deficient B_{12}.

Procedure: (42)

Without Intrinsic Factor

1. The patient is NPO 12 hours prior to exam.
2. Have the patient void and discard urine.
3. Give vitamin B_{12} tagged with radioactive cobalt by mouth.
4. Begin 24-hour urine collection.
5. 2 hours later, give dose of nonradioactive vitamin B_{12}.
6. Refrigerate urine during collection.
7. Send specimen to lab.

With Intrinsic Factor

1. The patient is NPO 12 hours prior to exam.
2. Have the patient void and discard the urine.
3. Give the patient vitamin B_{12} tagged with radioactive cobalt and intrinsic factor.
4. Begin 24-hour urine collection.
5. 2 hours later, give dose of nonradioactive vitamin B_{12}.
6. Refrigerate urine during collection.
7. Send specimen to lab.

Conditions Related to Increases

1. Not significant

Rationale

1. Normally the body receives much more B_{12} than it needs and excesses are excreted in the urine. If the body's requirements have been met, urinary excretion increases.

Conditions Related to Decreases

1. Malabsorption syndromes
   Sprue
   Intestinal bypass
   Enteritis
2. Pernicious anemia

3. Renal insufficiency
   Other medical conditions leading to impaired renal function, e.g.
      Diabetes
      Hypothyroidism
      Old age

Rationale

1. In these conditions there is defective absorption of B_{12} from the ileum and this may be due, in some situations, to surgical removal of the ileum.
2. In pernicious anemia there is a lack of production of intrinsic factor by the stomach, resulting in poor vitamin B_{12} absorption.
3. Impaired renal function delays B_{12} excretion.

Drug Influences: The following drugs may cause a decrease in serum and urine values of vitamin B_{12}. The drugs are listed alphabetically by generic name and divided into columns according to the effect of the drug. Examples of trade names are in parentheses.

Serum and Urine Decreases

Absorption impairment
   aminosalicylic acid (PAS)
   colchicine (ColBenemid)
   ethanol
   metformin
   neomycin
   oral contraceptives

Related Lab Studies: In the diagnosis of pernicious anemia:

   ↓ RBC (abnormal morphology)
   ↓ WBC
   ↓ platelets
   ↓ alkaline phosphatase
   ↑ indirect serum bilirubin
   ↑ LDH
   bone marrow aspiration (crowded red bone marrow but few normally developing RBCs)
   gastric analysis (absence of free hydrochloric acid after histamine injection) (42)

IMPLICATIONS FOR NURSING CARE
PRETEST: Factors related to the test
Nursing Diagnosis: Potential for injury related to changes in biochemical balance

Guide to assessment	Guide to planning and intervention	Guide to evaluation
Assess patient factors that may influence test results:		
1. Food and fluids	1. Place patient on NPO status from midnight until vitamin B_{12} has been given.	1. Food and fluids do not interfere with accurate lab results.
2. Comprehensive drug history (See Drug Influences)	2. Identify and report to physician and lab whether patient has had any diagnostic exams using radioactivity in the past 10 days: a. Report to the lab and physician drugs the patient is receiving that may influence lab results.	2. Diagnostic exams involving use of radioactive materials in past 10 days are identified and reported to appropriate people: a. Drugs patient is receiving that may influence lab results are identified and the appropriate people are notified.
3. Preexisting conditions (See Increases/Decreases)	3. Identify and note on lab slip any preexisting conditions.	3. Preexisting conditions of patient are identified and noted on lab slip.
4. Knowledge deficit	4. Explain test to patient: a. Define Schilling test (See Description). b. Describe procedure (See Procedure).	4. Patient demonstrates knowledge of test by defining test and stating procedure. 24-hour urine specimen is accurately collected.

Patient Preparation Checklist

1. √ NPO for 12 hours, or as ordered, prior to test.
2. √ No exams using radioactivity 10 days prior to test (See Drug Influences).
3. √ Influencing drugs noted and reported (See Drug Influences).
4. √ Preexisting conditions noted on lab slip (See Increases/Decreases).
5. √ Patient knowledge; explain test and procedure (See Description and Procedure).

CONSIDERATIONS FOR NURSING CARE RELATED TO ABNORMAL TEST RESULTS
POSTTEST: Factors related to the results of the test
Nursing Diagnosis: Alterations in biochemical balance

Guide to assessment	Guide to planning and intervention	Guide to evaluation
Assess patient factors that may be influencing test results.		
Nursing history and/or physical exam suggestive of:		
1. Pernicious anemia: Anemia Weakness Pallor Fatigue Palpitations Sore mouth Smooth, beefy red tongue Weight loss Indigestion Constipation or diarrhea Paresthesias in extremities Irritability Jaundice	1. Correct deficiency in vitamin B_{12} by: a. Administering vitamin B_{12} IM as ordered. b. Teaching patient the importance of continuing lifelong therapy of vitamin B_{12} injections. c. Administering iron salts as ordered.	1. The patient demonstrates correction of vitamin B_{12} deficiency as shown by decrease in symptoms. b. The patient will verbalize understanding of importance of and willingness to take injections on a continuing basis. c. Pernicious anemia is not complicated or precipitated by iron deficiency.
2. Malabsorption syndromes Sprue Intestinal bypass surgery Enteritis Gastrectomy Etc.	2. Promote decreased intestinal peristalsis and increased vitamin B_{12} absorption by: a. Maintaining NPO as ordered. b. Providing small, frequent meals with decreased fat and sugar; limiting fluids to between meals. c. Discouraging intake of iced or concentrated sugar drinks. d. Administering antibiotics, corticosteroids, antidiarrheals, bulk-forming laxatives, or calcium carbonate as ordered. e. Administering hyperalimentation as ordered.	2. The patient demonstrates decrease in frequency and volume of stools and increased consistency of stools.

Guide to assessment	Guide to planning and intervention	Guide to evaluation

3. Impaired renal function	3. Promote increased renal function by:
	  a. Administering diuretics as ordered.
	  b. Promoting fluid and electrolyte status with precise I&O and daily weights.
		3. The patient demonstrates improved renal function by balanced I&O and increased renal function.

Test: Sedimentation Rate

Abbreviation: ESR, Sed rate

Reference Values: *Westergren method*
                     Children   3–20 mm/hr
                     Men   0–15 mm/hr; over age 50   20 mg/hr
                     Women   0–20 mm/hr; over age 50   30 mg/hr
                     Values vary according to method used

Specimen: Whole blood

Description: The erythrocyte sedimentation rate (ESR) is a measure of the time it takes for erythrocytes to settle in a calibrated tube. The test is a nonspecific test that is elevated in inflammation. An elevated sedimentation rate is sometimes the first indicator of disease. Changes in the ESR are most often more significant than a single measurement. The test is ordered to follow the course of inflammatory or malignant disease or to aid in the diagnosis of hidden inflammation.

Procedure: (check with local lab)
                     1. No food or fluid restrictions.
                     2. At least 5 ml of blood is drawn from the patient.
                     3. Observe the puncture site for bleeding or evidence of hematoma.

Conditions Related to Increases

1. Marked elevations, e.g.
   Severe bacterial infections
   Cancers
   Collagen diseases, all
   Cirrhosis
   Severe renal disease
   Ulcerative colitis
   Viral pneumonia
   Macroglobulinemia
   Severe anemia
   Etc.
   Moderate elevations, e.g.
   Age, advanced
   Pregnancy, ectopic
   Oral contraceptives
   Menstruation
   Pregnancy, first trimester
   Infections, acute or chronic
   Nephritis
   Lead ingestion
   Coronary disease
   Destruction, cell and tissue
   Inflammatory diseases
   Etc.

Rationale

1. There are many conditions that cause elevations in the ESR. Anything that adds to the weight of cells will increase settling. Clumping or aggregation of cells, increased amounts of fibrinogen and globulin, and antibody formation all increase the sedimentation rate.

Conditions Related to Decreases	Rationale

1. Polycythemia, primary
   Sickle-cell anemia
   Congestive heart failure
   Cryoglobulinemia
	1. Decreases in the sedimentation rate occur with large cells (increased cell surface). Viscosity of the blood of decreased plasma proteins also slows the sedimentation rate. Sickle-cell blood is oxygenated before testing.

Drug Influences: The following drugs may influence test results. The drugs are listed alphabetically by generic name and divided into columns according to the effect of the drug. Examples of trade names are in parentheses.

The following drugs may cause an increase in test results:

Associated with SLE-like syndrome
   anticonvulsants
   procainamide

Cell aggregation
   dextran

Increased fibrinogen
   oral contraceptives

Miscellaneous
   methyldopa (Aldomet)
   methysergide (Sansert)
   penicillamine
   theophylline
   trifluperidol
   vitamin A

The following drugs may cause a decrease in test results:

Especially in rheumatoid patients
   aspirin
   corticotropin (ACTH)
   cortisone
   trimethoprim (Septra, Bactrim)

Miscellaneous
   ethambutol
   quinine

Related Lab Studies: Monitor response to treatment or progress of disease and adjust nursing care accordingly. See individual tests for information. Tests ordered depend on suspected diagnosis.
   CBC
   urinalysis
   ANA
   C-reactive protein
   cold agglutinins
   Rh factor

IMPLICATIONS FOR NURSING CARE
PRETEST: Factors related to the test
Nursing Diagnosis: Potential for injury related to changes in biochemical balance

Guide to assessment	Guide to planning and intervention	Guide to evaluation
Assess patient factors that may influence test results: 1. Comprehensive drug history (See Drug Influences)	1. Identify influencing drugs, note on lab slip, and consult with physician.	1. Patient's medications do not influence test results.
2. Preexisting conditions	2. Identify pertinent preconditions and note on lab slip.	2. Patient's preexisting conditions that may influence test results are identified on lab slip.
3. Hemolysis	3. Prevent hemolysis by: a. Not saturating skin with antiseptic. b. Not probing venipuncture site or leaving the tourniquet on too long. c. Not forcefully withdrawing specimen. Not withdrawing specimen too slowly. d. Not agitating or handling specimen roughly.	3. Patient's values are not influenced by hemolysis.
4. Need for specimen transport Need for test completion within 3 hours	4. Transport specimen to lab immediately to prevent falsely low reading. Notify lab tech. directly of specimen arrival.	4. Patient's values are not affected by specimen aging.
5. Knowledge deficit	5. Explain test to patient: a. Define ESR (See Definition). b. Explain procedure (See Procedure).	5. Patient demonstrates knowledge by defining test and stating procedure.

Patient Preparation Checklist

1. √ Comprehensive drug history; note interfering drugs on lab slip.
2. √ Pertinent preexisting conditions noted on lab slip.
3. √ Prevent hemolysis. See 3 above.
4. √ Speedy specimen transportation. See 4 above.
5. √ Patient knowledge; explain test to patient.

CONSIDERATIONS FOR NURSING CARE RELATED TO ABNORMAL TEST RESULTS
POSTTEST: Factors related to the result of the test
Nursing Diagnosis: Alterations in biochemical balance

Guide to assessment	Guide to planning and intervention	Guide to evaluation
Assess patient factors that may be influencing test results: 1. Abnormal test result	1. Initiate medical plan of care for underlying condition.	1. The patient demonstrates response to therapy by normal test value.

Test: Serum Protein Electrophoresis

Abbreviation: None

Reference Values:

Measurements in gm/dl

Age	Total	Albumin	Globulin	Gamma Globulin
Preterm	4.0–7.0	2.5–4.5	1.2–2.0	0.5–0.9
Newborn	5.0–7.1	2.5–5.0	1.2–4.0	0.7–0.9
1–3 months	4.7–7.4	3.0–4.2	1.0–3.3	0.1–0.5
3–12 months	5.0–7.5	2.7–5.0	2.0–3.8	0.4–1.2
1–15 years	6.5–8.6	3.2–5.0	2.0–4.0	0.6–1.2
Adults	6.6–7.9	3.3–4.5	A_1 0.2–0.4	0.5–1.6
			A_2 0.6–1.0	
			Beta 0.6–1.2	

Specimen: Serum

Description: Serum protein electrophoresis is a method of measuring the major blood proteins, albumin and globulin. It is achieved by using an electric field to separate the proteins according to size and electrical charge.

Albumin makes up the major portion of serum protein. Albumin plays an important role in total body water distribution and in transporting and storing low molecular weight substances. Globulins are categorized by electrophoretic activity. Alpha globulins (1 and 2) and beta globulin are known as transport or carrier proteins. Gamma globulins are antibodies and of utmost importance to the body's defense against disease. Gamma globulins also act as carrier proteins.

The test is done to identify serum protein abnormalities.

Procedure: (red top tube)
1. No food or fluid restrictions.
2. 1 ml–5 ml of blood is drawn from the patient.
3. Observe the puncture site for bleeding or evidence of hematoma.

Conditions Related to Increases

Rationale

The following is a discussion on the globulin fraction of serum proteins. For an in-depth discussion of the albumin fraction, turn to Albumin.

1. Gammaglobulinopathies, e.g.
   Alpha heavy chain disease
   Multiple myeloma
   Macroglobulinemia
   Muchain disease
   Hodgkin's disease

1. These conditions are uncommon in persons under the age of 30. The exact etiology is unknown. The increase in gamma globulins involves abnormal production of abnormal immunoglobulins from an abnormal proliferation of lymphoid cells.

Conditions Related to Decreases	Rationale

The following is a discussion on the globulin fraction of serum proteins. For an in-depth discussion of albumin fraction, turn to Albumin.

1. Hypogammaglobulinemia

2. Agammaglobulinemia

1. A condition resulting in decreased circulating immunoglobulins. The congenital form is usually from an atrophy of lymphoid tissue, and children may die during childhood from inconsequential infections. The acquired form is usually not manifested until adolescence or later.

2. In this very rare condition there is complete failure of immunoglobulin synthesis. This is a congenital defect.

Drug Influences: The following drugs may influence test results. The drugs are listed alphabetically by generic name and divided into columns according to the effect of the drug. Examples of trade names are in parentheses.

The following drugs may cause an increase in test results:

Drugs Affecting Gamma Globulin Fraction

Hypersensitive reaction
    aminopyrine; specific antibodies to drug
    hydantoin derivatives (Dilantin)
    tolazamide (Tolinase)
    tubocurarine (Tubocurarine Chloride)

Miscellaneous
    anticonvulsants; SLE-like syndrome
    asparaginase (Elspar)

The following drugs may cause a decrease in test results:

Hypersensitive reaction
    BCG vaccine

Immunosuppressive response
    methotrexate (Mexate)

The following drugs may cause an increase in test results:

Drugs Affecting Albumin Fraction

Drug sensitivity effect
    gallamine (Flaxedil)

The following drugs may cause a decrease in test results.

Hepatotoxic effect
    acetaminophen (Tylenol)
    asparaginase (Elspar)
    azathioprine (Imuran)
    cyclophosphamide (Cytoxan)
    heroin
    niacin (Nicotinex)

pyrazinamide (Tebrazid)
thorium dioxide

Hypersensitivity reaction
nicotinyl alcohol (Roniacol)
oxyphenisatin

Metabolic effect
estrogens (Premarin)
ethinyl estradiol (Estinyl)
mestranol (Enovid)

Miscellaneous
dextran, after infusion (Macrodex)

Related Lab Values: In suspected globulin deficiencies:

serum protein electrophoresis
Bence-Jones protein
bone marrow biopsy
calcium, serum
*serum immunoglobulins
*lymph node biopsy
WBC with differential
platelet count

IMPLICATIONS FOR NURSING CARE
PRETEST: Factors related to the test
Nursing Diagnosis: Potential for injury due to changes in biochemical balance

Guide to assessment	Guide to planning and intervention	Guide to evaluation

Assess patient factors that may influence test results:
1. Comprehensive drug history (See Drug Influences)
 	
2. Knowledge deficit
	1. Identify drugs that may influence test results and note them on lab slip.
	2. Explain test to patient:
	  a. Define test.
	  b. Explain procedure.
		1. Patient's drugs that may influence test results are noted on lab slip.
		2. The patient demonstrates knowledge by defining test and stating procedure.

*Not discussed in this book.

Patient Preparation Checklist

1. √ Influencing drugs noted on lab slip.
2. √ Patient knowledge; explain test to patient

CONSIDERATIONS FOR NURSING CARE RELATED TO ABNORMAL TEST RESULTS
POSTTEST: Factors related to the results of the test
Nursing Diagnosis: Alterations in biochemical balance

Guide to assessment	Guide to planning and intervention	Guide to evaluation
Assess patient factors that may be influencing test results. Nursing history and/or physical exam that is suggestive of:		

1. Signs and symptoms
   Frequent infections
   Chronic infections
   History of slow recovery from infection
   Family history of immunoglobulin deficiencies
	1. Recognize signs and symptoms of globulinopathy. Consult with physician.	1. Patient's symptoms of globulinopathy are identified.

2. Infant under 3 months
   Family history of immunoglobulin deficiencies
   Agammaglobulinemia
	2. Promote the maintenance of gamma globulin levels:
	  a. Provide sterile environment as needed.
	  b. Assist with bone marrow transplant or blood transfusions:
		2. Infant remains free of infection.

(1) 1–3 weeks post bone marrow transplant, foreign substance response:
    Fever
    Skin rash
    Hair loss
    Diarrhea
    Mucous membrane ulcers
    Hepatosplenomegaly
	(1) Watch for evidence of response to foreign substances (bone marrow transplant).
	  c. Administer gamma globulin as prescribed.
	  d. Initiate nursing measures to prevent infection.
	  e. Include family in all aspects of care as possible.
	  f. Make arrangements for genetic counseling as needed.	

Guide to assessment	Guide to planning and intervention	Guide to evaluation
2. Hypogammaglobulinemia	2. Protect patient from insult to immune system by: a. Initiating measures to protect patient from infection (Protective isolation measures). b. Give broad spectrum antibiotics as prescribed. Explain to patient need for continued use. c. Administer immunoglobulin cautiously, as prescribed.	2. The patient remains free of infection.
3. Monoclonal gammopathy	3. Suppress lymphoproliferative process by assisting with chemotherapy and/or radiotherapy.	

Test: Stained Blood Smear
Sickle-Cell Test
Sickledex
Hemoglobin Electrophoresis
Fetal Sickle-Cell Test

Abbreviation: None

Reference Values: For stained blood smear, Sickle-cell test, Sickledex: negative findings
For hemoglobin electrophoresis: negative for Hgb S or C
For fetal sickle-cell test: negative for DNA sickle-cell marker

Specimen: Whole blood

Description: Sickle-cell disease is an inherited disease that affects many races throughout the world. The term sickle-cell disease refers not only to sickle-cell anemia but also to sickle-cell hemoglobin C disease and sickle-cell-beta thalassemia. The population most affected by this disease in the United States is the black population, affecting about 1 in 600 live births. Sickle-cell anemia is an inherited disease affecting the hemoglobin of red blood cells. Within hemoglobin, DNA sends a message that changes the usual single amino acid valine to a polypeptide, glutamic. This change causes the red blood cell to change shape and molecular weight when in low oxygen concentrations. The cells become elongated and have a sickle shape to them. Even after full oxygenation many cells do not return to normal and remain irreversibly sickled cells. The cells become fragile and inflexible and are unable to move through microcirculation. The result is increased viscosity of the blood with vasoocclusion and hypoxia. The lack of oxygen causes more sickling to occur. Anemia occurs along with the sickling in homozygous HgbS (sickle-cell anemia) because of cell destruction. Sickle-cell crises occur with sudden severe sickling and anemia. Four types of crises have been described: thrombotic (also known as vasoocclusive or painful crises), splenic sequestration, aplastic, and hyperhemolytic.

Heterozygous HgbS, or sickle cell trait, while possessing one gene for the disease, generally experiences a benign clinical course. During periods of hypoxia, persons with sickle cell trait can experience sickling crises.

The purpose of sickle cell testing is to diagnose sickle cell disease or trait.

Procedure:

Stained Blood Smear

1. No food or fluid restriction.
2. A rubber band may be placed around finger to deoxygenate blood.
3. A fingerstick is performed.
4. A microscopic exam of the smear is done.

5. Sickled cells are seen if the patient has sickle-cell anemia. The process takes several hours.
6. Observe puncture site for bleeding.

Sickle-Cell Test

1. No food or fluid restrictions.
2. A finger stick is performed.
3. A microscopic exam is done of a deoxygenated drop of blood.
4. Sickled cells are seen if the patient has either sickle-cell disease or sickle-cell trait.
5. Observe puncture site for bleeding.

Sickledex

1. No food or fluid restrictions.
2. A fingerstick is performed.
3. A small amount of blood (0.02 ml) is placed in a test tube with a measured amount of precipitating reagent.
4. Sickle hemoglobin is present if the solution turns cloudy (either anemia or trait is present).
5. Observe puncture site for bleeding.

Hemoglobin Electrophoresis

(lavender top tube)
1. No food or fluid restrictions.
2. 0.5 ml–7 ml of blood is drawn from the patient. Cord blood samples from the newborn can also be used.
3. Hemoglobin molecules are separated by the movement of the molecules in an electrically charged system. Different molecules move at different rates and can be identified.
4. Sickled cells in major proportion indicates sickle-cell anemia. If there is a larger proportion of HgbA (normal hemoglobin) to HgbS, sickle-cell trait is diagnosed.
5. This test is done in combination with sickle-cell test or Sickledex.
6. Observe puncture site for bleeding or evidence of hematoma.

Fetal Sickle-Cell Test

1. Blood is drawn from both parents.
2. The mother is prepared for amniocentesis.
3. An amniocentesis is performed.
4. Enzymes are used to identify a DNA fragment that acts as a marker to indicate the presence of sickle-cell hemoglobin in amniotic cells.
5. Fetal blood is sampled if the DNA marker is not present in amniotic cells.
6. At this time this test is done only at large medical centers. Samples can be mailed to medical centers performing this test.

Conditions Related to Increases

1. Sickle-cell trait

2. Sickle-cell anemia

3. False positives
   Sickledex

Rationale

1. Hgb in this condition contains 30–45% of HgbS in total hemoglobin and 55–60% HgbA.
2. Hgb in this condition contains 80–90% HgbS and no HgbA.
3. After splenectomy, in patients with hemoglobin disorders that cause Heinz bodies or in patients with blood protein disorders, false positive may be seen.

Conditions Related to Decreases

1. False negatives
   Sickledex

Rationale

1. Blood transfusions within past 3 months. Infants under 3 months because of the inhibitory effect of fetal hemoglobin on sickle hemoglobin. Anemia (Hct ↓ 30%) will also cause a false negative.

Drug Influences: The following drugs may influence test results.
   The following drug may cause a positive test result:
      prostaglandin (Dinoprost)

   The following drugs may inhibit test results:
      phenothiazines; high doses

Related Lab Studies

In sickle cell crises
 CBC
 RBC morphology
   sickled cells
   polychromasia
   occasional nucleated red cell
   Howell-Jolly bodies
 WBC
 platelet count
 reticulocyte count
 *coagulation factor VIII
 Fibrinogen
 MCV
 iron, serum
 total iron-binding capacity (TIBC)

---

*Not discussed in this book.

Periodic routine check
CBC
reticulocyte count
platelet count
liver function studies
renal studies
uric acid, serum

IMPLICATIONS FOR NURSING CARE
PRETEST: Factors related to the test
Nursing Diagnosis: Potential for injury related to biochemical abnormality

Guide to assessment	Guide to planning and intervention	Guide to evaluation
Assess patient factors that may influence test results.		
1. Documented anemia of below 30% Hct	1. Note on lab slip patient's anemia.	1. Patient's lab values are not influenced negatively by anemia.
2. Age: 3 months or below	2. Note patient's age on lab slip.	2. Patient's age does not influence testing method.
3. Blood transfusion within past 3 months	3. Note on lab slip if patient has had transfusion within past 3 months.	3. Patient's lab values are not influenced by recent blood transfusion.
4. Knowledge deficit	4. Explain test to patient: a. Define sickle-cell hemoglobin (See Description). b. Explain procedure (See Procedure).	4. The patient demonstrates knowledge by defining test, stating procedure, and asking pertinent questions.
5. Family or patient history of sickle-cell disease or trait	5. Make available genetic counseling.	5. The patient is able to make informed choices about pregnancies.

Patient Preparation Checklist

1. √ Interfering factors are noted on lab slip (See 1, 2, 3 above).
2. √ Patient knowledge; explain test to patient (See Description/Procedure).
3. √ Genetic counseling available as appropriate.

CONSIDERATIONS FOR NURSING CARE RELATED TO ABNORMAL TEST RESULTS
POSTTEST: Factors related to the results of the test
Nursing Diagnosis: Potential for injury related to biochemical abnormality

Guide to assessment	Guide to planning and intervention	Guide to evaluation
Assess patient factors that may be influencing test results.		
1. In U.S., black population	1. Encourage sickle-cell screening: a. Screen all unscreened black children for sickle-cell hemoglobin. b. Screen all siblings of child positive for sickle-cell hemoglobin. c. Make available genetic counseling.	1. Persons undetected for sickle-cell hemoglobin are screened and genetic counseling is made available as appropriate.
2. Precipitating factors a. Dehydration	2. Protect patient from crisis, as possible, by: a. Preventing dehydration: (1) Weigh patient daily. (2) Keep strict I&O record. (3) Do not depend on specific gravity to determine hydration status as patients do not concentrate urine adequately. (4) Keep IV fluid levels current by maintaining fluid rate. (5) Offer fluids frequently. (6) Offer a wide variety of oral fluid choices. (7) Use creative strategies for increasing the patient's oral fluid intake (especially in children). (8) Administer blood transfusions as prescribed. (9) Assist with exchange transfusions as necessary. (10) Teach patient and parents why and how to avoid dehydration.	2. The patient is prevented from crisis. The patient experiences no further sickling and trapped sickled cells are mobilized because the patient is no longer dehyrated.

Guide to assessment	Guide to planning and intervention	Guide to evaluation
b. Infection Fever	b. Preventing infection: (1) Teach patient how to take accurate temperature. (2) Teach patient to seek immediate medical care for fever over 101°F (38.3° C). (3) Teach patient to recognize signs and symptoms of infection. (4) Teach parent to seek medical care when a child looks ill. (5) Teach patient to keep immunizations current, to be immunized with pneumococcal vaccine, and to be aware of infections even though he or she has had immunizations. (6) Administer prophylactic penicillin to child under 2 years as prescribed. Teach parent the necessity of giving medication. (7) Encourage good dental care. (8) Teach parents first-aid for cuts and abrasions. (9) Stress necessity for careful hygiene. (10) Stress need to stay well-rested. (11) Encourage well-balanced diets; administer folic acid and supplemental minerals as prescribed. (12) Administer antibiotics such as cefamandole (Mandol) as prescribed.	b. The patient achieves protection against infection or diminishes the chance of infection.
c. Physical activity	c. Encouraging activity appropriate to patient's condition, and encouraging patient to rest when needed to prevent fatigue.	c. The patient maintains activity appropriate to condition.
d. Hypoxia Sickle-cell	d. Recognizing hypoxic situations:	d. The patient recognizes potentially hypoxic situa-

Guide to assessment	Guide to planning and intervention	Guide to evaluation
anemia Sickle-cell trait	(1) Tell patients not to travel to high altitudes or in unpressurized airplanes. (2) Be alert to medical conditions that cause hypoxia, such as cardiac or pulmonary disease, respiratory depression, shock, hypothermia.	tions.
e. Vasoocclusive crises ↓ Number of circulating sickle cells Recurrent debilitating painful crisis	e. Assisting with exchange transfusion to suppress production of red blood cells to decrease the number of sickle cells.	e. The patient's HgbS is below 30%.
f. Antisickling agents, e.g. Sodium cyanate	f. Give antisickling agents as prescribed.	f. The patient experiences fewer crisis episodes.
3. Patient education	3. Promote patient health and quality of life by educating patients/parents: a. Advise where to go for genetic counseling. b. Explain about sickle-cell hemoglobin. c. Explain the difference between sickle-cell anemia and sickle-cell trait. d. Discuss precipitating factors and how to avoid them (See 2, above). e. Advise patients that special foods will not cure sickle-cell anemia. f. Advise patients to seek medical care for illnesses. g. Advise parents to teach their child's caregivers about condition.	3. The patient is able to discuss the pathophysiology, prevention, and symptoms of his or her condition.

Test:	Cytology, Microbiology Smears
Abbreviation:	None
Reference Values:	Negative
Specimen:	Cells or tissue
Description:	Smears are prepared by spreading a thin coating of a substance to be examined on a glass slide. It may be examined at this point or it may be stained. The slide is fixed by passing it through a flame. The slide is flooded with staining material, washed, and counterstained. Microbiological smears for Gram stain provides the examiner with knowledge about the number of bacteria, whether they are Gram-negative or Gram-positive, and their morphology.

Papanicolaou smears are cells prepared with a special stain for cytological study. The cells are studied for the early detection of cancer. Since 1954, Papanicolaou's method for reporting cytological smears has been used. Cytology reports read:

*Class I	Absence of atypical or abnormal cells
Class II	Atypical cytologic picture; no evidence of malignancy
Class III	Cytologic picture suggestive but not diagnostic of malignancy
Class IV	Cytologic picture strongly suggestive of malignancy
Class V	Cytologic picture diagnostic of malignancy

Procedure:

(Pap smear)

1. A speculum is inserted into vagina.
2. The cervix and vaginal tissues are observed.
3. Using an Ayre spatula, the cervix is scraped and the secretions are smeared on a glass slide. The smear is made by very gently smearing the cervical secretions in a single circular motion.
4. The slide is placed in a special fixative.
5. A smear is made of vaginal secretions. A cotton-tipped applicator is used to collect the specimen.
6. Place vaginal smear in special fixative.

Drug Influences: The following types of drugs will decrease test results:

antimicrobials; microbiological smears
douches; Pap smears
suppositories, vaginal; Pap smears

---

*From R. Douglas Collins, *Illustrated Manual of Laboratory Diagnosis*, (Philadelphia: J. B. Lippincott Company, 1975).

IMPLICATIONS FOR NURSING CARE
PRETEST: Factors related to the test
Nursing Diagnosis: Potential for injury related to changes in biochemical balance

Guide to assessment	Guide to planning and intervention	Guide to evaluation
Assess patient factors that may influence test results:		
1. Comprehensive drug history Microbiological smears	1. Obtain microbiological smear prior to antimicrobial therapy, if possible.	1. Patient's drug therapy does not interfere with test results.
2. Preexisting conditions	2. Note patient diagnosis or suspected diagnosis on lab slip.	2. The patient's preexisting conditions are noted on lab slip.
3. Papanicolaou (Pap)	3. Caution patient not to douche or use suppositories 24 hours prior to testing.	3. Patient's douching or vaginal suppositories do not interfere with test results.
4. Knowledge deficit	4. Explain test to patient.	4. The patient defines test.

Patient Preparation Checklist

1. √ Microbiological smear done prior to antimicrobial therapy.
2. √ Antimicrobial drugs noted on lab slip.
3. √ Note diagnosis or suspected diagnosis on lab slip.
4. √ No douching or vaginal suppositories 24 hours prior to Pap smear.
5. √ Patient knowledge; explain test to patient.

CONSIDERATIONS FOR NURSING CARE RELATED TO ABNORMAL TEST RESULTS
POSTTEST: Factors related to the results of the test
Nursing Diagnosis: Alterations in biochemical balance

Guide to assessment	Guide to planning and intervention	Guide to evaluation
Assess patient factors that may be influencing test results:		
1. Positive microbiological smear	1. Implement medical/nursing plan to treat microbiological condition.	1. The patient's microbiological smear is negative.
2. Positive Pap smear	2. Implement medical/nursing plan of care and support patient with positive Pap smear.	2. The patient is able to state understanding of condition and demonstrates willingness for appropriate treatment.

Test:	Sodium
Abbreviation:	Na
Reference Values:	Serum 135–145 mEq/L
	Urine 110–200 mEq/24 hours
	Sweat infant up to 40 mmol/L
	child up to 50 mmol/L
	adult up to 90 mmol/L
Specimen:	Serum, 24-hour urine collection
	Sweat

Description:

Sodium is the major cation found in the extracellular fluid. The average diet contains more than enough sodium for the body's needs. Sodium is absorbed through the gastrointestinal tract and excreted mainly through the kidneys. A small amount is lost in the feces and sweat. Sodium balance is controlled by aldosterone and functions in the body by maintaining normal osmolality of the extracellular fluid. The osmotic pressure created by sodium is the principal factor in the movement and volume of water. Sodium contributes to normal muscular irritability or excitability. Within the cellular compartment, sodium is a factor in numerous vital chemical reactions. Sodium in conjunction with chloride and bicarbonate plays a role in the acid-base balance of the body. The sodium serum level alone will not give a true picture of the body's sodium level. Since water moves with sodium in the body, sodium levels may appear low because of a dilutional effect. The patient's clinical picture and urine sodium levels must be included to determine true body levels. Serum and urine sodium levels are done to determine fluid and electrolyte balance and renal or endocrine disorders. Sweat concentrations of sodium are done to confirm the diagnosis of cystic fibrosis.

Procedure:

(red top tube)

Serum

1. No food or fluid restrictions.
2. 0.5–3 ml of blood is withdrawn from the patient.
3. Observe puncture site for bleeding or evidence of hematoma.

24-Hour Urine Collection

1. Collection container needs no preservative or refrigeration.
2. Collection.
   a. Discard first voided specimen.
   b. Begin timing.
   c. For next 24 hours place all voidings into specimen container immediately after voiding.
   d. Have patient void just prior to completion of 24 hours and put sample in collection bottle.
3. Record exact start and finish times on lab slip.
4. Send to lab.

Sweat

1. The test should be done by well-trained technicians.
2. Questionable results should be repeated.
3. In infants, the right leg is the area of choice. Otherwise, the flexor surface of the right forearm is used. *The chest is never used* (possibility of electrically induced cardiac arrest).
4. Analysis.
   a. Area is cleansed.
   b. A gauze pad with measured amount of pilocarpine solution and a gauze pad saturated with normal saline solution cover electrodes attached to the skin.
   c. The area is given minute electrical current charges every few seconds for 5 minutes (iontophoresis).
   d. The area is cleansed and dried and a weighed dry gauze covered by plastic is applied to the pilocarpine area and left in place 30–40 minutes.
   e. The gauze is carefully removed and placed in a weighing bottle.
   f. The difference in the weight of the gauze pad placed on the patient after iontophoresis gives the weight of the sweat specimen.
5. Any complaints of burning by the patient need immediate attention:
   a. *Stop* the test.
   b. Call technician immediately.

Conditions Related to Increases

Rationale

Serum

1. Cushing's disease
2. Aldosteronism
   Hypercorticoadrenalism
   Corticosteroid administration
3. Excessive perspiration
   Fever
   High environmental temperature
4. Watery diarrhea
5. Diabetes insipidus

1. In this condition there is excess production of ACTH, which causes increased levels of adrenocorticoid hormones leading to increased sodium retention.
2. Increased secretion of aldosterone causes decreased excretion of sodium by the kidneys.
3. Large losses of sweat result in loss of more water than sodium, causing elevated serum sodium levels.
4. Fluid loss exceeds sodium loss causing higher serum levels.
5. Lack of ADH secretion causes the excretion of a large amount of dilute urine that results in a state of dehydration and excessive concentration of sodium in the extracellular fluid.

6. Tracheobronchitis
   Hyperventilation
   Salicylate toxicity
   Head trauma
7. Tube feedings

6. Due to rapid breathing there is excessive insensible water loss through respiration.
7. Tube feedings usually contain high solute loads. In order to supply the kidney with the needed water volume for urinary excretion, there is increased water loss from the extracellular fluid.

8. Acute renal failure (anuria)

8. The kidneys are unable to excrete waste products, including sodium.

9. Saline-induced abortion
   Treatment of cardiac arrest with hypertonic sodium bicarbonate

9. Because of the rapid introduction of a large volume of hypertonic sodium chloride into the body, there is a resultant hypernatremia and a massive redistribution of body fluids (94).

Conditions Related to Decreases

Rationale

Serum

1. Addison's disease

1. Adrenal cortices no longer secrete aldosterone, so the body stores of sodium become depleted.

2. Burns

2. Large amounts of sodium are lost in the edema that forms at the burn site due to plasma leaking from damaged capillaries.

3. Paracentesis or thoracentesis

3. Sodium is lost from the body in the fluid removed during treatment.

4. Diarrhea

4. Severe diarrhea can lead to a daily loss of 5–10 L of fluids as well as large amounts of sodium, potassium, and bicarbonate. In cases of watery diarrhea, sodium *excess* may occur if fluid loss exceeds sodium losses.

5. Hypertrophic pyloric stenosis

5. Sodium is plentiful in gastric juices and prolonged vomiting will lead to a sodium deficit.

6. Salt-losing renal disorders
   Polycystic kidney disease
   Medullary cystic disease
   Interstitial nephritis
7. Excessive perspiration
   Fever
   High environmental temperatures

6. In these disorders kidney tubules lose their ability to reabsorb sodium, leading to a true reduction in total body sodium.
7. Loss of sodium in sweat can cause a decrease in serum sodium levels, especially if plain water is ingested in large amounts after profuse perspiration.

8. Syndrome of inappropriate secretion of ADH (SIADH) May be caused by:
   Pain
   Trauma, including surgery
   Anesthetics and narcotics
   IPPB treatments

8. In this syndrome there are increased levels of ADH that cause water retention and a dilutional effect on serum sodium levels.

9. Congestive heart failure
   Hepatic failure with ascites
   Acute/chronic renal failure

9. Body sodium may be normal or above normal but with the retained water there is a dilutional hyponatremia.

10. Pregnancy (last trimester)

10. Probably due to increased ADH secretion or increased secretion of oxytocin. Both of these hormones cause water retention and so the decreased serum sodium is probably related to dilutional causes.

11. Postobstructive diuresis

11. Removal of obstruction anywhere along the urinary tract results in decreased pressure on the renal parenchyma causing diuresis with excessive loss of water and sodium. The renal tubules lose their reabsorptive capacity during obstruction and it is one of the last functions to return after removal of pressure.

12. Hyperlipidemia

12. A high serum lipid concentration will displace the water content, lowering the amount of sodium in the total serum.

13. Diabetic acidosis

13. The combination of urinary sodium losses due to glucose diuresis, losses from vomiting, and sodium combining with ketonic anions for excretion results in low serum values (94).

14. Excessive tap water enemas

14. Tap water is hypotonic and absorbed by the bowel, resulting in dilution of extracellular fluid (32).

15. Starvation hyponatremia
    Sickle-cell syndrome

15. Because of chronic illness with persistent malnutrition and cellular destruction, there is chronic cellular hypoosmolality.

Conditions Related to Increases

Rationale

Urine

1. Diabetic acidosis

1. Glucose diuresis results in urinary losses of sodium, potassium, phosphate, and bicarbonate (94).

2. Addison's disease

2. The decrease in aldosterone results in decreased tubular reabsorption of sodium.

3. High dietary intake of salt

3. The body's regulating mechanism excretes the excess sodium to maintain equilibrium.

4. Salt-losing renal disease
   Medullary cystic disease
   Chronic pyelonephritis
   Polycystic disease
   Acute tubular necrosis

4. Kidney tubules lose their ability to reabsorb sodium.

5. Inappropriate secretion of ADH; may be caused by:
   Pain
   Trauma, including surgery
   Anesthetics and narcotics
   IPPB

5. Increased ADH causes greater water reabsorption without affecting electrolyte reabsorption, resulting in concentrated urine containing large amounts of sodium (45).

6. Postobstructive diuresis

6. The renal tubules lose their reabsorptive capacity during urinary tract obstruction and it is one of the last functions to return after removal of pressure on the renal parenchyma (93).

Conditions Related to Decreases

Rationale

Urine

1. Acute renal failure

1. When oliguria results from decreased perfusion of the kidneys, urine sodium levels will be low (89).

2. Primary aldosteronism and conditions associated with increased aldosterone secretion.
   Cirrhosis of the liver
   Congestive heart failure
   Shock

2. Hypersecretion of aldosterone causes excessive reabsorption of sodium and water.

3. Conditions of fluid loss exceeding sodium loss
   Diaphoresis
   Diuresis
   Hyperventilation
   Severe vomiting

3. The serum sodium levels will be normal or increased due to water loss in excess of sodium loss, but urinary sodium levels are low due to total body lack of sodium.

4. Physical exercise

4. Sodium excretion decreases during exercise because of secondary aldosteronism. Aldosterone encourages conservation of sodium and potassium excretion.

Conditions Related to Increases	**Rationale**

Sweat

1. Cystic fibrosis
2. Premenopausal women

1. An inherited disease of the exocrine glands that raises sodium levels in sweat.
2. Cyclic fluctuations have been reported in premenopausal women. These fluctuations peak 5–10 days prior to the onset of menses (11).

Conditions Related to Decreases	**Rationale**

Sweat

1. Conditions causing low electrolytes in the body, e.g.
   Exercise
   Adaptation to hot climate

1. Abnormal sweat test results have occurred in people with deficient electrolytes (11).

Drug Influences: The following drugs may cause an increase in sodium values. The drugs are listed alphabetically by generic name and divided into columns according to effect of the drug. Examples of trade names are in parentheses.

Serum

Mineralocorticoid effect
   anabolic steroids
   androgens
   prednisolone (Meticortelone)

Renal effect
   angiotensin
   clonidine (Catapres)
   corticosteroids
   diazoxide (Hyperstat)
   estrogens
   glucocorticoids
   mannitol
   methoxyflurane (Penthrane)
   methyldopa (Aldomet)
   mezlocillin, sodium (Mezlin)

   oral contraceptives
   oxyphenbutazone (Oxalid, Tandearil)
   phenylbutazone (Butazolidin)
   progesterone
   prolactin
   rauwolfia (Harmonyl, Raudixin)
   sodium bicarbonate
   tetracycline

Urine

Diuretic effect
   acetazolamide (Diamox)
   amiloride (Moduretic)
   ammonium chloride (Triaminicol)
   clopamide
   diuretics
   dopamine (Intropin)
   hydroflumethiazide (Diucardin, Saluron)

   isosorbide (Isordil, Sorbitrate)
   levodopa (Larodopa)
   lithium
   secretin
   tetracycline
   triamcinolone (Aristocort, Kenacort)

The following drugs may cause a decrease in sodium values:

Serum

Renal effect

ammonium chloride (Triaminicol)
amphotericin B (Fungizone, Mysteclin-F)
bendroflumethiazide (Naturetin, Rauzide)
cathartics
chlorothiazide (Diuril)
chlorpropamide (Diabinese)
chlorthalidone (Combipres, Hygroton)
dichlorphenamide
heparin

lithium
mannitol
meralluride
metolazone (Diulo, Zaroxolyn)
quinethazone (Hydromox)
spironolactone (Aldactone)
sulfates
triamterene (Dyrenium)
urea (Debrox, Gly-Oxide)
vasopressin (Pitressin)
vincristine (Oncovin)

Urine

Renal effect

aldosterone
anesthetic agents
angiotensin
corticosteroids
epinephrine
guancydine

insulin
levarterenol (Levophed)
lithium
prolactin
propranolol (Inderal)

Related Lab Studies: Monitor response to treatment or progression of disease and adjust nursing care accordingly. See individual tests for information.

aldosterone
creatinine, creatinine clearance
blood urea nitrogen
sweat test, chloride
hematocrit
osmolality, serum and urine
electrolytes (K, CO_2, Cl)
*renin

---

*Not discussed in this book.

IMPLICATIONS FOR NURSING CARE
PRETEST: Factors related to the test
Nursing Diagnosis: Potential for injury related to biochemical imbalance

Guide to assessment	Guide to planning and intervention	Guide to evaluation
Assess patient factors that may influence test results: 1. Comprehensive Drug History (See Drug Influences)	1. Report to laboratory and physician drugs the patient is receiving that may influence lab results.	1. Drugs the patient is receiving, or has received, that may influence lab results are identified and appropriate people notified.
2. Preexisting conditions (See Increases/Decreases) 3. Knowledge deficit	2. Record preexisting conditions on lab slip. 3. Explain to patient: a. Define sodium (See Description). b. Explain test procedure (See Procedure). c. Encourage parents to stay with child for support.	2. Patient's preexisting conditions noted on lab slip. 3. Patient demonstrates knowledge of test by defining test and stating procedure.

Patient Preparation Checklist

1. √ Influencing drugs are noted and reported (See Drug Influences).
2. √ Preexisting conditions noted on lab slip (See Increases/Decreases).
3. √ Patient knowledge; explain test and procedure (See Description and Procedure).

CONSIDERATIONS FOR NURSING CARE RELATED TO ABNORMAL TEST RESULTS
POSTTEST: Factors related to the results of the test
Nursing Diagnosis: Potential for injury related to changes in biochemical balance

Guide to assessment	Guide to planning and intervention	Guide to evaluation
Assess patient factors that may be influencing test results: Signs/symptoms of sodium excess: Thirst Poor skin turgor Dry, sticky mucous membranes Flushed, dry skin Rough, dry tongue	1. Implement plan of care to reduce sodium excess: a. Encourage oral fluids or administer salt-free IV solutions as ordered. b. Record intake and output from all sources: oral; nasogastric, wound drainage, diarrhea; estimate loss through diaphoresis, and	1. Patient demonstrates no signs or symptoms of dehydration: b. Accurate intake and output are recorded.

Guide to assessment	Guide to planning and intervention	Guide to evaluation
Eyeballs soft and sunken Loss of body weight Elevated temperature Apprehension Restlessness Concentrated urine Elevated hemoglobin/Hct	incontinence. c. Daily weight. d. Reduce high dietary intake of sodium. e. Implement medical plan to prevent loss of water from body such as antiemetics for vomiting; antidiarrheal agents for diarrhea; antipyretics for fever. f. Control environmental temperature.	c. Daily weight is recorded. e. Fluid output does not exceed intake. f. Environmental temperature is controlled to prevent diaphoresis.

2. Sodium excess
 	
a. Identify patients at risk of decreased thirst sensation or inability to respond to thirst:
   Elderly patients
   Infants
   Comatose patients
   Paralyzed patients
   Critically ill
b. Tube feeding (content and rate)
 	
d. Dietary history of high sodium intake
 	
e. History of strenuous exercise activity in high environmental temperatures.
	2. Implement plan of care to prevent sodium excess:
	a. Offer liquids at frequent intervals to patients with decreased thirst sensation or inability to request fluids.
	
	b. Insure proper water intake for patients receiving tube feedings containing high solutes.
	c. Record intake and output.
	d. Implement patient education related to foods high in sodium.
	e. Implement patient teaching related to cause and prevention of heat stress:
	   (1) Identify sodium and chloride increases.
	   (2) Replenish water losses as they occur.
	   (3) Discourage strenuous activity that produces excessive sweating during hot days.
		2. The patient demonstrates normal serum sodium:
		a. The patient with special needs is kept adequately hydrated.
		
		b. The patient's serum sodium is not increased due to inadequate water/solute ratio.
		c. The patient's fluid intake equals fluid output.
		d. The patient states dietary sources high in sodium that he should avoid.
		e. The patient explains cause and prevention of heat stress.

3. Assess for signs and symptoms of excessive sodium and water retention
   Weight gain
   Pitting edema
	3. Implement plan of care to reduce or prevent excessive sodium and water retention:
	a. Administer diuretics as ordered.
		3. The patient demonstrates reduced sodium/water retention by diminishing signs/symptoms of sodium/water retention.

Guide to assessment	Guide to planning and intervention	Guide to evaluation
Pulmonary edema Puffy eyelids Ascites Distention of neck veins	b. Restrict dietary intake of sodium. c. Record intake and output. d. Monitor blood pressure every 4 hours as ordered. e. Monitor IV flow rates carefully. f. Do not attempt to catch up an IV infusion that is behind schedule. Consult with physician first.	

4. Assess for signs and symptoms of low serum sodium:
  Weight loss or edema and weight gain
  Decreased skin turgor
  Hypovolemia
  Polyuria or oliguria
  Twitching
  Hyperirritability
  Mental disturbances
  Disorientation
  Convulsions
  Coma
  Hypotension
	4. Implement nursing care to correct low serum sodium:
	a. Detect and report signs/symptoms.
	b. Restrict water intake.
	c. Administer hypertonic solutions as ordered (only used in severe cases).
	d. Offer high-protein nutrition for patient with starvation low sodium.
	e. Implement medical plan to treat underlying causes.
		4. The patient's electrolytes are within normal limits and the patient does not demonstrate signs/symptoms of low serum sodium.

5. Identify patients with potential for water excess (See Decreases)	5. Implement nursing care to prevent water excess: a. Do not give excessive tap water enemas. b. Prevent fluid overload by IV fluids. c. Do not force fluids on patients with increased ADH secretion. d. Give bouillon or fruit juices for replacement of sodium and water as ordered. e. Irrigate nasogastric tubes with normal saline or as ordered. f. Administer isotonic ice chips to patients with nasogastric suction.	5. The patient's electrolytes remain within normal limits.
6. History of diabetes insipidus	6. Administer vasopressin as ordered and teach patient to monitor specific gravity.	6. The patient's urinary output is reduced. Patient demonstrates testing of urine for specific gravity.

Test:	Testosterone
Abbreviation:	None
Reference Values:	Female 30–95 ng/dl
	Male 300–1200 ng/dl
Specimen:	Serum

Description: Testosterone is a hormone formed in the Leydig cells of the testes and regulated by the interstitial cell-stimulating hormone (ICSH).* It is an androgen responsible for the development of secondary sex characteristics at puberty and the maintenance of these characteristics. At puberty, testosterone levels begin to rise, reaching adult levels about 18 years of age, and at about 40 years of age testosterone production begins to slow down.

The source of testosterone in women is from the ovaries and adrenal glands as well as conversion of peripheral testosterone precursors to testosterone. The action of testosterone in women is not well defined. Increased levels of testosterone in females cause excessive hair growth and virilization.

Testosterone levels are determined to aid in the diagnosis of gonadal disorders.

Procedure: (red top tube)
1. No food or fluid restrictions.
2. 0.5–10 ml of blood is withdrawn from the patient.
3. Observe puncture site for bleeding and evidence of hematoma.

Conditions Related to Increases

1. Polycystic ovaries (Stein-Leventhal syndrome)

2. Ovarian tumors, e.g.
   Arrhenoblastoma
   Gonadoblastoma
3. Adrenal tumors

4. Adrenal hyperplasia

Rationale

1. In this disease the stromal cells of the ovaries produce increased amounts of testosterone (26). There is also increased peripheral conversion of testosterone precursors to testosterone.
2. Increased ovarian production of testosterone.

3. Increased adrenal gland production of testosterone; there may also be increased conversion of peripheral testosterone precursors to testosterone in women. These increased levels are not suppressed with dexamethasone.
4. Due to the lack of certain enzymes there is decreased cortisol production. The lack of cortisol stimulates the release of ACTH that increases the re-

---

*Also known as luteinizing hormone.

5. Testicular tumors

lease of other adrenal steroids. Testosterone levels are suppressed when dexamethasone is administered.

5. Testosterone production may be increased in certain testicular tumors and may cause precocious sexual development.

6. Anterior pituitary tumors

6. Increased gonadotropin secretion due to a pituitary tumor may result in precocious sexual development or virilization because of increased testosterone (androgen) production.

Conditions Related to Decreases

1. Klinefelter's syndrome (primary hypogonadism)

Rationale

1. In this disease there may be inadequate testicular testosterone synthesis. Testes are small and firm, and Leydig cells may be clumped and hyperplastic.

2. Hypogonadism from trauma or infection

2. Trauma to the Leydig cells from infection, radiation, etc., may slowly decrease testosterone production.

3. Anterior pituitary hypofunction

3. Anterior pituitary trauma, surgery, or tumor may result in diminished interstitial cell-stimulating hormone (ICSH) release. This decreased release of gonadotropins results in decreased testosterone production.

4. Alcoholism

4. Chronic alcohol consumption increases the metabolism of testosterone and other steroids by increasing their water solubility that then allows for increased excretion through the kidneys (143).

5. Orchiectomy
   Testicular cancer
   Prostatic cancer

5. The decrease is due to diminished number or lack of Leydig cells.

Drug Influences: The following drugs may influence test results. The drugs are listed alphabetically by generic name and divided into columns according to the effect of the drug. Examples of trade names are in parentheses.

The following drugs may cause an increase in test results:

Effect in women
   barbiturates
   clomiphene (Clomid)

estrogens
oral contraceptives

Effect in men
   gonadotropin (Pergonal)

Increase, women
   clomiphene (Clomid)

Increase, men
   corticotropin
   gonadotropin (Pergonal)

The following drugs may cause a decrease in test results:

Decrease
   dexamethasone; in women
   diethylstilbestrol (Tylosterone)
   digoxin; in men
   ethanol; male alcoholics
   glucose
   halothane (Fluothane)
   spironolactone (Aldactone); in males

Related Lab Studies

*luteinizing hormone (ICSH, LH), serum/urine
*follicle-stimulating hormone (FSH), serum/urine
dexamethasone suppression test (DST)
17-KS
17-OHCS
estrogens, serum
*DHEA

IMPLICATIONS FOR NURSING CARE
PRETEST: Factors related to the test
Nursing Diagnosis: Potential biochemical imbalance

Guide to assessment	Guide to planning and intervention	Guide to evaluation
Assess patient factors that may influence test results:		
1. Comprehensive drug history, especially hormones (See Drug Influences)	1. Note interfering drugs on lab slip.	1. Patient's drug therapy does not interfere with test results.
2. Preexisting conditions (See Increases/Decreases) Age Sex	2. Note pertinent preexisting conditions, age, and sex on lab slip.	2. The patient's preexisting conditions, age, and sex are noted on lab slip.
3. Knowledge deficit	3. Explain test to patient: a. Define testosterone (See Description). b. Explain test to patient.	3. The patient demonstrates knowledge of the test by defining test and explaining procedure.

*Not discussed in this book.

Patient Preparation Checklist

1. √ Drug influences, especially hormone therapy, noted on lab slip (See Drug Influences).
2. √ Age, sex, pertinent preexisting conditions noted on lab slip (See Increases/Decreases).
3. √ Patient knowledge; explain test to patient (See Description/Procedure).

CONSIDERATIONS FOR NURSING CARE RELATED TO ABNORMAL TEST RESULTS

POSTTEST: Factors related to the results of the test

Nursing Diagnosis: Alterations in biochemical balance

Guide to assessment	Guide to planning and intervention	Guide to evaluation
Assess patient factors that may be influencing test results. Nursing history and/or physical exam suggestive of:		
1. Excessive testosterone	1. Encourage reduced testosterone levels by:	1. Patient testosterone levels return to normal:
a. Polycystic ovaries Amenorrhea Hirsutism Infertility	a. Administering clomiphene citrate as prescribed; explain drug to patient.	a. The patient's ovulatory cycle is reestablished.
b. Need for ovarian wedge resection	b. Initiating preoperative nursing care measures.	b. The patient resumes normal ovarian cycles post wedge resection.
c. Precocious sexual development Females: younger than 8 years Males: younger than 10 years	c. Being alert to possible disruption in hypothalamic-pituitary-gonadal axis and referring child and parents to physician for diagnosis.	c. The patient with precocious sexual development is referred for diagnosis.
d. Adrenal hyperplasia	d. Maintaining cortisol levels by: (1) Examining newborn infants for abnormal genitalia. (2) Administering cortisol as prescribed. (3) Reinforcing patient education concerning cortisol replacement. (4) Collecting evaluative urine test for androgens and glucocorticoids.	d. The patient's lab reports are within normal limits.

Guide to assessment	Guide to planning and intervention	Guide to evaluation

e. Tumors
    Adrenal
    Testicular
    Ovarian
    Anterior pituitary
	e. Encouraging correction of hypothalamic-pituitary-gonadal disruption. Initiate preoperative nursing care.	e. The patient's androgen-influencing tumor is removed.

f. Testosterone replacement	f. Being alert to signs of bladder retention in patients receiving testosterone replacement.	f. The patient does not experience bladder retention.
2. Decreased testosterone	2. Encourage increased testosterone levels:	2. Patient's testosterone levels are adequate:

a. Hypogonadism
    Past history of postpubertal orchitis
    ↓ Sperm count
    Small, soft testes
    ↓ Testosterone
	a. Administer testosterone preparation as ordered. (Long-acting in younger patients; short-acting in older patients.)	a. The patient receives testosterone replacement.

b. Hypophysectomy Anterior pituitary trauma	b. Replace testosterone as prescribed (See *a* above).	b. The patient's testosterone levels are adequate.
c. Alcoholism Impotence	c. Explain to chronic alcohol abuser, as appropriate, relationship of alcohol consumption and testosterone excretion.	c. The patient is able to state alcohol abuse/testosterone excretion relationship.
d. Need for testosterone replacement	d. Teach patient about testosterone replacement.	d. Patient states the reason for and administration and dosage of testosterone replacement.

Test: Theophylline Level

Abbreviation: None

Reference Values: *Therapeutic level*
Newborn, preterm   2–10 μg/ml
Children and adults   10–20 μg/ml

Toxic level
Newborn, preterm   over 13 μg/ml
Children and adults   over 20 μg/ml

Specimen: Serum

Description: Theophylline is a derivative of the naturally occurring xanthines found in plants. Theophylline produces a relaxation of smooth muscles, especially those of the bronchials; stimulates the central nervous system, including the medullary respiratory center; acts on the kidneys to produce diuresis; and stimulates cardiac muscle. Theophylline is readily absorbed after oral, rectal, or parenteral administration and is 90% metabolized in the liver with 10% of the drug excreted unchanged through the kidneys. The expected half-life in the adult is approximately 3–10 hours and in the preterm newborn 25–35 hours. The rate of metabolism is variable among individuals receiving the same amount of theophylline. Theophylline is felt to achieve its therapeutic effect in the lungs by competing with the enzyme phosphodiesterase in the breakdown of cyclic AMP. It is used in the treatment of respiratory disorders, especially those associated with bronchial constriction, newborn apnea, and Cheyne-Stokes respiration. The purpose of the test is to determine therapeutic level, monitor for toxic levels, and serve as a guide for dosage regulation. Although dyphylline (Lufyllin) is chemically a theophylline, blood levels cannot be measured by laboratory analysis (71, p. 362).

Procedure: (grey top tube)
1. Record theobromine or methylxanthine intake (See 2 and 4, Increases) or other interfering drugs on lab slip.
2. Determine if level is for trough value or peak serum concentrations. It may be for both:
   a. For trough value blood is drawn right before next dose due.
   b. Peak serum concentrations (34):
      Draw blood 1 hour after elixir ingestion.
      Draw blood 2 hours after conventional tablet administered.
      Draw blood 3–4 hours after sustained release tablet administered.
      Draw blood 1 hour after IV bolus dosage given.
3. Record dose, time of, and name of last theophylline given.

Conditions Related to Increases

1. Liver disease
   Congestive heart failure
   Pneumonia
   Respiratory failure

2. Theobromine intake

3. Renal disease

4. Dietary intake of methylxanthines

Rationale

1. Decreased functioning of the liver by disease prevents the normal breakdown of theophylline by hepatic microsomal oxidative enzymes, resulting in prolonged clearance from the body.

2. Theobromine is found in chocolate-containing candy, beverages, or medications. In using UV spectrophotometry, theobromine interferes with the test results. Two cups of strong cocoa may yield a theophylline equivalent of about 3 μg/ml (21).

3. Interference in excretion of theophylline via the kidneys can result in increased levels since 10% of the drug is excreted through the kidneys.

4. Methylxanthines, particularly caffeine, interfere with theophylline elimination by competing for common metabolic enzymes.

Conditions Related to Decreases

1. Smoking

2. Vigorous shaking of serum

Rationale

1. Smoking causes a faster plasma theophylline clearance and a shorter half-life, resulting in a need for larger doses to achieve therapeutic effect.

2. Lower levels occur due to oxidation of theophylline (21).

Drug Influences: The following drugs may affect the metabolism of theophylline or its excretion from the body. The drugs are listed alphabetically by generic name with examples of trade names in parentheses. The drugs are divided into columns according to their effect.

The following drugs may cause an increase in theophylline levels:

Decreased hepatic clearance
   caffeine
   erythromycin
   lincomycin
   troleandomycin (TAO)

Increased diuresis
   furosemide (Lasix)
   xanthine

Miscellaneous
   flu vaccine
   hexamethonium
   phenylbutazone
   sulfonamides
   theobromine

The following drugs may cause a decrease in theophylline levels:

Metabolic effect
   barbiturates

Related Lab Studies: Monitor effect of theophylline and possible interference with absorption.

   arterial blood gases (ABGs)
   BUN
   creatinine/creatinine clearance
   electrolytes (Na, K, Cl, CO_2)
   ALT (SGPT)
   alkaline phosphatase
   bilirubin

IMPLICATIONS FOR NURSING CARE
PRETEST: Factors related to the test
Nursing Diagnosis: Potential for injury to changes in chemical balance

Guide to assessment	Guide to planning and intervention	Guide to evaluation
Assess patient factors that may influence test results: 1. Diet history Recent ingestion of dietary methylxanthines and/or chocolate-containing candy, beverages, and medications.	1. Report ingestion of dietary foods that may interfere with lab results to the patient's physician and to the laboratory (See Increases 2 and 4).	1. Patient's lab results not misinterpreted because of recent dietary intake of methylxanthines and/or theobromines.
2. Comprehensive drug history	2. Report to lab and physician drugs the patient is receiving that may influence lab results:	2. Drugs patient is receiving do not interfere with test results. Blood specimens are drawn at the right time.
a. See Drug Influences	a. Order specimen to be drawn for peak levels or as ordered by physician.	
b. Note time, amount, and route of last dose of theophylline.	b. Order specimen to be drawn just prior to next scheduled dose for trough level or as ordered by physician.	
c. Note smoker/non-smoker	c. Record on lab slip time, amount, and route of last dose of theophylline and time specimen obtained.	

Guide to assessment	Guide to planning and intervention	Guide to evaluation
3. Preexisting conditions	3. Record preexisting conditions on lab slip.	3. Patient's preexisting conditions noted on lab slip.
4. Knowledge deficit	4. Explain test to patient: a. Define theophylline level (See Description). b. Explain test procedure (See Procedure).	4. Patient demonstrates knowledge of test by defining test and stating procedure.

Patient Preparation Checklist

1. √ Date, time, amount, and route of last dose of theophylline recorded on lab slip.
2. √ Influencing drugs and dietary intake noted and reported (See Drug Influences and 1 above).
3. √ Preexisting conditions noted on lab slip (See Increases/Decreases).
4. √ Time specimen drawn; record on lab slip.
5. √ Patient knowledge; explain test and procedure (See Description/Procedure).

CONSIDERATIONS FOR NURSING CARE RELATED TO ABNORMAL TEST RESULTS
POSTTEST: Factors related to the results of the test
Nursing Diagnosis: Alterations in biochemical balance due to drug toxicity

Guide to assessment	Guide to planning and intervention	Guide to evaluation
1. Assess for theophylline toxicity: Tachycardia Palpitations Headache Anorexia Nausea, vomiting Epigastric pain Diarrhea Nervousness Insomnia Irritability	1. Implement plan of care to correct theophylline toxicities: a. Discontinue or reduce amount of theophylline as ordered by physician. b. Record amount of dietary methylxanthines, especially caffeine. c. Restrict amount of dietary intake of methylxanthines if ordered by physician.	1. Patient demonstrates no signs or symptoms of theophylline toxicity.

Guide to assessment	Guide to planning and intervention	Guide to evaluation
Dizziness Hypotension Convulsions Arrhythmias Muscle twitching Fever Dehydration	d. Administer theophylline with a full glass of water or after meals to minimize gastric irritation that may cause nausea not related to the toxicity. e. Observe individuals with a history of smoking, or those who have recently quit, for signs of toxicity (See Decreases 1). f. Control life-threatening conditions of toxicity until excess theophylline excreted as ordered.	
2. Monitor for therapeutic effects of theophylline	2. Record observations of therapeutic effects of theophylline:	2.

a. Preterm newborns
  Apneic spells
  Altered lab values
    pCO_2
    pH
	a. Observe and record number and length of apneic episodes and monitor pCO_2 and pH levels if ordered.	a. Patient will demonstrate decrease in number of apneic episodes, increase in alveolar ventilation, arterial pCO_2 decrease, and increase in pH (46).

b. Children and adults with respiratory impairment
  Respiratory rate and character
  Pulse
  Output
	b. Record respiratory rate and quality every 4 hours or as ordered:
	(1) Auscultate lungs at least every 4 hours.
	(2) Record heart rate and quality at least every 4 hours.
	(3) Measure and record intake and output.
		b. Patient will demonstrate normal respiratory rate and pattern for age:
		(1) Normal breath sounds.
		(2) Normal pulse rate for age.
		
		(3) Increase in amount of urinary output.

3. Determine level of patient knowledge related to theophylline therapy	3. Implement patient education to prevent increases or decreases in theophylline levels: a. Teach name, dose, and desired effect of theophylline. b. Reinforce importance of not stopping or increasing the amount of theophylline prescribed by the physician. c. Teach signs and symptoms of toxicity to be re-	3. Patient will verbalize name, amount, and desired effect of theophylline: c. Patient will verbalize signs/symptoms of toxicity

Guide to assessment	Guide to planning and intervention	Guide to evaluation
	ported to physician. d. Alert patient to expect increased urinary output. e. If rectal suppository form of the drug is used, instruct patient that the rectum should be empty prior to insertion of suppository and report rectal irritation immediately.	to be reported to physician. e. The patient will state procedure for use of rectal suppository and report to physician rectal irritation.

Test:	Thrombin Time
Abbreviation:	TT
Reference Value:	10–15 seconds, within 3 seconds of control
Specimen:	Plasma
Description:	Thrombin functions as a catalyzing enzyme. Its presence is formed by the action of activated factor Xa (See Figure 1, Partial Thromboplastin Time, Activated) with the cofactor, plasma accelerator globulin (factor V), and phospholipids and calcium ions. Thrombin's action is to split fibrinogen to soluble fibrin. Fibrin is then made insoluble by the action of fibrin-stabilizing factor, factor XIIIa. The thrombin time (TT) is the amount of time needed for plasma to form fibrin once thrombin has been added to the specimen. This test, along with prothrombin time (PT) and activated partial thromboplastin time (APTT), forms the basis for coagulation screening. Thrombin time is also a tool used in the diagnosis of DIC, liver disease, and in monitoring heparin and antithrombotic enzyme therapy.
Procedure:	(blue top tube) 1. No food or fluid restrictions. 2. A vacuum blood tube is completely filled; the tube is gently tipped back and forth to mix the anticoagulant. 3. Observe the puncture site carefully for bleeding or evidence of hematoma.

Drug Influences: The following drugs may influence test results.
  The following drugs may cause an increase in test results:

Thrombin time increase; miscellaneous
  asparaginase
  heparin
  streptokinase
  urokinase

  See Fibrinogen for:

  Increases/Decreases
  Related Lab Studies
  Posttest Considerations

IMPLICATIONS FOR NURSING CARE
PRETEST: Factors related to the test
Nursing Diagnosis: Potential for injury related to predisposition for bleeding and/or thrombus formation

Guide to assessment	Guide to planning and intervention	Guide to evaluation

Assess patient factors that
may influence test results:

Guide to assessment	Guide to planning and intervention	Guide to evaluation

1. Comprehensive drug history (See Drug Influences)	1. Identify influencing drugs and note on lab slip:
	  a. Identify and note the following on lab slip:
	    (1) Name of anticoagulant.
	    (2) Route.
	    (3) Dosage.
	    (4) Time of last dosage.
		1. Patient's test value is not influenced by unidentified drug.

2. Preexisting conditions Known coagulation disorder. See Increases/Decreases	2. Identify preexisting conditions and note on lab slip.	2. Patient's conditions pertinent to lab test are noted on lab slip.

3. Hemolysis	3. Prevent hemolysis by:
	  a. Not saturating the skin with antiseptic.
	  b. Not probing venipuncture site or leaving the tourniquet on too long.
	  c. Not forcefully withdrawing specimen.
	  d. Not withdrawing specimen too slowly.
	  e. Not agitating or handling specimen roughly.
		3. Patient's values are not influenced by hemolysis.

4. Knowledge deficit: Patient	4. Explain test to patient:
	  a. Define test; anticoagulant monitoring or coagulation screening.
	  b. Explain procedure.
		4. The patient demonstrates knowledge by defining test and stating procedure.

5. Knowledge deficit: Staff	5. Be informed about coagulation studies and anticoagulant medication schedule. Patients on full heparin therapy are tested at least once a day.	5. The patient's coagulation time is not abnormal due to staff error.

Patient Preparation Checklist

1. √ Interfering medications.
2. √ Anticoagulant, dose, time noted on lab slip.
3. √ Pertinent preexisting conditions noted on lab slip.
4. √ Patient knowledge; explain test to patient.

Test:	Thyroid-Binding Globulin
Abbreviation:	TBG
Reference Values:	12–30 μg/100 ml (radioimmunoassay)
	Values vary with laboratory
Specimen:	Serum

Description: Thyroid-binding globulin (TBG) is the inter-alpha-globulin that binds thyroxine (T_4) and triiodothyronine (T_3) in plasma. While T_4 is bound about 90% to TBG, T_3 is less tightly bound. TBG functions as a carrier for T_4 and T_3 in transporting the inactive hormones. TBG measures the total serum-binding capacity for the thyroid hormones, and abnormalities of TBG are identified by this measurement.

Procedure: (red top tube)
1. No food or fluid restrictions.
2. Up to 5 ml of blood is drawn from the patient.
3. Observe puncture site for bleeding or evidence of hematoma.

Conditions Related to Increases

1. Hypothyroidism
   Pregnancy
   Chronic hepatic disease
   Porphyria, acute intermittent
   Genetic disorders
   Newborn

Rationale

1. The thyroid-binding proteins are important in the regulation of T_4 and T_3 plasma levels. Certain conditions and drugs increase TBG.

Conditions Related to Decreases

1. Steroids; anabolic and
     androgens
   Nephrotic conditions
   Hypoproteinemia
   Genetic disorders
   Advanced age
   Stress; major illnesses

Rationale

1. Thyroid-binding globulins are decreased in these conditions.

Drug Influences: The following drugs may influence test results. The drugs are listed alphabetically by generic name and divided into columns according to the effect of the drug. Examples of trade names are in parentheses.

The following drugs may cause an increase in test values:

Direct effect of drug
   diethylstilbestrol
   estradiol (Menaval-10, Estrace)
   estrone (Estrone Aqueous, Hormonin)
   phenothiazines (Thorazine, Prolixin, Trilafon, etc.)

Increased binding capacity
  epinephrine; after infusion
  estrogens
  oral contraceptives

Miscellaneous
  chlormadinone
  clofibrate (Atromid-S)
  estrogens
  oral contraceptives
  perphenazine (Etrafon, Trilafon)

The following drugs may cause a decrease in test results:

Direct effect of drug
  anabolic steroids
  androgens
  phenytoin (Dilantin)
  salicylates; large doses
  steroids; reduced synthesis

Related Lab Studies:

In hyperthyroidism

  ↑ T_4
  ↑ T_3
  ↓ TBG
  normal TSH

  ↓ cholesterol
  ↑ calcium
  ↑ phosphorus
  ↑ alkaline phosphatase

In hypothyroidism

  ↓ T_4
  ↓ T_3; may be normal
  ↑ TBG
  ↑ TSH in primary hypothyroidism
  ↓ TSH in secondary hypothyroidism
  ↑ cholesterol

IMPLICATIONS FOR NURSING CARE
PRETEST: Factors related to the test

Guide to assessment	Guide to planning and intervention	Guide to evaluation
	See Thyroxine (T_4) for Pretest information.	

CONSIDERATIONS FOR NURSING CARE RELATED TO ABNORMAL TEST RESULTS
POSTTEST: Factors related to the results of the test
Nursing Diagnosis: Alterations in biochemical balance

Guide to assessment	Guide to planning and intervention	Guide to evaluation
Assess patient factors that may be influencing test results:		
1. Conditions related to TBG variations (See Increases/Decreases)	1. Recognize conditions and consult with physician. Order T_4 and free thyroxine assay.	1. Patient conditions influencing test results are recognized.

See Thyroxine (T_4) for more Posttest information.

Test:	Thyroid-Stimulating Hormone or Thyrotropin
Abbreviation:	TSH
Reference Value:	Radioimmunoassay 0–10 μU/ml Values vary with laboratory
Specimen:	Serum

Description: Thyroid-stimulating hormone (TSH) is secreted in response to thyroid-releasing hormone (TRH) and circulating thyroid hormone levels. TSH, via the negative feedback system, controls the synthesis and release of the thyroid hormones, triiodothyronine (T_3), and thyroxine (T_4). TSH stimulates iodine trapping in the thyroid follicular cells, the organification of iodine into a tyrosine molecule, and the coupling of molecules into the thyroid hormones for their subsequent storage or release.

Measurement of TSH is an aid in the differential diagnosis of primary or secondary hypothyroidism and in the monitoring of drug therapy in the treatment of primary hypothyroidism.

Procedure: (red top tube)
1. No food or fluid restrictions.
2. Up to 5 ml of blood is drawn from the patient.
3. Observe puncture site for bleeding or evidence of hematoma.

Conditions Related to Increases

1. Hypothyroidism, primary
   Malnutrition
   Neonates
   Elderly
   Inadequate thyroid replacement therapy
   Iodine deficiency
   Excessive antithyroid therapy
2. Hydatidiform mole

Rationale

1. Low thyroxine (T_4) levels stimulate a feedback response of increased TSH release. Review description.

2. Human chorionic gonadotrophin probably stimulates thyroid activity.

Conditions Related to Decreases

1. Hypothyroidism, secondary

2. Hyperthyroidism

Rationale

1. In secondary hypothyroidism and hypothalamic hypothyroidism there is failure of hypothalamic stimulation for TSH release, which results in the TSH deficiency.
2. TSH is suppressed via the feedback system due to the excessive circulating thyroid hormone.

Refer to Thyroxine (T$_4$) for further information:
Related Lab Studies
Pretest Implications
Posttest Considerations

Drug Influences: The following drugs may influence test results. The following drugs may cause an increase in test results:

Increased TSH, miscellaneous
lithium; mechanism unclear
potassium iodide
thyrotropin-releasing hormone

The following drugs may cause a decrease in test results:

Decreased TSH, miscellaneous
aspirin; decreased release
corticosteroids
heparin; interferes with protein binding by thyroxine

See Thyroxine (T$_4$) for Pretest and Posttest information.

Test:	Thyroxine, Bound T_4
Abbreviation:	T_4 or BT_4
Reference Values:	*Radioimmunoassay* Cord blood 5.9–19.5 µg/dl 24 hours 11.4–21.0 µg/dl 6 weeks 9.9–18.3 µg/dl All others 5–12 µg/dl Values vary with laboratory
Specimen:	Serum

Description:

Thyroxine (T_4) is an iodine-containing amino acid synthesized and released by the thyroid gland in response to thyroid-stimulating hormone (TSH). T_4 is predominately extracellular and is 75% bound to thyroid-binding globulin (TBG). The remaining T_4 is bound to thyroid-binding prealbumin (TBPA) and albumin. Free thyroxine (FT_4), the active T_4, is about 0.03%. It is thought that bound T_4 serves as a prohormone to triiodothyronine (T_3). About 80% of T_4 is deiodinized in the liver and kidneys to T_3. The remaining T_4 is converted to reverse T_3 (rT_3), an inactive hormone.

Measurements of T_4 are done to evaluate thyroid disorder and to monitor response to treatment. In nearly all states newborns are screened for congenital hypothyroidism as part of the newborn errors of metabolism screen (along with PKU, etc.) done at birth and 3–4 weeks after birth.

The free thyroxine assessment (FTA) is a calculation of the ratio of bound thyroxine (T_4) to thyroid-binding globulin (TBG). From the calculation one may derive an estimation of free thyroxine in plasma. Free thyroxine (FT_4) is the metabolically active T_4. It is believed that the ratio of T_4:TBG is more useful than the single measurement of FT_4. Free thyroxine measurement is difficult and expensive to determine.

The FTA is another test to evaluate thyroid function. It is particularly useful if there is a thyroid-binding globulin abnormality.

Procedure:

(red top tube)
1. No food or fluid restrictions.
2. Up to 5 ml of blood is drawn from the patient. For newborns, follow heelstick procedure found with PKU testing.
3. Observe puncture site for evidence of bleeding or hematoma.

Conditions Related to Increases	Rationale

1. Hyperthyroidism
   Toxic diffuse goiter
   (Graves' disease)
	1. The increase is due to an increased number of circulating stimulators (antibodies) that are active on thyroid tissue. The theory is that these

antibodies copy thyroid-stimulating hormone action and stimulate an increase in T_4, T_3, FT_3, and FT_4.

2. Thyroiditis, subacute

2. This disease is thought to be caused by a virus. The increased T_4 secretion is due to extrusion of thyroid hormone from the inflamed gland. This is a transient condition.

3. Toxic nodular goiter (Plummer's disease)

3. Hypersecretion of thyroid hormones from the enlarged thyroid gland is the cause of the increase in this condition. The diseased gland functions autonomously.

4. Hydatidiform mole

4. The increase in T_4 levels in this condition is thought to be due to the excessive amounts of chorionic gonadotropin and this hormone has intrinsic thyroid-stimulating properties.

5. Pregnancy
Viral hepatitis
Certain drugs:
  Estrogens
  L-Thyroxine
  Perphenazine (Trilafon)
Newborn
Porphyria, acute intermittent

5. The protein mainly responsible for transport of T_4 is thyroid-binding globulin. Conditions that increase the binding capacity of serum T_4 will increase T_4 levels.

Conditions Related to Decreases

1. Primary hypothyroidism, e.g.
  Goiter
  Chronic thyroiditis
  Carcinoma of thyroid
  Antithyroid drug overdose
  Thyroidectomy

Rationale

1. Hypothyroidism is classified as either primary or secondary. Primary hypothyroidism is due to thyroid gland disease. Secondary hypothyroidism is due to a problem with TSH secretion. Because of destruction to the thyroid parenchyma from disease, radiation therapy or surgery, there is insufficient gland to synthesize and secrete adequate T_4.

2. Chronic debilitating illnesses

2. Diminished T_4 may also be caused by decreased thyroid-binding globulin capacity, for example, acute illness, chronic debilitating disease, or glucocorticoid excess.

3. Secondary hypothyroidism, e.g.
   Pituitary tumors
   Postpartum pituitary necrosis
   Hypophysectomy, etc.

3. This kind of hypothyroidism is due to a problem with TSH secretion. This may be caused by destruction to the anterior pituitary or from hypothalamic hypothyroidism. The latter condition is caused by a TSH deficiency resulting in a lack of synthesis of thyroid-releasing hormone. There is often a concomitant cortisol deficiency in secondary hypothyroidism.

4. Congenital hypothyroidism

4. This condition is caused by the partial or complete lack of the thyroid gland at birth; or the gland is present but unable to synthesize or release thyroxine; or it may be caused by maternal antithyroid therapy during pregnancy.

Drug Influences: The following drugs may influence test results. The drugs are listed alphabetically by generic name and divided into columns according to the effect of the drug. Examples of trade names are in parentheses.

The following drugs may cause an increase in test results:

Increased T4 levels, miscellaneous
   levothyroxine (Synthroid, Levoid, L-Thyroxine Sodium)
   methadone

Increase binding capacity
   estrogens
   oral contraceptives
   perphenazine (Trilafon)
   progestins

The following drugs may cause a decrease in test results:

Displaces thyroxine from binding sites
   barbiturates
   chlorpropamide (Diabinese)
   clofibrate (Atromid-S)
   heparin
   penicillin
   phenytoin (Dilantin)
   steroids
   tolbutamide (Orinase)

Depresses thyroid function
   cobalt
   cortisone
   ethionamide (Trecator-SC)
   iodides
   levothyroxine (Synthroid)
   liothyronine (Cytomel, Ro-Thyronine)
   lithium
   methimazole (Tapazole); excessive doses
   oxyphenbutazone (Oxalid, Tandearil)
   resorcinol (Resorcin); on denuded skin
   thiouracils (Propylthiouracil); excessive doses

Decreases synthesis
   salicylates
   sulfonamides

Miscellaneous
  reserpine (Serpasil)

Related Lab Studies:

In hyperthyroidism:

↑ T_4
↑ T_3
↓ TBG
normal TSH

↓ cholesterol
↑ calcium, serum
↑ phosphorus
↑ alkaline phosphatase

In hypothyroidism:

↓ T_4
↓ T_3; may be normal
↑ TBG
↑ TSH in primary hypothyroidism
↓ TSH in secondary hypothyroidism
↑ cholesterol

IMPLICATIONS FOR NURSING CARE
PRETEST: Factors related to the test
Nursing Diagnosis: Potential for injury related to changes in biochemical balance

Guide to assessment	Guide to planning and intervention	Guide to evaluation
Assess patient factors that may influence test results: 1. Comprehensive drug history (See Drug Influences)	1. Withhold drugs that may influence test results as prescribed. Note influencing drugs that must be continued on lab slip. If test is to monitor drug therapy, patient should continue prescribed thyroid preparation.	1. Patient's drugs do not interfere with test values.
2. Preexisting conditions (See Increases/Decreases) Patient is newborn	2. Identify preexisting conditions and note on lab slip.	2. Patient's preexisting conditions are noted on lab slip.

3. Knowledge deficit	3. Explain test to patient:
	  a. Define thyroid function.
	  b. Explain procedure.
		3. Patient demonstrates knowledge by defining test and stating procedure.

Patient Preparation Checklist

1. √ Interfering drugs; either withhold or note on lab slip.
2. √ Preexisting conditions and if patient is newborn. Note on lab slip.
3. √ Patient knowledge; explain test to patient (See Description/Procedure).

CONSIDERATIONS FOR NURSING CARE RELATED TO ABNORMAL TEST RESULTS
POSTTEST: Factors related to the results of the test
Nursing Diagnosis: Alterations in biochemical balance

Guide to assessment	Guide to planning and intervention	Guide to evaluation
Assess patient factors that may be influencing test results. Nursing history and/or physical exam suggestive of:		
1. Hyperthyroidism Signs and symptoms Nervousness Irritability Restlessness Resting pulse ↑ 90 Low heat tolerance Diaphoresis Fine hand tremor Exophthalmos Increased appetite with weight loss Muscle weakness Cardiac involvement Amenorrhea	1. Initiate nursing measures to decrease T$_4$ secretion: a. Recognize signs and symptoms of hyperthyroidism. b. Refer patient to physician.	1. The patient experiences euthyroid status as demonstrated by decreasing pulse rate and normal thyroid blood studies.
2. Hyperthyroidism a. Propylthiouracil Methimazole Iodine therapy b. Radioiodine therapy	2. Block the synthesis and release of T$_4$ by: a. Giving antithyroid medications as prescribed. Explain to patient action of drugs. b. Explaining to patient action of radioiodine therapy. (1) Stress need for follow-up thyroid evaluations. (2) Detect early signs of hypothyroidism. Consult with physician. (3) Withhold iodine preparations prior to radio-iodine therapy.	2. Patient's thyroid studies return to normal.
3. Thyroidectomy	3. Prepare patient for surgery by: a. Giving antithyroid drugs as prescribed. b. Giving iodine preparations as prescribed. c. Explaining to patient preparation for surgery may take 2–3 months.	3. The patient is euthyroid prior to surgery.

Guide to assessment	Guide to planning and intervention	Guide to evaluation

4. Thyroiditis, subacute	4. Promote decreased inflammation of thyroid gland by:
	  a. Encouraging rest and diminished stress.
	  b. Giving steroids, as prescribed, for inflammation.
		4. The patient achieves euthyroid status as demonstrated by lab values.

5. Hydatidiform mole	5. Prepare patient for surgery.	5. The patient's T_4 level returns to normal after removal of hydatidiform mole.
6. Thyroid crisis	6. Prevent increased thyroid hormone secretion in thyroid crisis by:	6. The patient's clinical condition improves.

a. Signs and symptoms
    Hyperpyrexia
    Dehydration
    Extreme irritability
    Severe tachycardia
    Delirium
	a. Detecting signs and symptoms of thyroid crisis early. Consult with physician immediately.	

b. Precipitating factors
    Stress, physical, or psychic
    Poorly prepared patient prior to thyroidectomy
	b. Being aware of precipitating factors and consulting with physician.	

c. Antithyroid drugs:
    Sodium iodine
    Methimazole
    Propylthiouracil
	c. Administering antithyroid medication promptly and as prescribed.	

d. Precipitating condition	d. Carrying out medical treatment plan for underlying condition.	
7. Primary hypothyroidism	7. Initiate measures to achieve euthyroid state.	7. The patient demonstrates improvement by ↑ pulse rate, ↓ weight, loss of puffy appearance, improved neurological signs, and improved muscle tone. The patient remains euthyroid.

a. Signs and symptoms
    Intolerance to cold
    Low body temperature
    Weight gain
    Blood pressure low
    Skin becomes thick and dry
    Fatigue
    Constipation
    Poor memory
    Stolid mask-like face
    Hair thins/falls out
    Neurological and mental slowness
	a. Recognize signs and symptoms of hypothyroidism and refer to physician.
	  b. Administer thyroid hormones, such as levothyroxine sodium, as prescribed.
	  c. Teach patient about diseases and drugs and need to continue them for life.
	  d. Instruct patient in signs and symptoms of thyroid overdose (hyperthyroidism).	

Guide to assessment	Guide to planning and intervention	Guide to evaluation
8. Secondary hypothyroidism	8. Promote thyroid replacement: a. Administer cortisol replacement as prescribed. b. Administer thyroid replacement as prescribed. c. Explain drugs and therapy to patient. Stress need to take medication daily. d. Instruct patient in signs and symptoms of overdosage or underdosage of replacement drugs.	8. The patient is euthyroid.
9. Congenital hypothyroidism Signs and symptoms Lethargy Low food intake Long sleep periods Prolonged neonatal jaundice Infrequent bowel movements Mottling of skin at 2–3 weeks Hoarse cry Heart sounds of poor quality	9. Promote replacement of congenital deficient T$_4$ by: a. Administering gradually increasing doses of thyroid. b. Recognizing signs and symptoms of overdosage early (See 1 Posttest) and consulting with physician. c. Instructing parents in signs and symptoms of thyroid overdose. d. Instructing parents of absolute necessity in giving thyroid medication daily.	9. The patient grows normally mentally and physically without signs of thyroid overdose.

Test:	Triglycerides
Abbreviation:	None
Reference Value:	10–190 mg/dl Levels vary widely. Check with local lab.
Specimen:	Serum

Description: Triglycerides are produced in the liver and are esters of glycerol and fatty acids. They are mainly synthesized from carbohydrates. Fats and proteins may also be utilized for triglyceride production. The main function of triglycerides is as an energy source of metabolism. They are either used immediately after absorption or stored in adipose tissue. The main triglyceride transporters are chylomicrons and very low-density lipoproteins (VLDL). These lipoproteins are large molecule complexes that are carriers for insoluble lipids.

See Cholesterol.

Triglyceride levels are measured to evaluate coronary artery disease risk and lipid metabolism.

Procedure: (red top tube)
1. The patient should restrict food and fluids for 12–14 hours before the test.
2. The patient should eat a normal diet for 2 days prior to the test and should abstain from alcohol for 24 hours prior to testing.
3. Approximately 10 ml of blood is withdrawn from the patient.
4. Observe puncture site for evidence of bleeding or hematoma.

Refer to Cholesterol for discussion on:

Increases
Decreases
Related Lab Studies
Pretest Implications
Posttest Considerations

Drug Influences: The following drugs may influence test results. The drugs are listed alphabetically by generic name and divided into columns according to the effect of the drug. Examples of trade names are in parentheses.

The following drugs may cause an increase in test values:

Triglyceride increase

cholestyramine (Cuemid, Questran)	levothyroxine (Synthroid)
estrogens	mestranol
ethanol	oral contraceptives
glucocorticoids	phenformin; under starving conditions

The following drugs may cause a decrease in test values:

Therapeutic intent

cholestyramine (Cuemid, Questran)	dextrothyroxine (Choloxin)
clofibrate (Atromid-S)	nafenopin
colestipol	niacin

Miscellaneous

ascorbic acid; in atherosclerotic patients	metformin
asparaginase	methandrostenolone (Dianabol)
glucagon; lipids transferred to platelets	norethindrone
glyburide; in treated diabetics	oxandrolone (Anavar)
halofenate	oxymetholone (Adroyd, Anadrol)
heparin	sulfonylurea (Dymelor, Diabinese,
menotropins	Orinase, etc.)

Test:	Triiodothyronine
Abbreviation:	T$_3$
Reference Values:	Radioimmunoassay Newborn 30–100 ng/dl All others 100–220 ng/dl Values vary with laboratory
Specimen:	Serum
Description:	Triiodothyronine (T$_3$) contains three iodine atoms, and thyroxine (T$_4$) contains four. It is from the deiodinization of T$_4$ that about 80% of T$_3$ is derived. T$_3$ is metabolically very active. It is loosely bound to thyroid-binding globulin (TBG) and it has a plasma half-life of about 1 day compared to the 7-day half-life of thyroxine. Thyroid hormones stimulate energy production by increased oxygen consumption, heat production, and increased protein production. They are also involved in the growth and maturation of the body. T$_3$ measurements are done to evaluate thyroid function, especially in the diagnosis of T$_3$ toxicosis, and to monitor response to thyroid gland treatment.
Procedure:	(red top tube) 1. No food or fluid restrictions. 2. Up to 5 ml of blood is drawn from the patient. 3. Observe puncture site for bleeding or evidence of hematoma.

Conditions Related to Increases

Rationale

1. T$_3$ toxicosis

1. In this condition, T$_3$ is increased, but T$_4$ and free T$_4$ remain normal. T$_3$ toxicosis may occur with Graves' disease, early hyperthyroidism, after drug therapy, and in other primary hyperthyroid states.

2. Hyperthyroidism

2. T$_3$ is often elevated early in hyperthyroidism while T$_4$ measurements are still normal. It is a valuable tool in diagnosing this condition. T$_3$ is often normal in hypothyroidism, while T$_4$ is decreased.

    See Thyroxin (T$_4$) for further information. The tests are generally parallel except where indicated.

Test: Uric Acid

Abbreviation: Sometimes UA

Reference Values: *Serum*
Children   2.5–8.0 mg/dl
Men   4.3–8.0 mg/dl
Women   2.3–6.0 mg/dl
Urine   250–750 mg/24 hours

Description: Uric acid is the end product of purine metabolism and is mainly excreted in the urine. Uric acid levels are measured to aid in the diagnosis of gout.

Procedure: (red top tube)

Serum

1. Restrict food and fluids for 8 hours prior to test. Water is allowed. Food and fluids may not be restricted; check with local laboratory.
2. Approximately 10 ml of blood is withdrawn from the patient.
3. Observe puncture site for bleeding or evidence of hematoma.

24-Hour Urine Collection

1. No food or fluid restrictions.
2. Collection container is plain. Keep urine refrigerated during entire collection.
3. Collection.
    a. Discard first voided specimen.
    b. Begin timing.
    c. For next 24 hours place all voidings into specimen container immediately after voiding.
    d. Have patient void just prior to completion of 24 hours and put sample in collection bottle.
4. Record exact start and finish times on lab slip.
5. Send to lab immediately.

Conditions Related to Increases	Rationale
1. Primary gout	1. A hereditary disease mostly seen in males. This disease results in elevated serum uric acid from the body's increased production of uric acid, from a defect in renal excretion of uric acid, or from a combination of these. Lesch-Nyhan syndrome is a congenital form of gout that results in a lack of enzymes needed for purine metabolism with excess uric acid production.

2. Leukemias
   Polycythemia vera
   Malignant neoplasms

2. Secondary gout. Increased nucleoprotein catabolism from increased cell turnover will increase uric acid formation. Urine levels are also increased.

3. Drugs
   Diabetic ketoacidosis
   Glucose-6-phosphate dehydrogenase deficiency

3. See Drug Influences. Some drugs and organic acids such as lactic acid and hydroxybutyric acid compete with uric acid for renal tubular secretion.

4. Renal hypertension
   Glomerulosclerosis
   Chronic glomerulonephritis
   Eclampsia
   Lead poisoning
   Congestive heart failure

4. The increased serum uric acid is because of reduced renal clearance of uric acid. Urine uric acid is decreased.

5. Septicemia
   Pneumonia
   Manic depressive disorders
   Psychoses
   Cerebral vascular accident

5. Increased nucleoprotein catabolism in these conditions is probably responsible for the increase. Urine uric acid is also increased.

6. Normal neonate

6. Plasma, and consequently urine uric acid levels, are normally increased during the first few days of life. High levels are excreted and return to normal within the first week of life (34).

Conditions Related to Decreases

Rationale

1. Fanconi's syndrome
   Renal tubular degeneration

1. Diminished renal tubular reabsorption can cause decreased serum levels and increased urine uric acid levels.

2. Severe liver disease
   Congenital xanthine deficiency
   Allopurinol, excessive

2. Uric acid is formed from xanthine by the action of the enzyme, xanthine oxidase. A deficiency in the enzymes results in diminished uric acid formation.

Drug Influences: Many drugs may influence uric acid levels. The following drugs are some of the influencing drugs. They are listed alphabetically by generic name and divided into columns according to the effect of the drug. Examples of trade names are in parentheses.

The following drugs may cause an increase in test values:

Serum

Decreased urate clearance
   acetazolamide (Diamox)
   angiotensin
   aspirin (A.S.A., Aspergum)
   diuretics

ethoxyzolamide (Zarontin, Cardrase, Ethamide)
ibufenac

Increased catabolism
    azathioprine (Imuran)
    busulfan (Myleran)
    mercaptopurine (Purinethol)

    prednisone (Deltasone, Fernisone)
    vincristine (Oncovin)

Nephrotoxic effect
    capreomycin (Capastat Sulfate)
    methicillin (Azapen, Celbenin)

    mitomycin (Mutamycin)
    rifampin (Rifadin, Rimactane)

Urine

Uricosuric effect
    chlorpromazine (Chlorzine, Klorazine)
    clofibrate; weak effect (Atromid-S)
    corticotropins (Acthar, Cortigel-80)
    coumarin (Dicumarol, Panwarfin)

    glucose; infusions
    mannitol (Osmitrol)
    phenothiazines (Chlorpromazine, Compazine)
    probenecid (Benemid, Probalan)

Miscellaneous
    estrogen; men on therapy
    methotrexate (Mexate)
    thioguanine

The following drugs may cause a decrease in test values:

Serum

Uricosuric effect
    acetohexamide (Dymelor)
    aspirin (A.S.A., Aspergum)
    azathioprine (Imuran)
    chlorpromazine (Chlorzine, Klorazine)
    chlorprothixene (Taractan)
    cinchophen
    corticotropin (Acthar, Cortigel-80)

    coumarin (Dicumarol, Panwarfin)
    lithium (Eskalith, Lithane)
    mannitol (Osmitrol)
    mefenamic acid (Ponstel)
    phenothiazines (Chlorpromazine HCl tablets, Compazine)
    probenecid (Benemid, Probalan)

Urine

Decreases urate clearance
    acetazolamide (Diamox)
    azathioprine (Imuran)
    chlorthalidone (Hygroton)

    ethyl alcohol; during intake
    thiazides

Miscellaneous
    allopurinol (Lopurin, Zyloprim)

Related Lab Studies: In the diagnosis of gout:

    synovial fluid analysis
    *x-ray of bones
    CBC
    urinalysis
    ESR

---

*Not discussed in this book.

IMPLICATIONS FOR NURSING CARE
PRETEST: Factors related to the test
Nursing Diagnosis: Potential for injury related to changes in biochemical balance

Guide to assessment	Guide to planning and intervention	Guide to evaluation
Assess patient factors that may influence test results:		
1. Food and fluid restriction	1. Restrict food and fluids for 8 hours prior to serum uric acid. Water is allowed.	1. Patient's test values are not influenced by food or fluid intake.
2. Comprehensive drug history (See Drug Influences)	2. Identify drugs that may influence test results. Consult with physician. Note interfering drugs on lab slip.	2. Patient's test values are not influenced by medication. Medications are noted on lab slip.
3. Preexisting conditions (See Increases) Familial history of gout	3. Identify pertinent patient information; note on lab slip and chart. Consult with physician.	3. Patient's preexisting conditions are noted on lab slip.

4. Knowledge deficit	4. Explain test to patient:
	   a. Define uric acid (See Description).
	   b. Explain procedure (See Procedure).
		4. The patient demonstrates knowledge by defining test and stating procedure.

Patient Preparation Checklist

1. √ Food and fluids are restricted.
2. √ Influencing drugs; note on lab slip.
3. √ Preexisting conditions; note on lab slip.
4. √ Patient knowledge; explain test.

CONSIDERATIONS FOR NURSING CARE RELATED TO ABNORMAL TEST RESULTS
POSTTEST: Factors related to the results of the test
Nursing Diagnosis: Alterations in biochemical balance

Guide to assessment	Guide to planning and intervention	Guide to evaluation
Assess patient factors that may be influencing test results. Nursing history and/or physical exam that is suggestive of:		

1. Acute gout
  Signs and Symptoms
    ↑ Fever
    Sudden severe joint pain, especially:Toes, feet, ankles, knees, wrists, elbows
    ↑ WBC
    ↑ ESR
    Pain relief with colchicine
	1. Identify signs and symptoms of acute gout. Consult with physician.	1. Patient receives treatment for acute gout symptoms. Uric acid level returns to normal.

2. Chronic gout
  Complaints of arthritis
  Swollen, red, painful joints
  Presence of urate deposits about joints or ears (tophi)
  Symptoms in 1
	2. Identify signs and symptoms of chronic gout. Consult with physician.	2. Patient receives treatment for chronic gout symptoms. Uric acid returns to normal.

3. Gout
  a. Drug therapy
    allopurinol (Zyloprim)
    probenecid (Benemid)
    colchicine
    sulfinpyrazone (Anturane)
	3. Reduce uric acid levels:
	  a. Give antigout medications as prescribed:
	    (1) Give colchicine at first sign of symptoms.
	    (2) Continue medication prophylactically as prescribed.
	    (3) Avoid aspirin use when using uricosuric drugs.
	  b. Encourage liberal fluid intake to encourage urate output.
	  c. Encourage diet low in purine intake:
	    (1) Avoid organ meats and high-fat diet.	

Guide to assessment	Guide to planning and intervention	Guide to evaluation
	(2) Encourage high carbo-hydrate foods. (3) Avoid alcoholic beverages. d. Discourage sudden weight loss (See 3 Increases). Suggest slow weight loss program. e. Educate patient about how to reduce uric acid levels (*a* through *d* above).	

4. Kidney function
  Lab test
    Uric acid
    BUN
    Creatinine
	4. Prevent increased uric acid levels due to decreased kidney function:
	a. Keep accurate I&O records, daily weights.
	b. Encourage fluid intake.
	c. Attempt to maintain alkaline urine:
	  (1) Check urine pH.
	  (2) Give alkalinizing agents as ordered.
	  (3) Encourage diet high in alkaline ash: foods such as green vegetables, apples, oranges, melons, etc.
		4. Patient's kidney function tests remain normal.

5. Leukemia Chemotherapy	5. Control hyperuricemia from rapid cell turnover: a. Follow kidney function tests carefully. b. Give allopurinol as prescribed. c. Give sodium bicarbonate or acetazolamide as prescribed. d. Encourage fluid intake.	5. Patient's serum uric acid is normal.

Test:	Urinalysis		
Abbreviation:	Ua, U/A, UA		

Reference Values:

		Adult	*Child*
	Color	straw	straw
	Appearance (opacity, turbidity, clarity)	clear	clear
	Specific gravity	1.001–1.040 usual— 1.015–1.025	neonate— 1.012 infant— 1.001–1.020 usual— 1.003–1.010
	pH	4.5–8 usual is 6	neonate— 5.0–7.0
	Protein	negative	negative
	Glucose	negative	negative
	Ketones	negative	negative
	Occult blood	negative	negative
	Microscopic		
	WBC	0–4	0–4
	RBC	0–3	rare
	Bacteria	none	none
	Casts	rare hyaline cast	rare hyaline cast
	Crystals	few	few
	Epithelial cells	few	few

Specimen: Random urine

Description: Urine is constantly being formed in the kidneys. It is body fluid waste evolved from the blood through a process of ultrafiltration, reabsorption, and secretion. A urinalysis can be used to assess the status of kidney function, nutrition, and certain metabolic and systemic diseases. Parts of the urine test are done routinely by nurses as part of ongoing patient assessment.

Normal fresh urine has very little odor. What odor is present is not unpleasant but is slightly pungent. Urine volume varies with age. A one-day-old infant excretes about 50 cc of urine per day, and a middle-aged adult excretes an average of 1300–1700 cc of urine per day.

Routine urinalysis is best done on the first voided morning specimen. Random urines are sufficient for screening purposes.

Procedure:
1. No food or fluid restrictions are necessary.
2. The first voided specimen is generally the most desirable as it is most concentrated; it is not recommended for glucose testing. Random urine specimens are also suitable.

3. A clean catch urine specimen is usually preferred.

a. Cleanse meatus and surrounding genitalia with mild antiseptic solution.

b. Rinse meatus and genitalia thoroughly to prevent contamination of specimen with antiseptic.

c. Have patient begin initial urine flow.

d. Collect midstream urine flow in sterile container. Do not contaminate edges or inside of collection container.

e. Remove collector before urine flow stops.

f. Send to laboratory immediately.

4. The urine is collected in a clean container. The inside of the container should not be touched.

5. The urine is sent to the lab immediately. Examination of urine should be done within 1 hour of collection. Urine should be refrigerated until sent to lab.

Conditions Related to Increases	Rationale
1. Color darkens	1. Listed below are some causes of darker urine color.
a. Multiple colors	a. Drugs; see Drug Influences.
b. Darker color	b. Unclean collection containers.
c. Yellow-orange	c. Concentrated urine; some drugs.
d. Yellow-green or green-brown	d. Bilirubin. The urine may be dark green in severe obstructive jaundice; some drugs.
e. Dark brown or black	e. Hemoglobin in acid urine that has been standing for a period of time; urine containing the pigment melanin; with large doses of levadopa; possibly hair dyes. In dark-skinned patients with chronic intestinal obstruction, melanuria may be present. It is also seen in some patients with Addison's disease.
f. Red urine	f. Contamination from menstrual flow; from foods such as beets or rhubarb; from a number of drugs (See Drug Influences); hematuria; porphyria; lower urinary tract bleeding; candy and food dyes.
g. Bright yellow	g. Vitamin B_2 (riboflavin) or carotene.
h. Blue-green	h. From methylene blue found in some drugs, or Pseudomonas infection.

2. Appearance

2. Listed below are some causes of increased density of urine. Abnormal appearance should be examined microscopically.

a. Cloudy white

a. Usually due to phosphate precipitation in alkaline urine. May be seen in postprandial urine specimens. Pyuria may also be a cause. Other causes of general cloudiness are spermatozoa, fecal contamination, mucous threads, tissue, etc.

b. Opalescent

b. Fresh voided specimens should be transparent. Opalescence may indicate bacteria. If the opalescence is uniform, it is likely that it is due to postvoiding bacterial growth. Urine specimens should be refrigerated or sent to lab immediately to prevent this occurrence. Examination should be within 1 hour of collection.

c. Milky

c. From fat globules in urine seen in degenerative tubular disease, crush injuries, or lymphatic obstruction.

d. Smoky

d. Red blood cells.

e. Pink or white cloud

e. Caused by urates or uric acid. May be seen in postprandial urine specimens.

3. Specific gravity

3. Listed below are some of the causes of an increased specific gravity. An increase in specific gravity indicates kidney's ability to concentrate urine.

a. Dehydration

a. Patient has concentrated urine due to a lack of fluids.

b. X-ray dye
   Glucose
   Protein
   IV Albumin

b. Gives high specific gravity due to increased number of solutes in the urine.

c. Trauma
   Stress
   Postsurgery

c. The high specific gravity in these conditions is due to an increased secretion of antidiuretic hormone (ADH). ADH causes a decrease in urine volume.

d. Old, unrefrigerated specimen

d. Specific gravity will increase due to deterioration of specimen.

4. Alkaluria (pH ↑)

    a. Old, unrefrigerated specimen

    b. Respiratory alkalosis

    c. Metabolic alkalosis

    d. Renal tubular acidosis

    e. Diet

    f. Infection

    g. Drugs

    h. Bed rest

5. Protein

4. Listed below are some of the causes of increased urine pH.

    a. A urine specimen more than 1 hour old that is not refrigerated will begin to deteriorate. Bacterial contamination occurs that results in alkalinization, and so the pH increases. Ammonia smell becomes apparent.

    b. Increased excretion of bicarbonate causes the urine to be alkaline.

    c. The urine may be alkalotic. However, if there is potassium/chloride depletion, the urine may be slightly acid; this is because hydrogen ions are excreted and bicarbonate ions are reabsorbed.

    d. The urine remains relatively alkalotic in this disease because the tubules are unable to form ammonia and have decreased hydrogen ion excreting ability. The urine remains with a pH at 6–6.5 even after an acid loading test.

    e. Certain foods such as vegetables and citrus fruits may cause alkaline urine. After meals urine is alkaline (called alkaline tide) due to the increased release of gastric HCl. The urine returns to acid in a few hours. Vegetarians are more likely to have alkaline urine.

    f. Bacteria, especially those called urea-splitting, may cause an alkaline urine. Proteus and Pseudomonas are urea-splitting bacteria.

    g. Certain drugs induce alkaline urine. See Drug Influences.

    h. Immobilized patients show an increase in urine pH (27).

5. Listed are some of the causes of increased protein in the urine.

a. Electroshock
   therapy
   Mushroom
   poisoning
   Poison
   ivy/oak
   reaction

b. Dehydration
   Muscular exercise,
   strenuous
   Hemorrhage
   Salt depletion
   Febrile illnesses
   Emotional stress

c. Postural proteinuria

d. Kidney disease

a. The cause is from the nephrotoxic effect and the extent of the
   insult on the kidney glomeruli.

b. The cause of the proteinuria in
   these conditions is transient and
   probably due to the relative is-
   chemia to the kidney due to the
   adaption reaction to stress and/or
   dehydration. Proteinuria may last
   up to 72 hours after the strenuous exercise.

c. Also called orthostatic proteinuria, this condition is seen in
   young adults. It is thought to be
   caused by changes in kidney circulation due to exaggerated lor-
   dotic position. Generally, this is a
   benign condition showing small
   amounts of protein. To determine
   postural proteinuria, the patient's
   first voided specimen is tested for
   protein. Two hours later, after
   the patient has been standing
   and walking about, another urine
   specimen is tested for proteinuria. The patient may have postural proteinuria if the first urine
   specimen is negative for protein
   and the second urine specimen is
   positive. Patients with postural
   proteinuria should have repeated
   urine protein tests and be followed closely. A small percentage
   of patients develop significant
   renal disease.

d. Normally, protein is not found in
   the urine of healthy individuals.
   If it is found, it is usually albumin. Persistent proteinuria is an
   indication of renal disease. For
   the most accurate estimate of
   urine protein, a 24-hour urine
   collection is done.

(1) Protein
   excretion
   >4 g/
   24 hours

(1) Seen in nephrotic syndrome, glomerulonephritis (acute/chronic), lupus nephritis, amyloidosis, and in severe venous congestion of the kidneys (9, 11).

(2) Protein
   excretion
   0.5–4 g/
   24 hours

(2) Moderate amounts of proteinuria are seen in nephrotoxicities (toxins due to drugs, pathogens, chemicals, poisons, radiation, etc.), urinary tract infections, diabetic nephropathy, hematologic diseases, pyelonephritis with hypertension, renal tubular acidosis, Fanconi's syndrome, medullary cystic disease, and those diseases listed in (1).

(3) Protein
   excretion
   <0.5 g/
   24 hours

(3) Chronic pyelonephritis, polycystic diseases, renal tubular disease, orthostatic proteinuria, hematuria, and urinary tract infections may show a slight amount of urine protein. A negative urine test for protein does not rule out renal disease.

6. Glycosuria

6. Conditions showing glucose in the urine are:

a. Glycosuria with hyperglycemia

a. Diabetes mellitus, pituitary and adrenal disorders, pancreatic disease, hyperthyroidism, pheochromocytoma, disturbances of metabolism (burns, shock, emotional stress, MI, infection, fractures, etc.). From liver disease, glycogen storage disease, obesity, high carbohydrate diet, hyperalimentation too fast, pregnancy, and some drugs (See Drug Influences).

b. Glycosuria without hyperglycemia

b. Renal tubular dysfunction, with the kidney's inability to reabsorb glucose, results in glycosuria. Examples of some causes are drugs, poisons, pregnancy, congenital metabolic disorders, or Fanconi's syndrome.

7. Ketonuria

7. Ketonuria is seen in conditions that require the body to utilize increased amounts of fats for energy, resulting in increased ketone production. Examples of such conditions are uncontrolled diabetes mellitus, vomiting, diarrhea, starvation, conditions that increase the metabolic rate (cold, fever, exercise, hyperthyroidism), glycogen storage disease, ketogenic diets, and hypoglycemia. Urine containing phenylketones may show a false positive. See Drug Influences for list of drugs influencing ketone testing.

False positives

8. Occult blood (hemoglobinuria)

8. Test is for heme. This test is done as well as the microscopic exam. May be influenced by drugs. See Drug Influences.

a. Strenuous exercise

a. Seen following strenuous exercise due to the direct trauma to small vessels.

b. Artificial
   heart valves
   After frozen
   RBC
   transfusions
   Hemolytic
   uremic
   syndrome
   Thrombotic
   thrombocytopenic
   purpura
   Transfusion
   reaction
   Toxins
   Malaria
   Severe
   burns
   Hemolytic
   anemias

b. Hemoglobinuria is seen following hemolytic response.

c. Lupus
   erythematosus
   Viral
   infections
   Syphilis

c. The hemoglobinuria is seen in autoimmune disorders. These reactions are precipitated by cold.

d. Paroxysmal nocturnal hemoglobinuria

d. This is an acquired disease in which the red cell is susceptible

e. False positives

9. Microscopic exam

a. WBC

b. RBCs

(1) Renal disease

(2) Postrenal disease

(3) Extrarenal

c. Bacteria or yeast

to complement action hemolysis.

e. Hypochlorites (e.g., bleach) may cause a false positive.

9. The microscopic exam may be done on a drop of sediment or on a drop of well-mixed uncentrifuged urine.

a. WBCs are best identified in fresh urine. The white cells identified are principally neutrophiles. Normally only rare WBCs are seen. Increased numbers are in almost all renal and urinary tract diseases. Transient increases in WBCs may be seen during febrile illness and strenuous exercises. Large numbers of WBCs are indicative of infection.

b. An occasional RBC is all that is seen in a normal urine specimen. Increases can come from a variety of conditions.

(1) Renal disease is suspected as the source for RBCs in urine, especially if accompanied by red blood cell casts.

(2) RBCs are present, but proteinuria and red blood cell casts are missing. Examples are stricture, calculi, bladder infections, etc.

(3) RBCs may be found in urine from toxic drug reactions, hematologic disease, febrile illnesses, subacute bacterial endocarditis, invading tumors of the lower abdomen, and renovascular hypertension. Lordosis or strenuous exercise may cause a temporary increase in RBCs. Trauma from catheterization or from manipulating (pulling) catheter will also cause a temporary increase.

c. It is not unusual to see a few bacteria or yeast on microscopic exam. This is usually due to perineal contamination. If large num-

d. Cylindruria (increased casts)

d. The source of casts is from mucoproteins that precipitate and mold to the form of the lumina in which they originate. Normally there are no casts as there is trace to no protein in normal urine. Generally, the presence of casts in the urine indicates renal disease. The formation of casts is encouraged by urinary stasis, acid urine, increased solutes, and the presence of protein.

(1) Hyaline casts

(1) Increased numbers may be seen during febrile illnesses, after strenuous exercise, in orthostatic proteinuria, or following diuretic therapy. The casts are transient and do not necessarily mean renal disease. Hyaline casts are also seen in acute renal inflammatory disease, renal hypertension, heart failure, and diabetic renal disease.

(2) Red blood cell casts

(2) The presence of RBC casts generally indicates glomerular damage.

(3) White blood cell casts

(3) WBC casts are indicative of acute or chronic pyelonephritis.

(4) Granular casts

(4) These casts may be seen after strenuous exercise or during a totally carbohydrate diet. Generally these casts are indicative of serious renal disease. They may also be seen in lead poisoning or in viral diseases.

(5) Waxy casts

(5) The most serious casts are the broad waxy casts of end-stage renal disease. They are seen most often in patients with chronic renal failure.

The passage at the top of the right column continues: bers of bacteria are seen as well as leukocytes, infection is probably present. A nitrite dipstick may be done to identify the presence of bacteria.

e. Crystals

e. Crystals are found in normal urine and are usually of little clinical significance. A few very specific crystals are important. Cystine crystals are seen in patients with cystinosis, and may cause large renal calculi. Patients with severe liver disease may have tyrosine or leucine crystals. Some medications in high dosages also cause crystalluria, and these are probably identified as sulfonamide crystals. Normal alkaline urine crystals are:
Ammonium phosphates
Amorphous phosphates
Calcium carbonate
Calcium phosphate
Triple phosphates

f. Epithelial cells

f. A few epithelial cells are found in normal urine. Large numbers of epithelial cells are abnormal and may be indicative of renal tubular degeneration.

10. Odor

10. Deteriorating urine has a strong ammonia smell. Asparagus causes a very distinctive odor. Certain congenital metabolic conditions cause distinctive odors. PKU causes a mousey odor; maple syrup disease produces urine that smells like maple syrup. Pyuria has a very offensive odor.

11. Volume

11. Urine volume increases occur due to:
Increased fluid intake
Increased serum osmolality, especially increased glucose
Diuresis due to drugs, food, alcohol
Diminished ADH release
Renal damage

Conditions Related to Decreases

1. Color

Rationale

1. Dilution of the pigment urochrome will diminish the normal straw color of urine.

2. Specific gravity

    a. Diabetes insipidus

    b. Renal damage

    c. Cold urine

3. Aciduria ($\downarrow$ pH)

    a. Sleep

    b. Diet

    c. Acidosis
       Respiratory/
       metabolic

    d. Drugs

4. Protein

5. Glucose

6. Volume

2. Dilution of solutes with increased fluid volume decreases specific gravity.

    a. Due to lack of ADH, the kidneys produce excessive urine.

    b. Tubular damage may affect the kidneys' ability to concentrate urine.

    c. Urine right out of the refrigerator will have a falsely low specific gravity.

3. Listed below are some of the causes of decreased urine pH. Urinary pH should only be tested on fresh urine.

    a. A mild acidosis is experienced during sleep because of diminished respirations.

    b. The average adult diet causes a slightly acid urine of about pH 6. A diet high in meat protein and fruits (not citrus) decreases the pH. Vegetarian diets tend to increase pH.

    c. Conditions that cause metabolic or respiratory acidosis will cause acidic urine. For example, diabetes mellitus, dehydration, diarrhea, fever, respiratory conditions, ketogenic diets, etc.

    d. Certain drugs may cause acidic urine. See Drug Influences.

4. Causes of decreased proteinuria may be due to a very dilute specimen or false negatives induced by a very alkaline urine.

5. Falsely low glucose levels may be reported if directions for specific test are not followed carefully.

6. Urine volume decreases occur due to:
    Diminished water intake
    Loss of body water
    Decreased renal blood flow and ischemia
    Transfusion reactions
    Obstruction
    Increased ADH secretion
    Renal disease

Drug Influences: Many drugs influence the results of a urinalysis. Listed below are some of the drugs that may influence test results. The drugs are listed alphabetically by generic name and divided into columns according to the effect of the drug. Examples of trade names are in parentheses.

The following drugs may cause an increase in test results:

Color

Red or Pink

aniline dye (foods/candies)
danthron (Dorbane, Duolax)
deferoxamine mesylate (Desferal mesylate)
levodopa; red on voiding, then turns dark
phenolphthalein (Evac-Q-Kit, Sarolax)

phenolsulfonphthalein
phenothiazines; multicolored reaction
rifampin (Rifadin)
sulfobromophthalein

Orange, orange-red, or yellow-orange

cascara; in alkaline urine
chlorzoxazone (Flexaphen, Paraflex); orange to purple-red
ethoxazene (Serenium)

indandione anticoagulants (Miradon, Dipaxin, Hedulin)
phenazopyridine (Azodine, Pyridium)
sulfasalazine (Azulfidine)

Yellow

fluorescein, IV (Funduscein Injections)
quinacrine (Atabrine Hydrochloride)

riboflavin (vitamin B_2)

Green, green-blue

Doan's pills
indomethacin (Indocin)
methylene blue

triamterene (Dyazide, Dyrenium)

Brown, brown-red, or dark

antipyrine (Auralgan Otic Solution); may turn green in reflected light (9)
cascara; in acid urine
chloroquine (Aralen)
furazolidone (Furoxone)

iron preparations
metronidazole (Flagyl)
nitrofurantoin (Macrodantin)
sulfamethoxazole (Bactrim, Septra)

Appearance

Cloudy

carbonates
phosphates

x-ray contrast media; in acid urine

Specific Gravity

Increases, S.G.

albumin (Albumin, Albuconn)
dextran

glucose
x-ray contrast media

pH

Alkaline urine
acetazolamide (Diamox)
amphotericin B (Fungizone, Mysteclin-F)
epinephrine
mafenide (Sulfamylon Cream)
niacinamide (Albafort, Natalins)
parathyroid extract (Parathormone)
triamterene (Dyazide, Dyrenium)

Protein

Nephrotoxic effect
acetaminophen
acids; if ingested
amphotericin B
ampicillin
aspirin
bacitracin
capreomycin
carbon tetrachloride
cephaloridine
chlorpropamide
codeine
colistin
corticosteroids; chronic treatment of children
edetate (E.D.T.A.)
furosemide
gentamicin
gold
griseofulvin
heroin
kanamycin
methicillin
mithramycin
mitomycin
neomycin
polymyxin
probenecid
trimethadione
viomycin

False positives
acetazolamide
aminosalicylic acid
bicarbonates
chlorhexidine (Hibiclens, Hibitane Tincture)
phenazopyridine
x-ray contrast media

Glucose

Glycosuria
ammonium chloride (Triaminicol)
aspirin
carbamazepine (Tegretol)
chlorpromazine (Thorazine)
chlorthalidone (Hygroton, Combipres)
corticosteroids
dextrothyroxine (Choloxin)
lithium
phenothiazines (Chlorpromazine, Phenergan, Thorazine)
thiazides (Aquapres, HydroDiuril, Diuril)

False positive, Clinitest
ascorbic acid; in many antibiotics, also
cephalosporins (Ancef, Keflin)
chloramphenicol (Chloromycetin)
levodopa; large doses
metaxalone (Skelaxin)
nalidixic acid (NegGram)
probenecid (Benemid)
salicylates; high doses

False positive, Benedict's
aminosalicylic acid
chloral hydrate
chloramphenicol (Chloromycetin)
isoniazid (INH)
metaxalone (Skelaxin)
nalidixic acid (NegGram)
nitrofurantoin (Furadantin)
penicillin G; large doses

probenecid (Benemid)
streptomycin

False positive Clinistix, Diastix
   ascorbic acid; in many antibiotics
   levodopa
   phenazopyridine (Pyridium, Azo
     Gantanol)
   salicylates; in high doses
   tetracycline

False positive, Tes-tape
   ascorbic acid; in many antibiotics
   levodopa
   methyldopa (Aldomet)
   phenazopyridine (Pyridium, Azo
     Gantanol)
   tetracycline

Ketones

Ketonuria
   aspirin
   ethanol
   ether
   insulin; dose too high
   isoniazid

isopropanol; dose too high
metformin
niacin
phenformin
triclofos

False positives
   bromsulphalein (BSP dye)
   levodopa; ketostix or Phenistix
   phenazopyridine (Azo Gantanol,
     Pyridium); ketostix or ferric chloride
     test

phenolphthalein (Ex-Lax, Feen-A-Mint);
  Ketostix, Acetest, Rothera test
pyrazinamide (Tebrazid); ketostix,
  Acetest, Rothera test

Occult blood
   Hypochlorites (bleach)

Microscopic

RBCs ↑
   acetaminophen
   allopurinol (Zyloprim)
   aminosalicylic acid
   amphotericin B (Fungizone, Mysteclin-
     F)
   aspirin
   bacitracin (Neosporin, Polysporin)
   caffeine
   coumarin (Dicumarol, Panwarfin)
   gold (Myochrysine)
   indomethacin (Indocin)

kanamycin (Kantrex)
lipomul
mefenamic acid (Ponstel)
methenamine (Prosed, Trac Tabs)
methicillin
phenylbutazone (Butazolidin)
phytonadione (AquaMephyton)
polymyxin
sulfonamides
thiazides (Diuril, Aquapres)

WBCs ↑
   allopurinol (Zyloprim)
   ampicillin
   aspirin toxicity
   capreomycin (Capastat)

kanamycin
levodopa
methicillin

Casts
   amphotericin B (Fungizone, Mysteclin-
     F)
   aspirin toxicity

isoniazid (INH)
kanamycin
neomycin

bacitracin (Polysporin, Neosporin)
furosemide (Lasix)
gentamicin
griseofulvin (Fulvicin)

penicillin
polymyxin B
sulfonamides
trimethadione (Tridione)

Crystals; in acidic urine
  acetazolamide
  aminosalicylic acid
  ascorbic acid
  nitrofurantoin

theophylline (Theo-Dur)
thiazide diuretics (Diuril, HydroDiuril)

Cells
  acetaminophen
  aspirin
  caffeine
  calcitonin (Calcimar)

castor oil
cortisone; long-term treatment

The following drugs may cause a decrease in test values:

Cells
  acetaminophen
  aspirin
  caffeine
  calcitonin (Calcimar)

castor oil
cortisone; long-term treatment

Color ↓
  ethanol

S.G. ↓
  methoxyflurane (Penthrane)

Acid urine (pH ↓ *)*
  ammonium chloride (Triaminicol)
  ascorbic acid
  corticotropin (ACTH)
  diazoxide (Hyperstat I.V., Proglycem)

glucose
methenamine (Mandelamine, Urex,
  Hexalet)
metolazone (Diulo, Zaroxolyn)
niacin (Nicobid, Niacin)

Glucose ↓ *on testing*

Clinistix
  ampicillin
  ascorbic acid
  bisacodyl (Dulcolax)
  chloral hydrate
  diazepam (Valium)
  digoxin
  epinephrine
  ferrous sulfate
  flurazepam (Dalmane)
  furosemide (Lasix)
  levodopa
  phenobarbital
  prednisone
  secobarbital

Diastix
  ampicillin
  bisacodyl (Dulcolax)
  chloral hydrate
  diazepam (Valium)
  digoxin
  ferrous sulfate
  flurazepam (Dalmane)
  furosemide (Lasix)
  phenobarbital
  prednisone
  secobarbital
  vitamin preparations

vitamin preparations
Tes-Tape
   ascorbic acid

Related Lab Studies: Some of the related studies are listed below:
   urine culture
   BUN
   creatinine, creatinine clearance
   urine osmolality
   CBC
   electrolytes
   *PSP or PAH
   *radioisotope renogram
   *concentration test (e.g., Addis or Fishberg)
   *urine cytology
   *I.V.P.
   *K.U.B.
   *retrograde pyelogram
   *cystourethrography
   *renal angiography

IMPLICATIONS FOR NURSING CARE
PRETEST: Factors related to the test
Nursing Diagnosis: Potential for injury related to changes in biochemical balance

Guide to assessment	Guide to planning and intervention	Guide to evaluation
Assess patient factors that may influence test results: 1. Fluids	1. Do not force fluids.	1. Patient's test results are not diluted.
2. Comprehensive drug history	2. Note on lab slip drugs that may influence test results.	2. Patient's drugs that may influence test values are noted on lab slip.
3. Preexisting conditions (See Increases/Decreases)	3. Note preexisting conditions that may influence test results.	3. Patient's preexisting conditions that may influence test results are recorded.
4. Contaminants	4. Prevent contamination of specimen by:	4. Patient's test values are not influenced by contaminants.
a. Perineal	a. Performing or teaching patient the procedure for a clean catch midstream urine.	
b. From hands	b. Teaching patient to wash hands prior to collection and not to touch inside or edges of collection container.	

*Not discussed in this book.

Guide to assessment	Guide to planning and intervention	Guide to evaluation
c. Vaginal	c. Instructing female patient to insert a vaginal tampon if patient has interfering vaginal discharge.	
5. Nursing staff factors influencing test results. a. Old urine	5. Prevent false results due to staff mismanagement: a. Send urine to lab or refrigerate immediately after collection. Note time and date of collection.	5. Patient's lab values are not influenced by: a. Deteriorating specimen or
b. Use of dipstix, urinometer, refractometer, clinitest tablets, acetest tablets c. Double voiding Glucose testing d. pH testing	b. Use correct directions and color chart for test being performed. c. Have patient double void when testing for glucose; test both urine samples. d. Test pH on fresh specimen only, specimen after first morning voiding and between meals. Note diet.	b. Incorrect use of materials or c. False urine glucose result or d. False pH result.
6. Knowledge deficit	6. Explain test to patient: a. Define test (See Description). b. Explain procedure (See Procedure, hospital procedure manual, or any nursing fundamentals text).	6. Patient demonstrates knowledge by defining test and explaining procedure.
7. Knowledge deficit about urinary tract health.	7. Promote health of urinary tract by: a. Encouraging daily fluid intake. b. Encouraging adequate activity daily. c. Encouraging a balanced diet. d. Keeping genitalia clean and dry. e. Emphasizing to female patients to cleanse perineal area *from* meatus to rectum; emphasizing to male patients to cleanse area *from* scrotum to rectum. f. Discouraging use of chemical irritants during bath (bubble bath, bath crystals, etc.).	7. Patient's urinalysis is normal.

Patient Preparation Checklist

1. √ Note influencing drugs on lab slip (See Drug Influences).
2. √ Note preexisting conditions on lab slip.
3. √ Take measures to prevent contamination (See 4 above).
4. √ Correct procedure (See Procedure and 5 above).
5. √ Patient knowledge; explain test (See Description/Procedure).

CONSIDERATIONS FOR NURSING CARE RELATED TO ABNORMAL TEST RESULTS

POSTTEST: Factors related to the results of the test

Nursing Diagnosis: Alterations in biochemical balance

Guide to assessment	Guide to planning and intervention	Guide to evaluation
Assess patient factors that may be influencing test results.		
Nursing history and/or physical exam suggestive of:		
1. Abnormal urinalysis	1. Recognize and report abnormal findings.	1. Patient's abnormal findings are recognized and physician informed.
2. Specific gravity imbalances Hydration status	2. Promote specific gravity within normal limits by: a. Maintaining adequate hydration. b. Recognizing fluid retention in response to ADH secretion. c. Recognizing fluid loss from osmotic diuresis. d. Recognizing changes in I&O and daily weight values.	2. Patient's hydration status is normal for age.
3. Urinary pH changes a. Neonate Aged At-risk for acid-base imbalances	3. Manipulate pH to appropriate levels by: a. Testing pH 3–4 times per day.	3. a. At-risk patients do not experience acid-base imbalances.

Guide to assessment	Guide to planning and intervention	Guide to evaluation
b. Urinary tract infections Calcium renal stones Immobilized patients	b. Maintaining alkaline urine as appropriate to specific treatment or renal calculi prevention.	b. Patient's urine remains alkaline.
c. Urinary tract infections	c. Maintaining acid urine to prevent growth of urea-splitting bacteria.	c. The patient remains infection-free.
d. Renal tubular acidosis	d. Recognizing that urine pH does not drop below 6–6.5 and consulting with physician.	d. Patient's abnormal pH is recognized and physician consulted.
4. Proteinuria	4. Promote kidney function by:	4. Patient's proteinuria is negative to trace, and kidney function tests are normal.
a. Transient proteinuria	a. Recognizing and correcting transient proteinuria by: (1) Informing physician. (2) Replacing fluid volume. (3) Reducing fever. (4) Encouraging non-stressful environment.	
b. Postural proteinuria	b. Stressing the need for follow-up of orthostatic proteinuria to young adult patients.	
c. Kidney disease or at-risk	c. Encouraing maximum renal function: (1) Keep accurate I&O records and daily weights for assessment purposes. (2) Be alert to signs of edema. (3) Provide adequate fluid intake. (4) Prevent urinary tract infections (See 7 below). (5) Be alert to nephrotoxic agents from toxins due to drugs, pathogens, poisons, chemicals, and radiation, and remove offending agent. (6) Prepare and assist with dialysis as needed.	
d. Dilute urine and proteinuria	d. Prevent falsely low protein analysis by not testing	

Guide to assessment	Guide to planning and intervention	Guide to evaluation
	dilute urine. First morning specimen is best with specific gravity of at least 1.020.	
5. Glycosuria/hyperglycemia	5. Maintain blood glucose equilibrium: a. Recognize and report signs/symptoms of blood glucose imbalance. b. Test urine for glucose: (1) Choose correct testing material (See Drug Influences). (2) Follow product directions precisely. (3) Have patient double void and check both specimens. (4) Check urine before meals. (5) Teach the patient how to test urine and watch return demonstration. c. Recognize and report signs/symptoms of blood glucose imbalance. d. Recognize and report signs/symptoms of dehydration.	5. The patient's glucose equilibrium is maintained as shown by blood and urine glucose results.
e. Aged Pregnancy Females Obesity Hyperalimentation Disturbances of metabolism See 6, Increases	e. Be alert to patients at-risk.	
6. Ketonuria Conditions. See 7 Increases	6. Maintain sufficient glucose for energy utilization: a. Recognize and report signs/symptoms of ketoacidosis. b. Test urine for ketones: (1) Choose correct testing material (See Drug Influences). (2) Follow product directions precisely.	6. Patient is provided with sufficient glucose for energy utilization as shown by negative ketone testing.

Guide to assessment	Guide to planning and intervention	Guide to evaluation
	(3) Have patient double void; check both specimens. c. Recognize causes of false positives.	
7. Microscopic exam positive	7. Promote healthy environment for urinary tract: a. Encourage perineal hygiene (See Pretest 7). b. Recognize patients at risk for developing urinary tract infections. c. Initiate nursing care to prevent infection in debilitated patient: (1) Keep perineal area clean. (2) Catheterize patients using sterile technique. (3) Initiate nursing measures for catheterized patient. (4) Provide noncatheterized patient proper positioning to void. (5) Prevent urinary stasis by changing patient's position. (6) Provide dietary or drug induced acid urine as indicated. d. Maintain adequate fluid intake.	7. The patient is free of urinary tract disease.
e. ↑ WBC	e. Encourage fluids, report to physician, administer antibiotics.	
f. ↑ RBC	f. Localize source by checking for casts, drugs patient is receiving, trauma from catheterization, other possible source of bleeding.	
g. Bacteria	g. Determine if specimen is contaminated, obtain catch urine, observe for other signs of infection, inform physician, increase fluid intake if appropriate.	

Guide to assessment	Guide to planning and intervention	Guide to evaluation
h. Cylindruria	h. Recognize abnormal report (See Increases, 9 Microscopic Exam), bring to physician's attention.	
i. Crystals of Cystine Tyrosine Leucine Sulfonamide	i. Recognize abnormal crystal report and inform physician; prevent crystal formation by encouraging fluid intake and diet proper to type of calculi.	
j. Epithelial cells; large amount	j. Bring to attention of physician.	

Test:	Urobilinogen
Abbreviation:	None
Reference Values:	Men 0.3–2.1 Ehrlich U/2 hours Women 0.1–1.1 Ehrlich U/2 hours Random specimen 0.3–3.5 mg/100 ml
Specimen:	Urine

Description: Bilirubin joined by glucuronic acid in the liver becomes conjugated bilirubin. This conjugated bilirubin is excreted with bile into the small intestine. In the intestines it is reduced by bacterial enzymes to urobilinogen. Urobilinogen is mostly excreted by the intestine and gives feces its brown color. A small amount of urobilinogen is reabsorbed from the intestine and is reexcreted by the liver into the bile. Part of this reabsorbed urobilinogen is excreted in the urine. The peak hours of urobilinogen excretion are 1 P.M.–3 P.M.

This test is done to differentiate liver disease, hemolytic disease, and common bile duct blockage.

Procedure:

Random Urine

1. Collect fresh clean catch urine, preferably between 1 P.M. and 3 P.M.
    Protect specimen from light.
2. If testing with dipstick method, test immediately.
3. If sending to lab, send to lab immediately. Give to laboratory personnel and tell them what test is to be performed.
4. This test shows only the presence of urobilinogen, not the absence.

2-Hour Timed Collection

1. Have patient void at 1 P.M. (preferably). Discard urine.
2. At 3 P.M. collect clean catch urine.
    Protect specimen from light.
3. Send to lab immediately and hand to lab personnel, stating what test is to be done.

Conditions Related to Increases

1. Hemolytic diseases, e.g.
    Sickle-cell anemia
    Disorders of glutathione metabolism
    Acquired hemolytic anemia
    Hemolytic disease of the newborn
    Lead poisoning, etc.
2. Liver disease

Rationale

1. Increased hemoglobin breakdown increases intestinal urobilinogen, and subsequently, urine urobilinogen rises.

2. Often an early indicator of liver disease. The diseased liver is unable to reabsorb or reexcrete circulating urobilinogen.

Conditions Related to Decreases	Rationale
1. Obstruction of bile duct, e.g. Carcinoma of the head of the pancreas	1. With complete obstruction of the bile duct, no bilirubin enters the bowel. Consequently, no urobilinogen enters the urine.
2. Drugs	2. Certain drugs may decrease urobilinogen by reducing bacterial activity or decreasing enzyme activity.

Drug Influences: The following drugs may influence test results. The drugs are listed alphabetically by generic name and divided into columns according to the effect of the drug. Examples of trade names are in parentheses.

The following drugs may cause an increase in urine urobilinogen:

Hemolysis; any drug causing hemolysis
   antipyrine
   chloroquine (Aralen HCl, Chlorocon); in G-6PD deficiency
   methyldopa; autoimmune hemolytic anemia
   novobiocin; in G-6PD deficiency
   vitamin K; in G-6PD deficiency

Increased excretion
   acetazolamide (Diamox)
   sodium bicarbonate

Interferes with reagent
   aminosalicylic acid
   mandelate
   phenazopyridine (Azodine, Pyridium)
   phenothiazines
   sulfonamides

The following drugs may decrease test values:

Inhibits intestinal bacterial action
   antibiotics

Acidifies urine, decreases excretion
   ammonium salts
   ascorbic acid

Cholestatic effect
   androgens
   mepazine
   methimazole (Tapazole)
   oral contraceptives
   phenothiazines
   sulfonamides
   thiazides
   tolazamide (Tolinase)

Related Lab Studies:

bilirubin, serum and urine
AST (SGOT)
ALT (SGPT)
alkaline phosphatase
serum protein electrophoresis
prothrombin time
*BSP test
*thymol turbidity

IMPLICATIONS FOR NURSING CARE
PRETEST: Factors related to the test
Nursing Diagnosis: Potential for injury related to changes in biochemical balance

Guide to assessment	Guide to planning and intervention	Guide to evaluation
Assess patient factors that may influence test results: 1. Comprehensive drug history (See Drug Influences)	1. Identify drugs the patient is taking that may interfere with test result. Consult with physician. Note interfering drugs on lab slip.	1. Patient's test values are not influenced by medication.
2. Preexisting conditions (See Increases/Decreases)	2. Note pertinent preexisting conditions on lab slip.	2. Patient's preexisting conditions are noted on lab slip.
3. Knowledge deficit	3. Explain test to patient: a. Define test (See Description). b. Explain procedure (See Procedure).	3. Patient demonstrates knowledge by defining testing and stating procedure.
4. Care of specimen a. Exposed to light b. Specimen older than one-half hour	4. Protect specimen from oxidizing to urobilin by: a. Protecting specimen from light. b. Giving specimen to lab personnel immediately.	4. Patient's lab values are correct.
5. Fecal urobilinogen contamination	5. Protect specimen from fecal urobilinogen by collecting a clean catch urine.	5. Patient's lab values are correct.

*Not discussed in this book.

Patient Preparation Checklist

1. √ Interfering drugs; note on lab slip (See Drug Influences).
2. √ Preexisting conditions; note pertinent information on lab slip (See Increases/Decreases).
3. √ Patient knowledge; explain test to patient (See Description/Procedure).
4. √ Care of specimen. See 4 and 5 above.

CONSIDERATIONS FOR NURSING CARE RELATED TO ABNORMAL TEST RESULTS
POSTTEST: Factors related to the results of the test
Nursing Diagnosis: Alterations in biochemical balance

Guide to assessment	Guide to planning and intervention	Guide to evaluation
Assess patient factors that may be influencing test results. Nursing history and/or physical exam that is suggestive of:		
1. Liver disease Biliary obstruction Hemolytic disease	1. Implement medical plan to treat underlying cause of abnormal urobilinogen values.	1. The urobilinogen returns to normal.
See Bilirubin for complete discussion.		

Test:	Vanillylmandelic Acid
Abbreviation:	VMA
Reference Values:	1–12 months 1.40–15.0 mg/g creatinine
	1–2 years 1.25–8.0 mg/g creatinine
	2–5 years 1.50–7.5 mg/g creatinine
	5–10 years 0.50–6.0 mg/g creatinine
	10–15 years 0.25–3.25 mg/g creatinine (46)
	Adults 1.5–7.5 mg/24 hours
Specimen:	24-hour urine collection
Description:	Vanillylmandelic acid is a metabolite of the catecholamines epinephrine and norepinephrine. Catecholamines are hormones and amines produced in the brain, sympathetic ganglia, and the adrenal medulla. Catecholamines are almost completely metabolized before they appear in the urine so concentrations of VMA are higher than total catecholamine levels. Measurements of urinary VMA have the same physiological significance as catecholamine values and are performed primarily in the diagnosis of pheochromocytoma and neuroblastoma. VMA is usually measured with HVA (homovanillic acid is the metabolite of the catecholamine dopamine). Foods and drugs may produce falsely elevated VMA levels, so patients may be on a special regimen 2–3 days before the test is started.
Procedure:	1. Amine-rich foods may or may not be restricted. Check with local lab. If restricted, the foods include fruits, coffee, tea, and foods containing vanilla.
	2. Collection is in dark bottle that is acidified with hydrochloric acid.
	3. The urine should be refrigerated during entire collection.
	4. Collection.
	a. Discard first voided specimen.
	b. For next 24 hours, place all voidings into specimen container immediately after voiding.
	c. Have patient void just prior to completion of the 24 hours and put sample in collection bottle.
	5. Record exact start and finish times on lab slip.
	6. Send to lab immediately.

Conditions Related to Increases

Conditions Related to Increases	Rationale
1. Pheochromocytoma	1. This is a tumor of chromaffin tissue secreting increased amounts of catecholamines, resulting in increased production of VMA.
2. Neuroblastomas, ganglioneuromas, and ganglioblastomas	2. All are tumors arising in sympathetic or adrenal medullary tissue and producing increased amounts of catecholamines.

3. Carotid body tumor

3. The carotid bodies normally stimulate the sympathetic nervous system when oxygen concentration of the blood diminishes. The tumor may cause increased activation of this mechanism and pressure on the carotid sinus, which stimulates the sympathetic system.

4. Stress, e.g.
   Burns
   Surgery
   Childbirth
   Overwhelming infections
   Trauma, etc.

4. Stress causes an increased output of catecholamines, which break down into VMA.

5. Certain tumors, such as:
   Retinoblastoma
   Carcinoid tumors

5. Kinins (biologically active polypeptides) are physiologically active in carcinoid syndromes, and catecholamines are thought to act as mediators of the kinin system (51).

Drug Influences: The following drugs may influence test results. The drugs are listed alphabetically by generic name and divided into columns according to the effect of the drug. Examples of trade names are in parentheses.

The following drugs may cause an increase in test results:

Release of metabolites
   ajmaline
   epinephrine
   levarterenol (Levophed)

   rauwolfia
   reserpine

Interferes with lab method
   disulfiram (Antabuse)
   glyceryl guaiacolate (Robitussin)

   hydroxymandelic acid
   mephenesin (Tolserol)
   salicylates

Miscellaneous
   chlorpromazine (Thorazine)
   insulin; after insulin shock
   isoproterenol
   levodopa; slight

   lithium; slight
   methyldopa (Aldomet)
   nitroglycerin
   prochlorperazine (Compazine)

The following drugs may cause a decrease in test results:

Inhibition of metabolite formation
   disulfiram (Antabuse)
   imipramine
   isocarboxazid

   levodopa
   MAO inhibitors

Miscellaneous

clonidine (Catapres)
debrisoquin
guanethidine (Ismelin)
methyldopa (Aldomet)
morphine

phenothiazines (Thorazine, Prolixin,
 Compazine)
radiographic agents
reserpine (Serpasil)

Related Lab Studies: In diagnosis of pheochromocytoma or neuroblastoma:

↑ catecholamines
↑ homovanillic acid
  GTT (diabetic curve)
* histamine pressor test
* phentolamine pressor test
* tyramine pressor test

IMPLICATIONS FOR NURSING CARE
PRETEST: Factors related to the test
Nursing Diagnosis: Potential for injury related to changes in biochemical balance

Guide to assessment	Guide to planning and intervention	Guide to evaluation
Assess patient factors that may influence test results:		
1. Food and fluids	1. Do not schedule test while patient is NPO. Check with specific laboratory about food restrictions (See Procedure).	1. Food ingestion, or lack of, does not influence lab results.
2. Exercise and stress	2. Avoid excessive physical activity while 24-hour sample is being obtained. Avoid stressful situations during 24-hour sample collection time.	2. Lab results are not influenced by exercise or stress.
3. Comprehensive drug history (See Drug Influences)	3. Report drugs the patient is currently receiving that may influence lab results to the patient's physician and to the lab (drugs may be withheld as long as 72 hours prior to the exam). Instruct patient to avoid taking aspirin for 3 days prior to the exam.	3. Drugs patient is currently receiving that may influence test results are identified and proper people notified. Lab results will not be influenced by ingestion of nonessential drugs.
4. Preexisting conditions (See Increases/Decreases)	4. Record preexisting conditions on lab slip.	4. Patient's preexisting conditions are noted on lab slip.

5. Knowledge deficit	5. Explain test to patient:
	  a. Define vanillylmandelic acid (See Description).
	  b. Explain procedure (See Procedure).
		5. Patient demonstrates knowledge of test by defining test and explaining procedure. 24-hour urine collection is correct.

*Not discussed in this book.

Patient Preparation Checklist

1. √ Restricted foods omitted from diet for 3 days before exam.
2. √ Patient not NPO.
3. √ Decrease exercise and stress during 24-hour urine collection.
4. √ Influencing drugs noted and reported (See Drug Influences).
5. √ Preexisting conditions noted on lab slip (See Increases/Decreases).
6. √ Patient knowledge; explain test and procedure (See Description and Procedure).

CONSIDERATIONS FOR NURSING CARE RELATED TO ABNORMAL TEST RESULTS
POSTTEST: Factors related to the results of the test
Nursing Diagnosis: Alterations in biochemical balance

Guide to assessment	Guide to planning and intervention	Guide to evaluation
Assess patient factors influencing test results. Nursing history and/or physical exam suggestive of:		
1. Pheochromocytoma Neuroblastoma	1. Excessive catecholamine secretion is prevented by:	1. The patient demonstrates no excessive catecholamine secretion by:
	a. Protecting patient from excessive palpation of abdominal mass or manipulation of tumor by staff and students.	a. Being protected from excessive palpation by staff and students.
	b. Administering as ordered adjuvant chemotherapeutic drugs.	b. The patient receives medication ordered as scheduled.
2. Stress	2. Establishing a nonstressful environment for the patient with the patient's help.	2. The patient's VMA level is not increased due to stress.

Test:	Venereal Disease Research Laboratory
Abbreviation:	VDRL
Reference Value:	Nonreactive
Specimen:	Serum, CSF
Description:	Syphilis is a sexually transmitted disease caused by the spirochete *Treponema pallidum*. It is a disease that is easily treated. Lack of treatment can lead to serious health problems, however, and, in some cases, death.

The most common method of screening for syphilis is by use of the VDRL. The test identifies the antibody reagin. It takes about 10 days to 3 weeks for antibodies to form against the spirochete. The antibodies are demonstrated in the lab by their reaction with a lipid antigen. Tests are most useful in diagnosing primary and secondary syphilis. False positive VDRL results may occur. This test is useful as a screening test for syphilis and as a measure of response to therapy.

Another test that identifies reagin is called the rapid plasma reagin (RPR) test. It is rapidly becoming the more common test.

Procedure:

(red top tube)
1. Abstinence from alcohol for 24 hours is encouraged.
2. 10 ml of blood is withdrawn from the patient.
3. The serum is mixed with a lipid antigen. If the mixture causes flocculation, that is, island-like clumping, it is reactive. Serial dilutions of the serum are performed with the titer of antibody being the last visible dilution.
4. Observe puncture site for bleeding or evidence of hematoma.

Conditions Related to Positive Findings	Rationale
1. Syphilis	1. The test becomes positive after antibodies are formed against the spirochete and this takes about 10 days to 3 weeks. The test has variable results during tertiary syphilis. If syphilitic-like lesions are present, a positive VDRL is diagnostic of the disease.

2. Acute biologic false positives, e.g.
    Infectious mononucleosis
    Atypical pneumonia
    Chicken pox
    Rheumatic fever
    Subacute bacterial endocarditis
	2. False positive results caused by acute conditions other than syphilis. These are acute infectious diseases and the VDRL reverts to normal within 6 months.

3. Chronic biologic false positives, e.g.
   Malaria
   Leprosy
   Lupus erythematosus
   Hepatitis
   Rheumatoid arthritis

3. False positive results associated with conditions other than syphilis. The false positive reaction lasts more than 6 months.

Conditions Related to Decreases

Rationale

1. Nonreactive test

1. During the early stage of the disease, before antibodies have formed, the test may be nonreactive. If the history is positive, the test should be repeated in 2–3 weeks.

2. Successful therapy

2. After successful therapy for primary and secondary syphilis, test results usually revert to negative.

Drug Influences: Drugs apparently do not interfere with test results.

Related Lab Studies:

FTA-ABS

IMPLICATIONS FOR NURSING CARE
PRETEST: Factors related to the test
Nursing Diagnosis: Potential for injury related to changes in microbiological environment

Guide to assessment	Guide to planning and intervention	Guide to evaluation
Assess patient factors that may influence test results:		
1. Alcohol consumption	1. Advise patient not to drink alcoholic beverages for 24 hours prior to test as it interferes with test results.	1. Patient's lab values are not diminished by alcohol consumption.
2. Preexisting conditions (See Increases, 2 and 3)	2. Note preexisting conditions that might influence test results on lab slip.	2. Patient's conditions that may result in biologic false positives are noted on lab slip.
3. Hemolysis of specimen	3. Prevent hemolysis by: a. Not probing venipuncture site or leaving tourniquet on too long. b. Not forcefully withdrawing specimen. c. Not withdrawing specimen too slowly. d. Not agitating or handling specimen roughly. e. Not saturating skin with antiseptic.	3. Patient's test results are not influenced by hemolysis.

Guide to assessment	Guide to planning and intervention	Guide to evaluation

4. Knowledge deficit	4. Explain test to patient
	  a. Define test (See Definition).
	  b. Explain procedure (See Procedure).
		4. Patient demonstrates knowledge of test by defining test and explaining procedure.

5. Knowledge deficit
  Patient/public knowledge about sexually transmitted diseases (STD)
	5. Promote public awareness about STD by:
	  a. Being knowledgeable about the diseases.
	  b. Educating patients with STD about the diseases, diagnoses, and treatments.
	  c. Being knowledgeable about treatment facility options available (private and free clinics).
	  d. Informing patient that while condoms afford some protection against disease, there is still risk involved.
	  e. Informing patient that reporting the disease and case findings are important steps in preventing spread of disease.
	  f. Advising patient that treatment of known contacts of someone with diagnosed STD is a method of prevention.
	  g. Informing patients that infants of mothers with untreated syphilis are born with congenital syphilis.
	  h. Encouraging public education about STD.
		5. Statistics on STD improve.

Patient Preparation Checklist

1. √ No alcoholic beverages 24 hours prior to testing.
2. √ Note preexisting conditions on lab slip.
3. √ Prevention of hemolysis.
4. √ Patient knowledge about test; explain test to patient.
5. √ Patient/public knowledge about STD; inform patient/public.

CONSIDERATIONS FOR NURSING CARE RELATED TO ABNORMAL TEST RESULTS
POSTTEST: Factors related to the results of the test
Nursing Diagnosis: Alterations in microbiological balance

Guide to assessment	Guide to planning and intervention	Guide to evaluation
Assess patient factors influencing test results. Nursing history and/or physical exam suggestive of: 1. Syphilis	1. Establish treatment of disease: a. Refer to VDRL testing as appropriate. b. Administer antibiotics as prescribed. (Penicillin is drug of choice.) c. Follow patient response to therapy with follow-up VDRL or other tests or titers. d. See 5 Pretest.	1. Patient's positive test results revert to negative.

Test:	White Blood Cell Count and Differential
Abbreviation:	WBC, WBC diff.

Reference Values:

White blood cell count
1 day   7,000–35,000
1 week   4,000–20,000
1 month   6,000–18,000
3–5 months   6,000–17,000
6–11 months   6,000–16,000
1 year   6,000–15,000
2–10 years   7,000–13,000
11–15 years   5,000–12,000
Adults   4,300–10,000

Differential count
Neutrophiles   55%–70%
Lymphocytes   20%–40%
Monocytes   2%–8%
Eosinophiles   2%–4%
Basophiles   0.5%–1%

Specimen: Whole blood

Description: The white blood cell count (WBC) represents the total number of circulating leukocytes in the serum. The leukocytes are produced in the bone marrow and lymphatic tissue and enter the bloodstream, where they are transported to different areas of the body as they are needed. Hormones affect the production, storage, release, and disintegration of the WBC (8). The WBC indicates how the leukocytes are responding to various conditions of infection or inflammation. Increases in WBC help determine the presence of infection or inflammation and if there is need for further investigation. Decreases in WBC are most often caused by diseases, toxic reactions, or therapies (radiation, drugs) that suppress white blood cell formation.

In order to gain more specific information regarding the different cell types that comprise the leukocytes, a WBC differential is done in addition to the WBC. The differential determines the maturity of the cell and the percentage of the granulocytes (neutrophiles, eosinophiles, and basophiles) and the nongranulocytes (lymphocytes and monocytes) in the overall leukocyte count.* Overall, the differential provides specific information regarding the stage and severity of a disease or infection and the ability of the body to resist or overcome the infection. The specific functions of the five cell types are discussed in the following paragraphs.

---

*In order to interpret the differential accurately, the percentage value *and* the absolute value must be considered. The absolute value is determined by multiplying the percentage value of the individual cell grouping by the total WBC.

Neutrophiles ("segs," "polys," polymorphonuclear neutrophiles, PMN): These are the most numerous of the circulating leukocytes. Phagocytosis is the major mode of action. In the immature stages of development, the cells are referred to as "bands" or "stab" cells.† Neutrophiles are considered to be the body's primary line of defense against infection because they are the first cells to arrive at the inflammatory site. The counts are most often high in acute bacterial infections and whenever there is tissue damage.

Eosinophiles: Eosinophiles are phagocytic cells. They are normally found in the tissue in concentrations at least 100 times greater than in the blood and are primarily located in those tissues (skin, GI tract, lungs) that are regarded as "epithelial barriers to the outside world" (11). The function of eosinophiles is not completely understood. It is speculated that they detoxify foreign protein before it can cause damage to the body (11). Because they increase during allergic reactions and collect at sites of antigen-antibody reactions in the tissues, eosinophiles are associated with immune responses. They are also increased during the healing phase of inflammation.

Basophiles: These are the least numerous of the leukocytes. It is known that they release heparin and histamine. They play an active role in allergic and anaphylactic reactions and are associated with fibrinolysis in inflamed tissues (5). The cells are released during the healing phase of inflammation and during chronic inflammation.

Lymphocytes: Lymphocytes are receiving much attention in the area of immunology because they play a major role in immune reactivity.* They are present in early and late stages of the inflammation process and in chronic inflammation. Lymphocytes respond to what they consider foreign substances by an antigen reaction. They may also be responsible for storage of immunologic memory that causes subsequent exposure to an antigen to elicit an accelerated and increased response.

Monocytes: These cells form the second line of defense against infection. Through the process of phagocytosis they are able to engulf much larger and more numerous particles than those

---

†An increase in these immature cells is often described as a "shift to the left" since cell maturity is normally illustrated right to left, with the most immature cells being on the left. An increase in the number of bands indicates that the bone marrow is releasing cells that are not developed in order to try to keep up with the body's demand for neutrophiles. The WBC and the degree of this shift to the left help determine the severity of infection and the extent of the individual's resistance (5).

---

*The discussion of the categories of lymphocytes and their specific functions is not within the scope of this text.

acted on by neutrophiles. A major function is their ability to prepare tissue for healing and to combat chronic infection by removing injured and dead cells. Monocytes are able to ingest large protozoa such as fungi and parasites. Monocytes also have complex interactions with components of the immune system.*

Procedure: (lavender top tube)
1. No food or fluid restrictions.
2. A skin puncture or venipuncture is performed.
3. 0.5–5 cc of blood is collected from the patient.
4. Observe for bleeding at the puncture site or for evidence of hematoma.

Conditions Related to Increases (Leukocytosis)

Rationale

1. Physiologic conditions
   Pain
   Digestion
   Stress
   Exercise
   Diurnal rhythm
   Age (increase noted in newborns and infants; the normal adult values are usually reached about age 21) (8)
   Menstruation
   Pregnancy
   Labor

1. Stimulation for production and release of leukocytes is not clearly defined (21). In these conditions, the maximum level of WBC usually does not exceed twice the minimum normal level.

2. Hypovolemia, e.g.
   Dehydration
   Hemorrhage

2. This results in hemoconcentration which shows an overall rise in WBC.

3. Tissue damage, e.g.
   Burns
   Ulcers
   Carcinoma

3. An inflammatory response occurs in areas of tissue injury. This response increases the number of circulating leukocytes.

4. Neoplastic disorders of blood-forming organs
   Polycythemia vera
   Hodgkin's disease
   Leukemias
   Lymphomas

4. In these conditions, there is an abnormal proliferation and release of granulocytes and agranulocytes from the bone marrow or lymph system.

5. Infections (depending on cause and stage), e.g.
   Abscess
   Meningitis
   Appendicitis
   Tonsillitis

5. These conditions stimulate the bone marrow and lymph glands to increase the release of granulocytes and/or agranulocytes, resulting in an elevation of the WBC. Review WBC types in Description.

*Not discussed in this book.

Otitis media
Pneumonia
Peritonitis
Rheumatic fever
6. Parasitic infestations

6. Overall increase in WBC is mainly a result of increase in the monocytes. Eosinophiles increase in response to foreign protein.

7. Immune reaction, e.g.
   Allergic conditions
   Transfusion reaction
   Serum sickness
   Systemic lupus erythematosus
   Rheumatoid arthritis
   Hemolytic disease of the newborn

7. The immune system is stimulated as a result of antigen-antibody reactions. In the case of hemolytic disease of the newborn, this reaction is precipitated by the Rh factors in the blood of the fetus and the mother.

Conditions Related to Decreases

1. Agranulocytosis

Rationale

1. An acute blood dyscrasia in which neutrophiles cannot be formed. Usually due to drug toxicity or a hypersensitivity reaction. Also a term used to describe decreased granulocyte production present in other conditions.

2. Aplastic anemia

2. Condition in which the bone marrow is unable to produce any cells (RBCs, platelets, or WBCs). Results in agranulocytosis.

3. Some anemias
   a. Autoimmune hemolytic anemia (AIHA)
   b. Some megaloblastic anemias

3. a. In some cases of AIHA, leukopenia may develop if antileukocytic antibodies are also present.
   b. In some megaloblastic anemias where there is a vitamin B_{12} or folic acid deficiency, there may also be leukopenia because the B_{12} and folic acid are essential for nucleic acid metabolism, which is a necessary part of cellular maturation.

4. Hypersplenism (e.g., idiopathic thrombocytopenic purpura, cirrhosis)

4. Spleen becomes hyperactive and there is an increased destruction of WBCs.

5. Bone marrow depressants
   Toxic reactions
   Radiation therapy
   Antineoplastics
   Viral infections (herpes, measles, influenza, viral pneumonias, chickenpox, rabies, colds)

5. All may cause bone marrow depression leading to a decreased WBC.

Ingestion of mercury or other heavy metals or exposure to benzene or arsenicals

6. Myxedema

6. There is sometimes a coexisting B_{12} and folic acid deficiency in hypothyroidism (see 3b).

7. Overwhelming bacterial infections

7. May be referred to as a degenerative shift when the body cannot respond sufficiently to mature leukocytes. One would see immature neutrophiles and a decreased total WBC.

Drug Influences: Many drugs affect the WBC. Listed below are some of the drugs that may influence test results. The drugs are listed alphabetically by generic name and divided into columns according to the effect of the drug. Examples of trade names are in parentheses.

The following drugs may cause an increase in WBC:

Causes leukocytosis
amphotericin B
atropine; in children
belladonna
carbamazine
chloramphenicol; after bone marrow depression
colchicine
copper; in poisoning
digitalis; rare

epinephrine; with neutrophilia
erythromycin
mercury compounds
oxyphenbutazone (Tandearil)
phenylbutazone (Butazolidin)
prednisolone
tetracycline
thiothixene (Navane)

Eosinophilia
allopurinol (Zyloprim)
aminosalicylic acid (PAS)
ampicillin
capreomycin (Capastat)
cephalothin (Keflin)
chlorpropamide (Diabinese)
cloxacillin
desipramine (Norpramin)
gold
iodides

kanamycin
methicillin
methyldopa (Aldomet)
nalidixic acid (NegGram)
novobiocin (Albamycin)
phenothiazines
phenytoin (Dilantin)
triamterene (Dyrenium)
trifluperidol
vancomycin

Miscellaneous
acids
anesthetics
corticotropin
imipramine (Tofranil)
levodopa
lithium; may double
methysergide (Sansert)

niacinamide
oral contraceptives
pilocarpine; splenic contraction
quinine; splenic contraction
strychnine
sulfonamides (Sulfamylon, Azulfidine, Sulamyd, etc.)

The following drugs may cause a decrease in test results:

May cause aplastic anemia

diphenylhydantoin (Dilantin)
ethotoin (Peganone)
gold compounds

mephenytoin (Mesantoin)
methsuximide (Celontin)
trimethadione (Tridione)

May cause pancytopenia

busulfan (Myleran)
chloramphenicol (Chloromycetin)
dactinomycin (Actinomycin D)

mefenamic acid (Ponstel)
mitomycin (Mitomycin-C)
primidone (Mysoline)

Agranulocytosis

acetazolamide (Diamox)
chlordiazepoxide (Librium)
chloroquine (Aralen)
indomethacin (Indocin)
isoniazid; rare (INH)
lincomycin
mercaptopurine (6-MP, 6-
  Mercaptopurine)
methimazole (Tapazole)
methotrexate

oxyphenbutazone (Tandearil)
phenylbutazone (Azolid, Butazolidin)
primaquine
propylthiouracil
quinidine
sulfonamides (Sulfamylon, Azulfidine,
  Sulamyd)
thiazides (Diuril, Enduron, Hydro-
  Diuril)

Leukopenia, miscellaneous

allopurinol (Zyloprim)
ampicillin
asparaginase
azathioprine (Imuran)
barbiturates
capreomycin (Capastat)
carbenicillin
chlorambucil (Leukeran)
clofibrate (Atromid-S)
colchicine
cyclophosphamide (Cytoxan)
diazepam (Valium)
diazoxide (Hyperstat I.V.)
doxorubicin (Adriamycin)
floxuridine
flucytosine (Ancobon)
fluorouracil (5-FU)
griseofulvin (Fulvicin-U/F)

hetacillin
hydroxychloroquine (Plaquenil Sulfate)
hydroxyurea (Hydrea)
levodopa (L-dopa)
melphalan (Alkeran, L-Pam)
metronidazole (Flagyl)
oxacillin (Prostaphlin, Bactocill)
pipobroman (Vercyte)
procarbazine (Matulane)
quinine
rifampin (Rifadin)
thioguanine (Thioguanine, TG)
thiotepa (Thiotepa)
uracil mustard
vinblastine (Velban)
vincristine (Oncovin)

Related Lab Studies: Monitor response to treatment or the progression of disease and adjust nursing care accordingly. See individual tests for information.

hematocrit
hemoglobin
RBC morphology
culture and sensitivity studies
bone marrow aspiration
urinalysis

IMPLICATIONS FOR NURSING CARE
PRETEST: Factors related to the test
Nursing Diagnosis: Potential for injury related to changes in biochemical balance

Guide to assessment	Guide to planning and intervention	Guide to evaluation
Assess patient factors influencing test results:		
1. Comprehensive drug history (See Drug Influences)	1. Consult with physician about and inform lab of drugs the patient is receiving that may influence WBC.	1. The patient's pertinent drug history is discussed with physician and lab.
2. Preexisting conditions (See Increases/Decreases)	2. Record preexisting conditions on lab slip.	2. The patient's preexisting conditions are noted on lab slip.
3. Knowledge deficit	3. Explain test to patient: a. Define WBC (See Description). b. Explain procedure (See Procedure).	3. The patient demonstrates knowledge of test by defining test and stating procedure.

Patient Preparation Checklist

1. √ Drug history (See Drug Influences).
2. √ Preexisting conditions and note on lab slip (See Increases/Decreases).
3. √ Patient knowledge; explain test to patient (See Description/Procedure).

CONSIDERATIONS FOR NURSING CARE RELATED TO ABNORMAL TEST RESULTS
POSTTEST: Factors related to the results of the test
Nursing Diagnosis: Alterations in biochemical balance

Guide to assessment	Guide to planning and intervention	Guide to evaluation
Assess patient factors that may be influencing test results:		

1. Fluid balance
   I&O
   VS
   Skin turgor
   Mucous membranes
   Weight loss or gain
	1. Demonstrate fluid balance by:	1. The patient's WBC is not influenced by fluid imbalance:

Guide to assessment	Guide to planning and intervention	Guide to evaluation
	a. Recording accurate I&O.	a. Fluid output is approximately equal to intake.
	b. Monitoring VS.	b. VS do not show evidence of hyper- or hypovolemia.
	c. Monitoring weight.	c. Patient's body water status remains stable.
	d. Recording assessment data.	d. Assessments are recorded.
2. Nursing history and physical exam suggestive of:	2. Monitor patient status (objective and subjective data) carefully for the purposes of:	2. Physician is consulted regarding assessments that may indicate:
a. Unnecessary treatments and medications.	a. Recognizing and reporting when treatment which affects WBC is no longer required.	a. Medications and treatments affecting WBC may no longer be necessary.
b. Uncontrolled disease conditions affecting WBC.	b. Monitoring disease conditions which, if not controlled, will lead to increases or decreases in WBC.	b. Disease conditions affecting WBC are controlled.
3. Quality of nursing care and physical findings Use of aseptic technique Patient knowledge VS Hydration status WBC values Responses to medications and therapies Skin condition Respiratory status	3. Facilitate decreases in WBC by: a. Maintaining good aseptic technique. b. Administering medications (e.g., immunosuppressives, antineoplastics, antibiotics) as ordered. c. Instructing patient in methods of avoiding infection and/or controlling infection. d. Informing physician of any allergic responses or adverse reactions to drugs or other treatments. e. Maintaining hydration. f. Maintaining good respiratory and integumentary status. g. Providing good nursing care specific to disease conditions present or probable.	3. Elevated WBC values will decrease. Conditions leading to increases or decreases are recognized and reported.

Reference Bibliography

1. Aspinall, Mary Jo, *Decision Making for Patient Care, Applying the Nursing Process*, New York, Appleton-Century-Crofts, 1981.

2. Baldonado, Ardelina A., and Stahl, Dulcelina Albano, *Cancer Nursing, Nursing Outline Series*, Garden City, N.Y., Medical Examination Publishing Co., Inc., 1978.

3. Brunner, Lillian Sholtis, and Suddarth, Doris Smith, *The Lippincott Manual of Nursing Practice* (3rd ed), Philadelphia, J. B. Lippincott Co., 1982.

4. Burgess, Audrey, *The Nurse's Guide to Fluid and Electrolyte Balance* (2nd ed), N.Y., McGraw-Hill Book Co., 1979.

5. Byrne, C. Judith et al, *Laboratory Tests*, Menlo Park, Ca., Addison-Wesley Publishing Co., 1981.

6. Campbell, Claire, *Nursing Diagnosis and Intervention in Nursing Practice*, N.Y., John Wiley & Sons, 1978.

7. Collins, Douglas R., *Illustrated Manual of Laboratory Diagnosis* (2nd ed), Philadelphia, J. B. Lippincott Co., 1975.

8. Fischbach, Frances, *A Manual of Laboratory Diagnostic Tests*, Philadelphia, J. B. Lippincott Co., 1980.

9. Friedman, Richard et al, *Effects of Disease on Clinical Laboratory Tests, Journal of the American Association for Clinical Chemists*, Vol. 26, No. 4, 1980.

10. Halsted, James A., *The Laboratory in Clinical Medicine, Interpretation and Application*, Philadelphia, W. B. Saunders Co., 1976.

11. Henry, John B., *Todd-Sanford Clinical Diagnosis by Laboratory Methods* (16th ed), Philadelphia, W. B. Saunders Co., 1979.

12. Henry, Richard; Cannon, Donald C.; and Winkleman, James W., *Clinical Chemistry, Principles and Techniques* (2nd ed), Hagerstown, Md., Harper & Row Publishers, 1974.

13. Holley, James W. (ed), *Enzymology, An Educational Program*, Indianapolis, mabbheim boeringer, Bio-Dynamics/bmc, 1980.

14. Leavell, Byrd Stuart, and Thorup, Oscar Andreas, *Fundamentals of Clinical Hematology* (4th ed), Philadelphia, W. B. Saunders Co., 1976.

15. Martin, Eric W., "Hazards of Errors in Clinical Laboratory Testing," in *Hazards of Medications* (2nd ed), Philadelphia, J. B. Lippincott Co., 1978.

16. Methany, Norma, and Snively, W. D., *Nurses' Handbook of Fluid Balance* (3rd ed), Philadelphia, J. B. Lippincott Co., 1979.

17. Price, Sylvia Anderson, and Wilson, Lorraine McCarty, *Pathophysiology, Clinical Concepts of Disease Processes* (2nd ed), N.Y., McGraw-Hill Book Co., 1982.

18. Tilkian, Sarko M.; Conover, Mary Boudreau; and Tilkian, Ara G., *Clinical Implications of Laboratory Tests* (2nd ed), St. Louis, C. V. Mosby Co., 1979.

19. Sheen, Anitra Peebles, *Breathing Life into Medical Writing*, St. Louis, C. V. Mosby Co., 1982.

20. Sodeman, William A., and Sodeman, Thomas A., *Sodeman's Pathologic Physiology, Mechanisms of Disease* (6th ed), Philadelphia, W. B. Saunders Co., 1979.

21. Sonnenwirth, Alex C., and Jerrett, Leonard, *Gradwohl's Clinical Laboratory Methods and Diagnosis* (8th ed), St. Louis, C. V. Mosby Co., 1980.

22. Thomas, Clayton (ed), *Taber's Cyclopedic Medical Dictionary* (13th ed), Philadelphia, F. A. Davis Co., 1977.

23. Vaughn, Victor et al, *Nelson Textbook of Pediatrics* (11th ed), Philadelphia, W. B. Saunders Co., 1979.

24. Wallach, James, *Interpretation of Diagnostic Tests* (3rd ed), Boston, Little, Brown and Co., 1978.

25. White, Abraham et al, *Principles of Biochemistry* (6th ed), N.Y., McGraw-Hill Book Co., 1978.

26. Widman, Frances K., *Clinical Interpretation of Laboratory Tests* (8th ed), Philadelphia, F. A. Davis Co., 1979.

27. Young, D. S.; Pestaner, I. C.; and Gibberman, V., *Clinical Chemistry Effects of Drugs on Clinical Laboratory Tests, Journal of the American Association for Clinical Chemists*, Vol. 21, No. 5, 1975.

28. Yura, Helen, and Walsh, Mary B., *The Nursing Process, Assessing, Planning, Implementing, Evaluating* (3rd ed), N.Y., Appleton-Century-Crofts, 1978.

29. Western Region Laboratory Procedures Inc., *Laboratory Procedures, Western Region Service Manual*, The Upjohn Company, Woodland Hills, Ca., 1981.

30. Barrett, James T., *Basic immunology and its medical application* (2nd ed), St. Louis, C. V. Mosby Co., 1980.

31. Jones, Dorothy A.; Dunbar, Claire Ford; and Jirovec, Mary Marmoll, *Medical-Surgical Nursing, A Conceptual Approach*, N.Y., McGraw-Hill Book Co., 1978.

32. Luckman, Joan, and Sorensen, Karen Creason, *Medical-Surgical Nursing, A Psychophysiologic Approach* (2nd ed), Philadelphia, W. B. Saunders Co., 1980.

33. Finegold, Sidney M.; Martin, William J.; and Scott, Elvyn G., *Baily and Scott's Diagnostic Microbiology* (5th ed), St. Louis, C. V. Mosby Co., 1978.

34. Meites, Samuel (ed), *Pediatric Clinical Chemistry* (2nd ed), Washington, DC, The American Association for Clinical Chemistry, Inc., 1981.

35. Graham, Gary, and Kenny, Margaret A., "Changes in Transcutaneous Oxygen Tension During Blood-Gas Sampling," *Clinical Chemistry*, Vol. 26, pp 1860–1863 (1980).

36. Batsakis, John G., "Serum Alkaline Phosphatase, Refining and Old Test For The Future," *Diagnostic Medicine*, Vol. 5, No. 3, pp 25–33 (May/June 1982).

37. Shaw, Leslie M., "Keeping Pace With a Popular Enzyme, GGT," *Diagnostic Medicine*, Vol. 5, No. 3, pp 59–78 (May/June 1982).

38. Lente, Frederic Van, "Case of the Month, Rediscovering C-Reactive Protein," *Diagnostic Medicine*, Vol. 5, No. 3, pp 95–96 (May/June 1982).

39. Tietz, Norbert W. (ed), *Fundamentals of Clinical Chemistry* (2nd ed), Philadelphia, W. B. Saunders Co., 1976.

40. Williams, R. H. (ed), *Textbook of Endocrinology* (6th ed), Philadelphia, W. B. Saunders Co., 1981.

41. Pritchard, J. A., and MacDonald, P. C., *Williams Obstetrics* (16th ed), N.Y., Appleton-Century-Crofts, 1980.

42. *Diagnostics* (The Nurse's Reference Library), Springhouse, Pa., Nursing '81 Books, Intermed Communication, Inc., 1981.

43. Stark, J. L., "BUN/CREATININE Your Keys to Kidney Function," *Nursing '80*, Vol. 10, No. 5, pp 33–38 (May 1980).

44. Macleod, John (ed), *Davidson's Principles and Practice of Medicine* (12th ed), N.Y., Churchill Livingstone, 1977.

45. Guyton, A. G., *Textbook of Medical Physiology* (5th ed), Philadelphia, W. B. Saunders Co., 1976.

46. Biller, Jeffery A., and Yeager, Andrew M. (eds), *The Harriet Lane Handbook* (9th ed), Chicago, Year Book Medical Publishers, Inc., 1981.

47. Scipein, Gladys et al, *Comprehensive Pediatric Nursing* (2nd ed), N.Y., McGraw-Hill Book Co., 1979.

48. Phipps, Wilma J.; Long, Barbara C.; and Woods, Nancy Fugate, *Medical-Surgical Nursing, Concepts and Clinical Practice*, St. Louis, C. V. Mosby Co., 1979.

49. Werner, Sidney, and Ingbar, Disney, *The Thyroid* (4th ed), N.Y., Harper and Row Publishers, Inc., 1978.

50. Brooke, Michael, *A Clinician's View of Neuromuscular Diseases*, Baltimore, Williams and Wilkins Co., 1977.

51. Conn, Howard, and Conn, Rex Jr., *Current Diagnosis*, Philadelphia, W. B. Saunders Co., 1980.

52. Isselbacher, Kurt; Adams, Raymond; Braunwald, Eugene; Petersdorf, Robert G., and Wilson, Jean D., *Harrison's Principles of Internal Medicine*, N.Y., McGraw-Hill Book Co., 1980.

53. Ingalls, Joy and Solerno, M., *Maternal and Child Health Nursing*, St. Louis, C. V. Mosby Co., 1975.

54. Sleisinger, Marvin, and Fordtran, John, *Gastrointestinal Disease*, Philadelphia, W. B. Saunders Co., 1978.

55. White, Thomas; Sarles, Henry; and Benhamore, J., *Liver, Bile Ducts and Pancreas*, N.Y., Grune and Stratton, 1977.

56. Brunner, Lillian Sholtis, and Suddarth, Doris Smith, *Textbook of Medical-Surgical Nursing* (4th ed), Philadelphia, J. B. Lippincott Co., 1980.

57. Given, Barbara A., Simmons, Sandra J., *Gastroenterology in Clinical Nursing* (3rd ed), St. Louis, C. V. Mosby Co., 1979.

58. McConnell, Edwina, "Meeting the Special Needs of Diabetics Facing Surgery," *Nursing '76*, pp 30–37 (June 1976).

59. Whaley, Lucille, and Wong, Donna L., *Nursing Care of Infants and Children*, St. Louis, C. V. Mosby Co., 1979.

60. Smith, Donald R. (ed), *General Urology* (10th ed), Los Altos, Ca., Lange Medical Publications, 1981.

61. *Monitoring Fluid and Electrolytes Precisely* (Nursing Skillbook), Horsham, Pa., Intermed Communications, Inc., 1979.

62. Williams, Sue Rodwell, *Nutrition and Diet Therapy* (4th ed), St. Louis, C. V. Mosby Co., 1981.

63. Netter, Frank D., *The CIBA Collection of Medical Illustrations, Vol 7, Respiratory System*, CIBA Pharmaceutical Co., 1979.

64. Gellis, Sydney, and Kagan, Benjamin, *Current Pediatric Therapy*, Philadelphia, W. B. Saunders Co., 1980.

65. Phillips, Raymond E., *Cardiovascular Therapy: A Systematic Approach, Vol. 1, Circulation*, Philadelphia, W. B. Saunders Co., 1979.

66. Beeson, Paul; McDermott, Walsh; and Wyngaarder, James B., *Cecil Textbook of Medicine* (15th ed), Philadelphia, W. B. Saunders Co., 1979.

67. Lane, Gere, and Pierce, Anne Griswold, "When Persistence Pays Off Resolving the Mystery of Unexplained Electrolyte Imbalance," *Nursing '82*, pp 44–47 (Jan. 1982).

68. Kozak, Jr., Peter, "Factors That Influence Theophylline Metabolism," *The Western Journal of Medicine*, Oct. 1979.

69. Brenner, Barry M., and Stein, Jay H. (eds), *Acid-Base and Potassium Homostasis, Contemporary Issues in Nephrology*, Vol. 2, N.Y., Churchill Livingstone, 1979.

70. Hollister, Leo E. (ed), *1981 Year Book of Drug Therapy*, Chicago, Year Book Medical Publishers, Inc., June 1981.

71. Weiner, Matthew et al, *Clinical Pharmacology and Therapeutics in Nursing*, N.Y., McGraw-Hill Book Co., 1979.

72. Jones, Rosamond, and Baillie, Eivor, "Intravenous Aminophylline in Apnoea of Prematurity Based on Pharmacokinetic Studies," *Archives of Disease in Childhood*, March 1979, Vol. 54, pp 190–193.

73. Modell, Walter (ed), *1980 Drugs of Choice*, St. Louis, C. V. Mosby Co., 1980.

74. Gilman, Alfred et al, *Goodman and Gilman's The Pharmacological Basis of Therapeutics* (6th ed), N.Y., Macmillan Publishing Co., Inc., 1980.

75. Rylance, George, and Moreland, Terence, "Drug Level Monitoring In Paediatric Practice," *Archives of Disease in Childhood*, February 1980, Vol. 55, pp 89–98.

76. Michaels, Rhoda M. (ed), *Nurses' Drug Alert*, N.Y., M. J. Powers & Co., Vol. 5, No. 5, May 1982, p 33.

77. Hendeles, Leslie; Weinberger, Miles; and Bighley, Lyle, "Disposition of Theophylline After a Single Intravenous Infusion of Aminophylline," *American Review of Respiratory Disease*, Vol. 118, 1978, pp 97–103.

78. Davi, Maria J. et al, "Physiologic Changes Induced by Theophylline in the Treatment of Apnea in Preterm Infants," *The Journal of Pediatrics*, Jan. 1978 Vol. 92, No. 1, pp 91–95.

79. Tucker, Susan Martin et al, *Patient Care Standards* (2nd ed), St. Louis, C. V. Mosby Co., 1980.

80. Falconer, Mary W. et al, *The Drug The Nurse The Patient* (6th ed), Philadelphia, W. B. Saunders Co., 1978.

81. Sorkin, Michael I., "Hyperkalemia—Causes, Management and Prevention," *Consultant*, July 1980, pp 25–32.

82. *Managing I.V. Therapy* (Nursing Photobook), Horsham, Pa., *Nursing '80 Photobook Series*, Intermed Communications, Inc., 1980.

83. Wright, Thomas R., and Murray, Margie, "Potassium Problems: Which Patient's In Danger," *RN*, June 1982, pp 57–62.

84. Felver, Linda, "Understanding the Electrolyte Maze," *American Journal of Nursing*, Sept. 1980, pp 1591–1595.

85. Zelechowske, Gina Pugliese, "Hidden Killer: Malignant Hyperthermia," *Nursing '77* Sept. 1977 p 35.

86. Knochel, James P., "Potassium Deficiency: Causes, Complications, and Treatment," *Consultant* March 1980, pp 139–149.

87. Maxwell, Morton and Kleeman, Charles R. (eds), *Clinical Disorders of Fluid and Electrolyte Metabolism* (3rd ed), N.Y., McGraw-Hill Book Co., 1980.

88. Idelson, Beldon A., "Renal and Hepatic Edema: Causes and Management," *Consultant*, May 1980, pp 90–96.

89. *Diseases* (The Nurses' Reference Library), *Nursing '81 Books*, Horsham, Pa., Intermed Communications, Inc., 1981.

90. Aspinall, Mary Jo, "A Simplified Guide to Managing Patients With Hyponatremia," *Nursing '78*, Dec. 1978, pp 32–35.

91. Watson, Jeannette E., *Medical-Surgical Nursing and Related Physiology* (2nd ed), Philadelphia, W. B. Saunders Co., 1979.

92. Jackle, Mary, and Rasmussen, Claire, *Renal Problems A Critical Care Nursing Focus*, Bowie, Md., Robert J. Brady Co., 1980.

93. Vogel, Connie Higgins, "Keeping Patients Alive In Spite of Postobstructive Diuresis," *Nursing '79*, March 1979, pp 50–56.

94. *Monitoring Fluid and Electrolytes Precisely* (Nursing Skillbook), Horsham, Pa., Intermed Communication, Inc., 1979.

95. Papper, Solomon, *Clinical Nephrology* (2nd ed), Boston, Little, Brown and Co., 1978.

96. *AMA Drug Evaluations* (4th ed), prepared by AMA Department of Drugs, American Medical Association, Chicago, Ill., 1980.

97. Williams, William J. et al, *Hematology* (2nd ed), N.Y., McGraw-Hill Book Co., 1977.

98. Shafer, Jean Al, *Marrow Morphology Workshop Manual*, published by Oregon Joint Spring Seminar, AOMT, OSSAMT, PSCM, Portland, Ore., May 1981.

99. Dunne, Roberta S., and Perez, Rosanne C., "Reye's Syndrome: A Challenge not limited to Critical Care Nurses," *Issues in Comprehensive Pediatric Nursing*, July/Aug. 1981, Vol. 5, No. 4.

100. McCulloch, James, "Assessment of Thyroid Function," *Nursing Mirror*, February 17, 1981, p 34.

101. Yao, Yulin, "A Current View of Thyroid Function Tests," *Hospital Practice*, Sept. 1981, pp 149–164.

102. Schatz, Irwin J., "The Coagulation of Blood Disorders and Drugs," *Emergency Medicine*, March 15, 1981, pp 24–35.

103. Campbell, Charles E., and Herten, R. Jeffrey, "VD to STD: Redefining Venereal Disease," *American Journal of Nursing*, Sept. 1981, pp 1629–1635.

104. Loebl, Suzanne; Spratto, George; and Wit, Andrew, *The Nurse's Drug Handbook*, N.Y., John Wiley & Sons, 1977.

105. Corbett, Jane Vincent, *Laboratory Tests in Nursing Practice*, N.Y., Appleton-Century-Crofts, 1982.

106. Treseler, Kathleen Morrison, *Clinical Laboratory Tests, Significance and Implications*, Englewood Cliffs, N.J., Prentice-Hall Inc., 1982.

107. Pagana, Kathleen Deska, and Pagana, Timothy James, *Diagnostic Testing and Nursing Implications a case study approach*, St. Louis, C. V. Mosby Co., 1982.

108. *Physicians' Desk Reference*, Oradell, N.J., Medical Economics Company, 1981.

109. *Nursing '81 Drug Handbook*, Horsham, Pa. (Nursing '81 Books), Intermed Communications, Inc., 1981.

110. Glasser, Lewis, "Cells in Cerebrospinal Fluid," *Diagnostic Medicine*, Mar./Apr. 1981, pp 33–50.

111. Vichinsky, Elliott P., and Lubin, Bertram H., "Sickle Cell Anemia and Related Hemoglobinopathies," *Pediatric Clinics of North America*, Vol. 27, No. 2, May 1981, pp 429–448.

112. Sullivan, Drew W., and Glader, Bertil E., "Erythrocyte Enzyme Disorders in Children," *Pediatric Clinics of North America*, Vol. 27, No. 2, May 1981, pp 449–461.

113. *The Laboratory in Pediatric Practice (The Pediatric Clinics of North America)*, Philadelphia, W. B. Saunders Co., Nov. 1980, Vol. 27, No. 4.

114. McCarthy, Joyce, "Somogyi Effect, Managing Blood Glucose Rebound," *Nursing '79*, Feb. 1979, pp 39–41.

115. Rosenbloom, Arlan, and Hunt, Sarah, "Prognosis of impaired glucose in children with stress hyperglycemia, symptoms of hypoglycemia, or asymptomatic glucosuria," *The Journal of Pediatrics*, Vol. 101, No. 3, Sept. 1982, pp 340–344.

116. Hite, Anna Morris, "Clinical Estimation of the Renal Threshhold for Glucose in Persons with Diabetes Mellitus," *Nursing Research*, Vol. 31, No. 3, May/June 1982, pp 153–158.

117. Rosenbloom, Arlan; Kohramn, Arthur; and Sperling, Mark, "Classification and diagnosis of diabetes mellitus in children and adolescents," *The Journal of Pediatrics*, Vol. 98, No. 2, Aug. 1981, pp 320–323.

118. Fredholm, Nancy Zilinsky, "The Insulin Pump: New Method of Insulin Delivery," *American Journal of Nursing*, Nov. 1981, pp 2024–2026.

119. McCarthy, Joyce, "Diabetic Nephropathy," *American Journal of Nursing*, Nov. 1981, pp 2030–2034.

120. Cavalier, Jacqueline, "Crucial Decisions in Diabetic Emergencies," *RN*, Nov. 1980, pp 32–37.

121. Marchiondo, Kathleen, "The Very Fine Art of Collecting Culture Specimens," *Nursing '79*, Apr. 1979, pp 34–43.

122. Thompson, Marie Ann, "Managing The Patient With Liver Dysfunction," *Nursing '81*, pp 101–107.

123. Martelli, Mary Elizabeth, "Teaching Parents About Reye's Syndrome," *American Journal of Nursing*, Feb. 1982, pp 260–263.

124. Grow, Donna, "Reye's Syndrome," *Nursing '81*, Nov. 1981, pp 156–158.

125. Berg, Mary J. et al, "Acceleration of the Body Clearance of Phenobarbital by Oral Activated Charcoal," *The New England Journal of Medicine*, Sept. 9, 1982, pp 642–644.

126. Glasser, Lewis, "Body Fluids III, Tapping the Wealth of Information in CSF," *Diagnostic Medicine*, Jan./Feb. 1981, pp 23–32.

127. Yip, Ray, and Nelson, Peter, "Hemoglobin concentration of children with sickle cell trait," *The Journal of Pediatrics*, Vol. 99, No. 2, Aug. 1981, pp 257–258.

128. Sullivan, Drew W., and Glader, Bertil E., "Erythrocyte Enzyme Disorders in Children," *Pediatric Clinics of North America*, Vol. 27, No. 2, May 1980, pp 449–461.

129. Schreiber, Alan D., "Immunohematology," *JAMA*, Vol. 248, No. 11, Sept. 17, 1982, pp 1380–1382.

130. Claypool, Janet M., "Rubella Protection for Maternal Child Health Care Providers," *MCN*, Vol. 6, No. 1, 1981, pp 53–56.

131. Miller, Suzanne J., "Nursing Care of the Lead Burdened Child: a Problem Oriented Approach," *Pediatric Nursing*, Vol. 7, No. 5, 1981, pp 47–52.

132. Dewees, Cornelia B., "Hematologic Disorders in Pregnancy," *The Nursing Clinics of North America*, Philadelphia, W. B. Saunders Co., Vol. 17, No. 1, Mar. 1982, pp 57–67.

133. Kelber, Sr. Mary, "Plasma Renin Activity," *Nursing '82*, Apr. 1982, p 140.

134. Mar, Dexter D., "Drug-Induced Hepatotoxicity," *American Journal of Nursing*, Jan. 1982, pp 124–126.

135. Clark, Barbara Ann, "Getting Those Blood Samples Right," *RN*, Dec. 1981, pp 36–42.

136. Harris, Elizabeth, "The Dexamethasone Suppression Test," *American Journal of Nursing*, May 1982, pp 784–785.

137. Stokes, Peter E., "The Dexamethasone Test, A Measure of HYPAC Function—

its use in Psychiatry: Part I," *Directions in Psychiatry*, St. Vincent's Hospital and Medical Center of New York, Lesson 17, 1982.

138. Brown, Walter Armin, "The Dexamethasone Suppression Test: Clinical Applications," *Psychosomatics*, Vol. 22, No. 11, Nov. 1981, pp 951–955.

139. Jensen, Margaret Duncan; Benson, Ralph C.; and Bobak, Irene M., *Maternity Care The Nurse and the Family* (2nd ed), St. Louis, C. V. Mosby Co., 1981.

140. Hicks, Eileen, "Obstetrical Emergencies, A Systematic Approach for Nursing Intervention," *Nursing Clinics of North America*, Vol. 17, No. 1, Mar. 1982, pp 79–84.

141. Harper, Rita et al, "Fetal movement, biochemical and biophysical parameters and the outcome of pregnancy," *American Journal of Obstetrics and Gynecology*, Vol. 141, No. 1, Sept. 1, 1981, pp 39–42.

142. Romney, Seymour L. et al, *Gynecology and Obstetrics, The Health Care of Women* (2nd ed), N.Y., McGraw-Hill Book Co., 1981.

143. Kushner, Jeffrey, "Ethanol—The Social Drug," *American Journal of Medical Technology*, Vol. 47, No. 3, Mar. 1981, pp 197–199.

144. Hurwitz, Linda S., "Nursing Implications of Selected Pediatric Endocrine Problems," *Nursing Clinics of North America*, Philadelphia, W. B. Saunders Co., Vol. 15, No. 3, Sept. 1980, pp 525–529.

145. Hoffman, Jeanette T. Taitaino, "Ectopic Hormone Production in Cancer," *Nursing Clinics of North America*, Philadelphia, W. B. Saunders Co., Vol. 15, No. 3, Sept. 1980, pp 505–509.

146. Hoffman, Jeanette T. Taitaino, and Newbry, Thelma Bond, "Hypercalcemia in Primary Hyperparathyroidism," *Nursing Clinics of North America*, Philadelphia, W. B. Saunders Co., Vol. 15, No. 3, Sept. 1980, pp 469–581.

147. Beland, Irene, and Passos, Joyce Y., *Clinical Nursing, Pathophysiological and Psychosocial Approaches*, N.Y., Macmillan Publishing Co., Inc., 1981.

148. Beacham, Daniel Winston, and Beacham, Woodward Davis, *Synopsis of Gynecology*, St. Louis, C. V. Mosby Co., 1982.

149. Berg, Mary J. et al, "Acceleration of the Body Clearance of Phenobarbital by Oral Activated Charcoal," *The New England Journal of Medicine*, Sept. 9, 1982, pp 642–644.

150. Kuntz, Robert E., "Parasites of Children in the United States," *Pediatric Nursing*, Nov./Dec. 1979, pp 12–17.

151. Ismail, A. A. A., "Biochemical Monitoring of High-risk Pregnancies," *Medical Laboratory Sciences*, 1982, pp 305–309.

152. Longberry, Joan, "Hemostasis: Part I Screening Tests to Evaluate Abnormal Hemostasis," *American Journal of Medical Technology*, Vol. 48, No. 2, Feb. 1982, pp 99–105.

153. Randolf, Virginia Sullivan, "Four Clinical Chemistry Analyses for Pediatric Patients: Glycosylated Hemoglobin, Free Bilirubin, Sweat Electrolytes, Neonatal Thyroxine," *American Journal of Medical Technology*, Vol. 48, No. 1, Jan. 1982, pp 15–20.

154. Randolf, Virginia Sullivan, "Considerations for the Clinical Laboratory Serving the Pediatric Patient," *American Journal of Medical Technology*, Vol. 48, No. 1, Jan. 1982, pp 7–11.

155. Sweetwood, Hannelore, "Acute Respiratory Insufficiency," *Nursing '77*, Dec. 1977, pp 24–31.

156. "Preventing Thromboembolic Disease with Aspirin," *Nurses' Drug Alert*, Vol. VI, No. 10, Oct. 1982, p 76.

157. Shrake, Kevin, "The ABC's of ABG's," *Nursing '79*, Sept. 1979, pp 26–33.

158. *Bio-Science Handbook* (12th ed), Van Nuys, Ca., Bio-Science Laboratories, 1979.

159. Alexander, Mary M., and Brown, Marie Scott, *Pediatric History Taking and Physical Diagnosis for Nurses* (2nd ed), N.Y., McGraw-Hill Book Co., 1979.

160. Kim, Mi Ja, and Moritz, Derry Ann, *Classification of Nursing Diagnoses*, N.Y., McGraw-Hill Book Co., 1982.

161. Bruce, Joan A., and Snyder, Marie E., "The Right and Responsibility to Diagnose," *The American Journal of Nursing*, Apr. 1982, pp 645–646.

162. Lunney, Margaret, "Nursing Diagnosis: Refining the System," *The American Journal of Nursing*, Mar. 1982, pp 456–459.

163. Purushotham, Devamma, "Nursing Diagnosis: a vital component of the nursing process," *The Canadian Nurse*, June 1981, pp 46–48.

164. Morris, Judith L., "Nursing Diagnosis—A Focus for Continuing Education," *The Journal of Continuing Education in Nursing*, Vol. 13, No. 3, 1982, pp 33–36.

Appendix A: Glossary

Acidosis   Lowered pH caused by respiratory carbonic acid increase or metabolically decreased bicarbonate.
Metabolic acidosis: pH $\downarrow$ pCO_2 $\downarrow$ CO_2 content $\downarrow$
Respiratory acidosis: pH $\downarrow$ pCO_2 $\uparrow$ CO_2 content $\uparrow$
(See Alkalosis)

Adenoma   A tumor of glandular epithelium.

Adjuvant   Something that assists, especially a drug that enhances or hastens the action of a primary drug.

A/G Ratio   Ratio of albumin to globulin which gives proportion of the two proteins.

Aggregation   Clumping together.

Agranulocytosis   Extremely low white blood cell count with very few neutrophiles.

Aldosteronism, Primary   Syndrome of arterial hypertension caused by an oversecretion of aldosterone by an adrenal adenoma or adrenal hyperplasia, low renin, potassium wastage, and sodium retention. Aldosterone concentrations of 40 mg/dl are found in patients with primary aldosteronism.

Aldosteronism, Secondary   Results from nonadrenal disease in which both adrenal glands are stimulated, producing increased aldosterone secretion (9, p. 453).

Alkalemia   Metabolic or respiratory alkalosis.

Alkalosis   Increased pH. From a metabolically caused bicarbonate increase or respiratory carbonic acid loss.
Metabolic alkalosis: pH $\uparrow$ pCO_2 $\uparrow$ CO_2 content $\uparrow$
Respiratory alkalosis: pH $\uparrow$ pCO_2 $\downarrow$ CO_2 content $\downarrow$
(See Acidosis)

Anemia   Term implying low red blood cell count, low hemoglobin or hematocrit.

Antibody   Protein substances, specific immunoglobulins, developed by the body in response to the presence of an antigen; it interacts only with the antigen which induced its synthesis.

Anti-DNA Test   Measures antinative DNA antibody levels in a serum sample to confirm diagnosis of SLE.

Antigen   Substances that stimulate formation of antibodies.

Auer Bodies   Structures found in the cytoplasm that are rod-shaped. These bodies are found in myeloid types of leukemia.

Axotemia   Nitrogenous substances in the blood, usually urea.

Bands   Immature neutrophiles, also called stab cells.

Barr Bodies   The X chromatin mass which can be stained with any nuclear stain to screen for abnormal sexual development. Found in normal females but not in males.

Base Excess/Base Deficit   A method of reporting all the buffer ions in the serum. A decrease in buffer ions is a base deficit; an increase is called a base excess. Normal is in range of $-2mEq$ to $+2mEq$.

Beriberi   Thiamine deficiency associated with malnutrition.

Carbonic Anhydrase   A catalyzing enzyme present in red blood cells that catalyzes H_2O and CO_2 to form carbonic acid or in the reverse action.

Carina   A structure that has at its center a projecting ridge.

Choledocholithiases   Calculi in common bile duct.

Circadian Rhythm   Biological rhythm occurring at approximately 24-hour intervals.

Colloidal Osmotic Pressure   Pressure which prevents the fluid of the plasma from leaking out of the capillaries into the interstitial spaces (45).

Complement System   A system of protein molecules, the sequential interactions of which produce biological effects on surface membranes, on cellular behavior, and on the interaction of other proteins. At least 11 different proteins circulate in normal plasma, each inactive by itself but predestined to play a specific function once the activation sequence begins. Activation can begin with IgG or IgM antigen-antibody reactions or following contact with aggregated IgA, with certain naturally occurring polysaccharides or lipopolysaccharides, or with activation products of the coagulation or kallikrein systems.

CrCl   Creatinine Clearance.

Cryoglobulinemia   An abnormal protein in the blood that in cold temperatures forms a gel.

Cyclic AMP   A biochemical second messenger that facilitates neuromuscular transmission.

Cysts   In parasitic infestations, cysts enclose larval forms of some intestinal parasites. It is the inactive stage of disease.

Deamination   Removal of amino acids from amino groups.

Deiodinization   As in the conversion of thyroxine (T_4) to triiodothyronine (T_3); one or more ions are removed.

DHEA   Dehydroepiandrosterone, a steroid precursor produced in fetal adrenal cortex.

Diurnal Rhythm   Opposite of nocturnal, pertaining to that which happens in the daytime.

Ectopic Hormone   Hormone secretion outside of normal secreting tissue.

Electrophoresis   A laboratory method for separating and measuring normal and certain abnormal hemoglobins. It separates materials, such as proteins, based on the movement of charged particles suspended in a liquid under the influence of an electrical current.

Enteral   Within the intestine.

Extravasation   The escaping of fluid into surrounding tissue.

Fanconi's Syndrome   A proximal tubular enzymatic defect that may cause the loss of unabsorbed substances such as amino acids, glucose, and phosphates into the urine. The defect may be acquired or inherited.

Felty's Syndrome   Hyperplasia of lymph nodes associated with splenomegaly in a patient with rheumatoid arthritis.

Flocculation   The formation of the white portion of a floating island or a fluid or culture containing whitish shreds of mucus.

Follicular Phase   Begins with the first day of menses and continues until ovulation.

G-6PD   Glucose-6-phosphate dehydrogenase deficiency.

Glycogenolysis   Conversion of glycogen from glucose.

Glycolytic Enzyme   An enzyme which catalyzes the hydrolysis of sugars (22).

Gluconeogenesis   The process of forming glycogen from noncarbohydrate sources such as fats or protein.

Granulocyte   A granular white blood cell containing specific cytoplasmic granules (neutrophilic, basophilic, or eosinophilic).

Heinz Bodies   Masses of denatured hemoglobin. Heinz bodies are produced in response to oxidative stress such as exposure to toxic agents, in patients with G-6PD, genetically unstable hemoglobin, and from thalassemia.

Hemagglutination   The clumping of red blood cells.

Hemagglutination Inhibition   Prevention of the clumping of red blood cells by interaction or blocking of the antibody or virus which would otherwise cause hemagglutination.

Hematopoiesis   The formation and maturation of blood cells.

Hemoconcentration   ↑ in the number of red blood cells because of ↓ in volume of plasma.

Hemolysis   Red blood cell destruction with the release of hemoglobin.

Hemostasis   Prevention of blood loss.

Henderson-Hasselbalch Equation   To maintain normal pH at 7.4, the ratio of bicarbonate (HCO_3) and carbonic acid (H_2CO_3) must be 20:1. This is maintained by the kidneys regulating bicarbonate, while respiration regulates carbonic acid.

Heterozygous   Possessing functionally or structurally different genes on corresponding areas of paired chromosomes.

Homozygote   An individual developed from genetically identical gametes and thereby possessing like pairs of genes for any hereditary characteristic.

Homozygous   When an organism has all germ cells transmitting identical genes as a result of inbreeding.

IgA   Immunoglobulin A.

IgG   Immunoglobulin gamma G.

IgM   Immunoglobulin M.

Immunofluorescent Method   Detection of antibodies by using special proteins labeled with fluorescein (22).

Immunoglobulin   One of a family of closely related though not identical proteins which are capable of acting as antibodies (22).

Intrahepatic Cholestasis   Simulating posthepatic cholestasis.

Isoenzyme   Fraction of fractionated enzyme.

Kinins   A general term for a group of polypeptides that are very active biologically.

Limbic System   A group of brain structures in the cerebrum that are interconnected. These structures include frontal lobe cortex, temporal lobe, thalamus, hypothalamus, circuitous neuron pathways. Limbic system is responsible for regulation of emotions.

Luteal Phase   Begins with the formation of the corpus luteum and ends with the cessation of its endocrinologic function.

Nematodes   A class of the phylum Nemathelminthes, which includes the true roundworms or threadworms, many species of which are parasitic. The sexes usually separate and development usually is direct and simple (22).

Nucleoprotein   The combination of one of the proteins with nucleic acid to form a conjugated protein found in cell nuclei.

16-OHDHEA   16-Hydroxydehydroepiandrosterone, a steroid precursor produced in fetal adrenal cortex.

Organification of Iodine   When iodine is incorporated into a tyrosine molecule called monoiodotyrosine.

Osteoblast   A cell of mesodermal origin which is concerned with the formation of bones.

Paget's Disease   Osteitis deformans.

pCO_2   Partial pressure of carbon dioxide. Indicates alveolar ventilation.

pH   Measures acidity and alkalinity.

Phagocytosis   Ingestion and digestion of bacteria and particles by phagocytes.

Phosphorylation   When an enzyme catalyzes the formation of glucose-1-phosphate from glycogen.

Pica   A perverse appetite and craving for substances not suitable for consumption, such as starch, dirt, plaster, and ashes. It is a condition seen in pregnancy, chlorosis, hysteria, helminthiasis, and in certain pychoses.

Plasma The fluid portion of lymph and unclotted blood. It does not contain red blood cells.

pO$_2$ Partial pressure of oxygen; measures oxygen tension.

Polychromatophilia Presence of RNA in red blood cell. Indicates RBC is young. Implies reticulocytosis. Seen most clearly in hemolysis or in acute blood loss.

Protozoa Single-celled animals with a body composed of one or more nuclei surrounded by cytoplasm and contained within a limiting cell membrane.

Radioimmunoassay (+ technique) A very sensitive method of determining the concentration of substances, particularly the proteins in hormones, in blood plasma. The procedure is based on the competitive inhibition of binding of radioactively labeled hormones to a specific antibody. Concentrations of protein in the picogram range can be measured by using this technique (22).

Radio-tagged Hormone In addition to a specific hormone, the laboratory uses a small amount of radioactive material to tag a measured amount of the antigen.

Reticuloendothelial System System comprised of lymph nodes, bone marrow, connective tissue, liver, and spleen. Applies to cells that are able to phagocytose particles (cell fragments, bacteria, etc.).

Serum The fluid portion of clotted blood; a fluid found when clotted blood is left standing long enough for the clot to shrink. Does not contain fibrinogen.

Shift to the Left Cell maturity is normally illustrated right to left, with the most immature cells being on the left. An increase in immature cells is therefore referred to as a "shift to the left."

Sniffing Position Slightly elevated shoulders, head extended at junction of spine and skull by moving the chin up and back (15).

Stab cell Immature neutrophile, also called band.

Thyrotropin Thyroid-stimulating hormone (TSH).

Torr The pressure of 1 mm of mercury under standard conditions of atmospheric pressure and temperature.

Trematodes A parasitic flatworm, a fluke, belonging to the class Trematoda.

Trophozoite The active feeding stage in the growth of a protozoa.

Appendix B: Table of Values

Abbreviations of measurements used in values

d, dl, dL   deciliter = ¹⁄₁₀ of a liter or 100 ml

g, gm   gram = ¹⁄₁₀₀₀ of a kilogram or 1000 mg

G%   grams in 100 ml

IU   international units

l, L   liter = 1000 ml

mcg, μg   micrograms = ¹⁄₁₀₀₀ milligram

mEq, meq   milliequivalent

mg   milligram

mg%   milligrams in 100 milliliters

mIU   milliinternational unit = ¹⁄₁₀₀₀ of IU

ml   milliliter = ¹⁄₁₀₀₀ of a liter

mm³   cubic millimeter

mm Hg   millimeters of mercury

mOsm   milliosmoles

ng   nanogram, ¹⁄₁₀₀₀ of a microgram (1000 ng = 1 microgram)

pg   picogram, ¹⁄₁₀₀₀ of a nanogram

SI   international system

μ   micron, micrometer

μg   microgram, ¹⁄₁₀₀₀ of a milligram

Reference Values

Values vary with laboratory.

Acid Phosphatase (ACP)	Adults:
	0.13–0.63 U/l
	0.0–0.8 IU/l
	Children:
	Newborn–2 weeks 10.4–16.4 King-Armstrong units/ml
	2 weeks–13 years 0.5–11.0 King-Armstrong units/ml

Alanine Aminotransferase (Serum Glutamic Pyruvic Transaminase) (ALT, SGPT)	Infant	below 54 U/L
	Child	1–30 U/L
	Adult	0–48 U/L
Albumin	Premature	2.5–4.5 g/dl
	Full-term newborn	2.5–5.0 g/dl
	1–3 months	3.0–4.2 g/dl
	3–12 months	2.7–5.0 g/dl
	1–15 years	6.5–8.6 g/dl dye binding
	Adults	3.8–5.0 g/dl dye binding
Albumin/Globulin Ratio (A/G Ratio)	1.5:1–2.5:1	
Aldolase (ALS)	Adult	2–8μ/L
	Newborn	up to 4× adult level
	Child	up to 2× adult level

Aldosterone

Plasma:
  Sodium intake   10 mEq/day
  Fasting, recumbent   12–36 ng/dl
  2 hours later, upright   17–137 ng/dl
  Sodium intake   100–200 mEq/day
  Fasting, recumbent   3–9 ng/dl
  2 hours later, upright   4–30 ng/dl
Urine:
  Sodium intake
  10 mEq/day 20–80 mcg/24 hours
  100–200 mEq/day 3–19 mcg/24 hours
  ↑ 200 mEq/day 2–12 mcg/24 hours

Alkaline Phosphatase (ALP)

Adults 20–90 IU/l @ 30°C
Children
  Newborn 50–165 μ/l
  Child 20–150 μ/l

Ammonia (NH$_3$)	Newborn	90–150 μg/dl
	0–2 weeks	70–129 μg/dl
	> 1 month	20–79 μg/dl
	Infant–child	29–80 μg/dl
	Adult	< 50 μg/dl

Amylase (AMS)

Serum:
  Adults 60–180 Somogyi units/dl
          5–81 IU/L
  Children 45–200 dye u/dl
          80–180 Somogyi units/d1
Urine:
35–260 Somogyi units/hr

Antinuclear Antibodies Fluorescent Screening Procedure (ANA, FANA)	negative (titer below 1:20)

Antistreptolysin O Test (ASO, ASL)

For ASO titers:

Age	*Normal upper limits*
Under 5 years	85 Todd U
School age	170 Todd U
Adults	125 Todd U

Check specific method and values with local lab.

Arterial Blood Gases (ABGs)

Arteriopuncture:
pH 7.35–7.45
pCO_2 35–45mm Hg
pO_2 75–100mm Hg
Skin puncture (arterialized):

pH	
Newborn	7.33–7.49
2 days–1 month	7.32–7.43
1 month	7.34–7.43
2 months–1 year	7.34–7.46
Child and adult	
Male	7.35–7.45
Female	7.36–7.44
pCO_2	
Newborn	26.8–40.4
2 months–2 years	26.4–41.2
Child and adult	
Male	36.2–46.2
Female	33.1–43.1
pO_2	
Newborn	unreliable
Child and adult	80–105

Transcutaneous pO_2 monitoring in infants 50–110 mm Hg

HCO_3 *(venous blood)*	
Premature	18–26 mmol/L
Full-term infant–2 years	20–26 mmol/L
2 years–adult	22–26 mmol/L

Base excess/deficit

CO_2 *content (Venous blood)*	
Cord blood	15.0–20.2 mmol/L
Child	18.27 mmol/L
Adult	24–35 mmol/L

Aspartate Amino-transferase (Serum Glutamic Oxaloacetic Transaminase) (AST, SGOT)	1–3 days		16–74 U/L
	< 6 months		20–43 U/L
	6 months–1 year		16–35 U/L
	1 year–5 years		6–30 U/L
	5 years–adult		19–28 U/L
	Adult	Male	8–46 U/L
		Female	7–34 U/L

Barbiturate Screen	Toxic levels associated with coma and shock	
	Short-acting barbiturates	3 mg/dL
	Intermediate-acting barbiturates	4 mg/dL
	Long-acting barbiturates	8–10 mg/dL

Bence-Jones Protein (BJP)	Negative		

Bilirubin	Cord		< 1.8 mg/dl
	24 hours	Premature	1–6 mg/dl
		Full-term	2–6 mg/dl
	48 hours	Premature	6–8 mg/dl
		Full-term	6–7 mg/dl
	3–5 days	Premature	10–15 mg/dl
		Full-term	4–12 mg/dl
	1 month–adult		1 mg/dl
	Conjugated		< 0.4 mg/dl

Bleeding Time	Template method—below 8 minutes; values vary with laboratories and method used

Blood Urea Nitrogen (BUN)	Adults	6–20 mg/dl
	Premature 1 week	3–25 mg/dl
	Newborn	4–18 mg/dl
	Infant-child	5–18 mg/dl

Body Fluid Analysis	*Gastric Fluid*	
	Abnormal is either marked hypersecretion or anacidity	
	Fasting residual volume	20–100 ml
	pH	< 3.5
	Basal acid output (BAO)	0–6 mEq/hr
	Maximum acid output (MAO) after histamine stimulation	5–40 mEq/hr
	BAO/MAO ratio	<0.4
	Pleural Fluid Analysis	
	Less than 20 ml	

Seminal Fluid

Liquefaction	within 20 minutes
Sperm morphology	> 70% normal, mature spermatozoa
Sperm motility	> 60%
pH	> 7.0 (average 7.7)
Sperm count	60–150 million
Volume	1.5–5.0 ml

Synovial Fluid

Glucose	70–100 mg/dl
WBC	0–200 μl
Neutrophiles	< 25%
Fibrin clot	absent
Mucin clot	abundant
Viscosity	high
Volume	< 3.5 ml

Bone Marrow Aspiration Biopsy

Normal Values	*Normal*
Cellularity	Normal
Megakaryocytes and platelet formation	Normal
Granulocytic cells	Normal
Neutrophilic	⎫ ⎧ any
Eosinophilic	⎬ ⎨ abnormality
Basophilic	⎭ ⎩ specified
Erythroid cells	
Maturation	Normoblastic
Activity	Normal
M:E ratio	
Birth	1.85:1
2 weeks	11:1
1–20 months	5.5:1
1–20 years	2.95:1
Adult	4:1

Other Cells	*Children*	*Adults*
Lympho-cytes	3.0–17.0%	2.7–24%
Plasma cells	0–2.0%	0.1–1.5%
Reticulum cells	0.2–2.0%	0.1–2.0%

Calcium (Ca)

Premature	< 1 week	6.0–10.0 mg/dl
Full-term	< 1 week	7.0–12.0 mg/dl
Child		8.0–11.0 mg/dl
Adult		8.9–10.1 mg/dl

Catecholamines	Plasma:	less than 1 μg/L
	Urine:	0–18 μg/dl per random sample (total catecholamines)
	Below 1 year	up to 20 μg/dl 24 hours
	1–5 years	up to 40 μg/dl 24 hours
	6–15 years	up to 80 μg/dl 24 hours
	Above 15 years	up to 100 μg/dl 24 hours

These are representative of total catecholamine levels.

Cerebral Spinal Fluid (CSF)	Pressure:	
	Newborn	80–110 mm H_2O
	Infant/child	< 200 mm H_2O
	Adult	50–180 mm H_2O
	Appearance:	Clear, colorless
	Protein:	
	Preterm	65–150 mg/dl
	Term	20–170 mg/dl
	Child	5–40 mg/dl
	Adult	15–45 mg/dl
	Glucose:	
	Preterm	24–63 mg/dl
	Term	34–119 mg/dl
	Child	40–80 mg/dl
	Adult	50–80 mg/dl
	⅔ of blood glucose	
	Cell count:	
	Preterm	0–25
	Term	0–22
	All others	0–5

Chloride (Cl)	Serum:	
	Newborn	96–106 mEq/L
	Child	95–105 mEq/L
	Adults	95–105 mEq/L
	Urine:	
	110–254 mEq/L/24 hour urine	
	Sweat:	
	10–35 mEq/L	
	> 60 mmol/L considered diagnostic for cystic fibrosis	

Cholesterol	Full term	50–120 mg/dl
	1–2 years	70–190 mg/dl
	2–16 years	135–250 mg/dl
	Adult	120–330 mg/dl

	HDL-Cholesterol	
	Female	mean 55 mg/dl
	Male	mean 45 mg/dl
	LDL-Cholesterol	
	Female	mean 131.1 mg/dl
	Male	mean 135.5 mg/dl

Clotting Time — 5–15 minutes

Cold Agglutinins — Less than 1:16

Complete Blood Count (CBC)

Hematocrit (Hct)		*Hemoglobin*
Newborn	57–68%	17–21 g/dl
1 week	46–62%	15–20 g
1 month	31–41%	11–14 g
3–5 months	30–36%	10–12 g
1 year	29–41%	11–13 g
2–10 years	36–41%	11–13 g
Adult		
Male	40–54%	14–18 g
Female	37–47%	12–16 g

Red blood cell count (RBCs)

Newborn	4.4–5.8 million/µl
2 months	3–3.8 million/µl
Children	4.6–4.8 million/µl
Adults	
Male	4.5–6.2 million/µl
Female	4.2–5.4 million/µl

White blood cell count and differential
(WBC with diff.)

Newborn	7,000–35,000
1 week	4,000–20,000
1 month	6,000–18,000
3–5 months	6,000–17,000
6–11 months	6,000–16,000
1 year	6,000–15,000
2–10 years	7,000–13,000
11–15 years	5,000–12,000
Adult	4,300–10,000
Neutrophiles	55–70%
Lymphocytes	20–40%
Monocytes	2–8%
Eosinophiles	2–4%
Basophiles	0.5–1%

Values vary with laboratory.

Coombs' Tests

Direct	Negative
Indirect	Negative

Cortisol	Cortisol	7 A.M.–9 P.M. 5–25 µg/dL
		4 P.M.–6 P.M. 2–13 µg/dL
	(DST)	Less than 5 µg/dL any sample
	(ACTH stimulation test)	more than 18 µg/dL or 2 to 3× baseline value

Creatine phosphokinase (CK, CPK)	Newborn	30–100 µ/l
	Child	15–50 µ/l
	Adult	
	Male	23–99 µ/l
	Female	15–57 µ/l
	Isoenzymes:	
	CPK-BB	None
	CPK-MB	0–7 IU/l
	CPK-MM	5–70 IU/l

| C-Reactive Protein (CPR) | Negative | |

Creatinine (Cr, CrCl)	Serum:	
	1–18 months	0.2–0.5 mg/dl
		0.3–0.8 mg/dl
	2–12 years	0.5–1.2 mg/dl
	13–20 years	0.8–1.5 mg/dl
	Adults	
	Urine:	
	*Children	0.7–1.5 gm/24 hours
	Adult	
	Male	1.0–2.0 gm/24 hours
	Female	0.8–1.8 gm/24 hours
	*very age-dependent; check with local lab	

| Cultures | Normal flora or no growth | |

| Digoxin Level | Therapeutic level | 0.8–2 ng/ml |
| | Toxic level | Over 2 ng/ml |

| Dilantin (phenytoin) | Therapeutic level | 10–20 µg/ml |
| | Toxic level | Over 20 µg/ml |

| Estriol (E_3) | Serum: | |
| | Levels depend upon week of gestation. Range during pregnancy is 6–34 ng/ml, showing a gradual rise. Serial tests are required for comparison. | |

Urine:
Levels depend upon week of gestation. Range during last 6 weeks of pregnancy is 10–24 mg/day. Serial tests are required for comparison.

Ethanol	Negative	Different states have different laws governing legal blood alcohol limit for operating a motor vehicle. Generally, 0.05–0.10% is considered intoxicated.
Fecal Fat	Below 7 g/24 hours	
Fibrinogen	Newborn	160–300 mg/dl
	Child and Adult	200–400 mg/dl
Fluorescent, Treponemal Antibody Absorption Test (FTA-ABS)	Negative	
Folic Acid	2–14 ng/ml	

Gamma-Glutamyl Transpeptidase (GGTP or GGT)	Males 12–38 milliunits/ml 4–23 IU/liter	Females 9–31 milliunits/ml 3.5–13 IU/liter

Glucose (FBS, 2° PP)	Premature infant	30–80 mg/dl
	Full-term infant	40–90 mg/dl
	Child-adult	60–115 mg/dl

Glucose-6-Phosphate Dehydrogenase Deficiency (GPD or G-6PD)	Values are dependent upon laboratory method. Check with your local lab for appropriate value.

Hematocrit (Hct)	Newborn	57–68%
	1 week	46–62%
	1 month	31–41%
	3–5 months	30–36%
	1 year	29–41%
	2–10 years	36–40%
	Adult	
	Male	40–54%
	Female	37–47%

Hemoglobin (Hgb)	Newborn	17–21 gm/dl
	1 week	15–20 gm/dl
	1 month	11–14 gm/dl
	3–5 months	10–12 gm/dl
	1 year	11–13 gm/dl
	2–10 years	12–15 gm/dl
	Adult	
	Male	14–18 gm/dl
	Female	12–16 gm/dl
Hepatitis B Surface Antigen (Hb$_s$Ag)	Negative	
17-Hydroxycortico-Steroids (17-OHCS)	Children to 16 years	3.1 ± 1.0 mg/M²/24 hours
	Adults	
	Male	4.5–12 mg/24 hours
	Female	2.5–10 mg/24 hours
5-Hydroxyindoleacetic Acid (5-HIAA)	2–10 mg/24 hours 60–100 mEq/24 hours	

Iron, Iron-Binding Capacity (TIBC)		Iron (μg/dl)	Iron-Bind-ing Capac-ity	% Sat.
	Newborn	20–157	59–175	65
	6 weeks–3 years	20–115	250–400	10–55
	3–10 years	53–119	250–400	20–55
	Adult	87–279	250–400	20–55

Ketones	Serum:	Negative
	Urine:	(random sample) Negative

17-Ketogenic Steroids (17-KGS)	Under 1 year		< 1 mg/d
	1 year–10 years		1 mg/d/year of age
	Adults	Male	Female
	Under 70	5–23	3–15
	Over 70	3–12	3–12

17-Ketosteroids (17-KS)	Under 1 year	< 1 mg/24 hours
	1–4 years	< 2 mg/24 hours
	5–8 years	< 3 mg/24 hours
	9–12 years	approx. 3 mg/24 hours
	13–16 years	near adult levels
	Adults	
	Male	8–18 mg/24 hours
	Female	5–15 mg/24 hours
	Over 65 years	4–8 mg/24hours

Lactic Dehydrogenase (LDH)	Birth	290–501 U/L
	1 day–1 month	185–404 U/L
	1 month–2 years	110–244 U/L
	< 4 years	60–170 U/L
	3–17 years	85–165 U/L
	Adult	30–90 U/L
	LDH isoenzymes:	% total
	LD_1 heart	24–34
	LD_2 heart, RBC	35–45
	LD_3 muscle	15–25
	LD_4 liver, trace muscle	4–10
	LD_5 liver, muscle	1–9
Lead Levels (PbB, PbU)	Serum:	
	Children	< 30 mcg/dl
	Adults	< 40 mcg/dl
	Urine:	
	less than 80 mcg/liter/24 hour urine collection	
Lipase	less than 1.5 μ/ml or 32–80 μ/l	
Lupus Erythematosus Cell Preparation (LE prep)	negative (at least two LE cells needed for positive test)	
Magnesium (Mg)	Serum:	
	Newborn	1.52–2.33 mEq/l
	Child	1.4–1.9 mEq/l
	Adult	1.3–2.5 mEq/l
	Urine 24 hour collection:	6.0–8.5 mEq/24 hours
Mean Corpuscular Hemoglobin (MCH)	Newborn	32–34 pg
	All others	27–31 pg
Mean Corpuscular Hemoglobin Concentration (MCHC)	Newborn	30–34 gm/dl
	1 month	33–37 gm/dl
	All others	32–36 gm/dl
Mean Corpuscular Volume (MCV)	Newborn	110–128 μm^3
	1 month	93–109 μm^3
	Thereafter	82–101 μm^3
Mono Tests	Negative	
Occult blood	Negative	
O_2 Saturation	94–100%	

Osmolality	Serum:	270–300 mOsm/L
	Urine:	
	Infant	50–645 mOsm/kg
	Child/adult	50–1400 mOsm/kg
	Serum/urine ratio:	above 1.0 but less than 3.0

| Ova and Parasites (O and P) | None |

| Partial Thromboplastin Time, Activated (APTT) | from 16 to 40 seconds |

| Phenylalanine, Serum (PKU) | < 4 mg/dl |

Phosphate	Newborn	4.0–10.5 mg/dl
	1 year	4.0–6.8 mg/dl
	5 years	3.6–6.5 mg/dl
	Adult	2.5–4.5 mg/dl

| Pinworms | Negative |

| Platelet (Thrombocyte) Count | 150,000–400,000/μl |

Porphyrins	Uroporphyrins	Women	1–22 μg/24 hours
		Men	0–42 μg/24 hours
	Coproporphyrins	Women	1–57 μg/24 hours
		Men	0–96 μg/24 hours
	PGB (Porphobilinogen)		1.5 μg/24 hours

Potassium (K)	Serum	Below 10 days of age	3.5–7.0 mEq/L
		All other ages	3.5–5.5 mEq/L
	Urine	Children and Adults	25–100 mEq/24 hours

Pregnancy test (beta subunit hCG)	Serum
	< 3 mlU/ml nonpregnant
	Pregnancy values vary with gestation.
	Urine	Negative

Progesterone	Males	< than 100 ng/dl	
	Females	Follicular phase	< 150 ng/dl
		Luteal phase	> 400 ng/dl
		Pregnancy	> 800 ng/dl

| Prothrombin Time (PT) | From 9 to 12 seconds | |

Red Blood Cell Count (RBC)	Newborn	4.4–5.8 million/μl
	2 months	3–3.8 million/μl
	Child	4.6–4.8 million/μl
	Adult	
	Male	4.5–6.2 million/μl
	Female	4.2–5.4 million/μl

Reticulocyte Count (Retic Count)	Newborn	1.8–4.6%
	1 month	0.1–1.7%
	Infants	0.4–2.7%
	Children	0.5–1.0%
	Adults	
	Male	0.8–2.5%
	Female	0.8–4.1%

| Rheumatoid Arthritis Factors (RAF) | Negative |

Rh Factor — About 85–90% of the population is Rh positive.
About 10–15% of the population is Rh negative.

Rubella Titer (HI or HAI test) — Titers above 1.8 indicate immunity.

Salicylates	Negative	
	Therapeutic range (3 hours after dose)	
	Children up to 10	25–30 mg/dl
	Thereafter	20–25 mg/dl
	Toxic	
	Up to age 60	> 30 mg/dl
	After age 60	> 20 mg/dl

Schilling Test — 24-hour urine:
Greater than 8% radioactive B_{12} excreted in 24 hours

Sedimentation Rate (ESR) Westergren method	Children	3–20 mm/hr
	Men	0–15 mm/hr
	Over age 50	20 mm/hr
	Women	0–20 mm/hr
	Over age 50	30 mm/hr
	Values vary with method used.	

Serum Protein
Electrophoresis   Measurements in gm/dl

Age	Total	Albumin	Globulin	Gamma Globulin
Preterm	4.0–7.0	2.5–4.5	1.2–2.0	0.5–0.9
Newborn	5.0–7.1	2.5–5.0	1.2–4.0	0.7–0.9
1–3 mos.	4.7–7.4	3.0–4.2	1.0–3.3	0.1–0.5
3–12 mos.	5.0–7.5	2.7–5.0	2.0–3.8	0.4–1.2
1–15 yrs.	6.5–8.6	3.2–5.0	2.0–4.0	0.6–1.2
Adults	6.6–7.9	3.3–4.5	A_1 0.2–0.4	0.5–1.6
			A_2 0.6–1.0	
			Beta 0.6–1.2	

Sickle-Cell Tests		
Stained blood smear	Negative Finding
Sickle-cell test	Negative Finding
Sickledex	Negative Finding
Hemoglobin electro-phoresis	Negative for Hgb S or C
Fetal sickle-cell test	Negative for DNA sickle-cell marker

Smears	Negative

Sodium (Na)		
Serum	135–145 mEq/l
Urine	110–200 mEq/24 hours
Sweat	Infant up to 40 mmol/L
	Child up to 50 mmol/L
	Adult up to 90 mmol/L

Testosterone		
Female	30–95 ng/dl
Male	300–1200 ng/dl

Theophylline Levels		
Therapeutic level:	
Child and adult	10–20 μg/ml
Newborn, preterm	2–10 μg/ml
Toxic level:	
Child and adult	over 20 μg/ml
Newborn, preterm	over 13 μg/ml

Thrombin Time   10–15 seconds
± 3 seconds of control

Thyroid-Binding
Globulin (TBG)   12–30 μg/100 ml

Thyroid-Stimulating
Hormone (TSH)   0–10 μU/ml

Thyroxine (T_4)		
Cord blood	5.9–19.5 μg/dl
24 hours	11.4–21.0 μg/dl
6 weeks	9.9–18.3 μg/dl
All others	5–12 μg/dl

Thyroxine free assessment is calculation of T_4 and TBG ratio

Triglycerides	29–154 mg/dl	
Triiodothyronine (T_3)	Newborn	30–100 ng/dl
	All others	100–220 ng/dl
Uric Acid	Serum:	
	Children	2.5–8.0 mg/dl
	Men	4.3–8.0 mg/dl
	Women	2.3–6.0 mg/dl
	Urine:	
	250–750 mg/24 hours	

Urinalysis (Ua, U/A, UA)		*Adult*	*Child*
	Color	Straw	Straw
	Appearance (opacity, turbidity, clarity)	Clear	Clear
	Specific gravity	1.001–1.040; Usual 1.015–1.025	Neonate 1.012 Infant 1.001–1.020, Usual 1.003–1.010
	pH	4.5–8; Usual is pH 6	Neonate 5.0–7.0
	Protein	Negative	Negative
	Glucose	Negative	Negative
	Ketones	Negative	Negative
	Occult blood	Negative	Negative
	Microscopic		
	WBC	0–4	0–4
	RBC	0–3	Rare
	Bacteria	None	None
	Casts	Rare hyaline cast	Rare hyaline cast
	Crystals	Few	Few
	Epithelial Cells	Few	Few

Urobilinogen	Ehrlich U/2 hours	
	Male	0.3–2.1
	Female	0.1–1.1
	Random	0.3–3.5 mg/100 ml

Vanillylmandelic Acid (VMA)	1–12 months	1.40–15.0 mg/gm creatinine
	1–2 years	1.25–8.0 mg/gm creatinine
	2–5 years	1.50–7.5 mg/gm creatinine
	5–10 years	0.50–6.0 mg/gm creatinine
	10–15 years	0.25–3.25 mg/gm creatinine
	Adults	1.5–7.5 mg/24 hours

Venereal Disease Research Laboratory (VDRL)	Nonreactive	
White Blood Cell Count and Differential (WBC with diff)	Newborn	7,000–35,000
	1 week	4,000–20,000
	1 month	6,000–18,000
	3–5 months	6,000–17,000
	6–11 months	6,000–16,000
	1 year	6,000–15,000
	2–10 years	7,000–13,000
	11–15 years	5,000–12,000
	Adult	4,300–10,000
	Neutrophiles	55–70%
	Lymphocytes	20–40%
	Monocytes	2–8%
	Eosinophiles	2–4%
	Basophiles	0.5–1%

Index